अष्टाङ्गहृदयम्
सूत्रस्थानम्

वैद्य जनार्धन वि हेब्बार्

|| Jai Guruji ||

I, Dr. Janardhana V. Hebbar, dedicate this book at the holy feet of Sri Guruji – Swami Vivekananda and my spiritual Guru, Dr. A. Chandrashekhara Udupa MBBS, FAGE, Managing Director, Divine Park Trust (R), Saligrama, Udupi. (www.divinepark.org)

He guides, He energizes, He shows the path,
He holds my hand and makes me walk!

क्रम-सूची

Ashtanga Hridaya is written by Acharya Laghu Vagbhata.

Sections and specialties of Ashtanga Hridaya:

Ashtanga Hridaya is a more simplified version of Ashtanga Sangraha. It comprises 6 sections and 120 chapters.

Sutra Sthana – In this section the basic principles of Ayurveda, daily regimen (dinacharya), seasonal regimen (ritucharya), diet and dietetics, etc are explained. It comprises of **30 chapters**

Shareera Sthana – In this section, concepts and details of Ayurvedic embryology, anatomy, physiology etc are discussed. This section comprises **6 chapters.**

Nidana Sthana – In this section discussion of the aetiology, pathology, signs and symptoms, prognosis of diseases etc are dealt with. These topics are dealt in **16 chapters.**

Chikitsa Sthana – In this section, the line of treatment of many diseases, medicines and diet towards healing of those diseases, patient care etc is detailed. Chikitsa Sthana has **22 chapters** dealing with these topics.

Kalpa Sthana – In this section formulations and methods pertaining to elimination therapies i.e. Panchakarma are dealt. Elimination therapies or shodhana treatments are Vamana (therapeutic emesis), Virechana (therapeutic purgation), Vasti (herbal enemas, decoction and oil) and Nasya (nasal medication). Kalpa Sthana comprises 6 chapters.

Uttara Sthana – This section deals with chapters dedicated to the discussion of other 7 branches (all the above said sthanas dealing with Kaya Chikitsa). Uttara Sthana comprises of **40 chapters** and is dedicated to 7 branches of Ayurveda as below mentioned:

Bala Roga – 3 chapters

Graha – 4 chapters

Urdhwanga Chikitsa – 17 chapters

Shalya Chikitsa – 10 chapters

Damshtra Chikitsa – 4 chapters

Jara – 1 chapter

Vrisha – 1 chapter

Ashtanga Hridayam was translated into almost all Indian languages. It was also translated into Arabic during the reign of Harun-al-Rashid (773-808

AD), into Tibetan language during the reign of king Krhrison-dehu (755-797 AD) and into German by Luise Hilgenberg and Willibald Kirfel in 1941.

Commentaries on AshtangaHridayam –

More than 30 commentaries were said to be written on Ashtangahrudayam, most of them are either lost, partly available or remaining M.S.S in the libraries. Only 6 are available partly or fully in printed form.

Sarvanga Sundari – only fully available best commentary on Ashtang Hruday, written by Arunadatta, son of Mriganka Datta belonging to Bengal region. His date is estimated to be around 12th or 13th century AD

Ayurveda Rasayana – written by Hemadri (not available completely), lived around 1260 – 1310 AD

Padartha Chandrika – written by Chandranandana (10th century AD)

Hridaya Bodhika or Hridaya Bodhini – written by Sridasa Pandita (14th century)

Tatwa Bodha – written by Shivadas Sen, commentary for Uttara Tantra (1457 – 1474 AD)

Dr Raghuram YS M.D(Ayu).

1

आयुष्कामीयमध्यायम्
(ayushkamiyam adhyayam)

Prayer:

रागादिरोगान् सततानुषक्तानशेषकायप्रसृतानशेषान् |
औत्सुक्यमोहारतिदाञ्जघान योऽपूर्ववैद्याय नमोस्तु तस्मै |१|

Salutations to the unique and rare Physician, who has destroyed, without any residue all the diseases like Raga (lust, anger, greed, arrogance, jealousy, selfishness, ego), which are constantly associated with the body, which is spread all over the body, giving rise to disease, delusion and restlessness. This salutation is done to Lord Dhanwantari.

Pledge by the author(s):

अथात आयुष्कामीयमध्यायं व्याख्यास्यामः| (गद्यसूत्रम्)||१||
इति ह स्माहुरात्रेयादयो महर्षयः| (गद्यसूत्रम्)|२|

Maharshi Atreya and the other sages pledge that henceforth they will be explaining the chapter named Ayushkameeyam.

The word meaning of Ayush is life; kameeyam means the quest for. Hence Ayushkameeyam means the quest for life.

Purpose of life:

आयुःकामायमानेन धर्मार्थसुखसाधनम्|
आयुर्वेदोपदेशेषु विधेयः परमादरः||२||

To achieve the purpose of life, that is
1. Dharma – following the path of righteousness,
2. Artha – earning money in a legal way,
3. Kama – fulfilling our desires,
4. Moksha – achieving salvation,

One should concentrate on having a long life. To learn the science of Ayurveda, which explains how to achieve this purpose, 'obedience' (Vidheya) is the most important quality.

Origin of Ayurveda:

ब्रह्मा स्मृत्वाऽऽयुषो वेदं प्रजापतिमजिग्रहत्|
सोऽश्विनौ तौ सहस्राक्षं सोऽत्रिपुत्रादिकान्मुनीन्||३||
तेऽग्निवेशादिकांस्ते तु पृथक् तन्त्राणि तेनिरे|

Lord Brahma, remembering Ayurveda, taught it to Prajapathi, he in turn taught it to Ashwini Kumaras (twins), they taught it to Sahasraksha (Lord Indra), he taught it to Atri's son (Atreya Punarvasu) and other sages, they taught it to Agnivesha and others and they (Agnivesa and other disciples) composed treatises, each one separately.

Ashtanga Hridaya – a concise textbook:

तेभ्योऽतिविप्रकीर्णेभ्यः प्रायः सारतरोच्चयः||४||
क्रियतेऽष्टाङ्गहृदयं नातिसंक्षेपविस्तरम्|

From those Ayurvedic text books, which are too elaborate and hence very difficult to study, only the essence is collected and presented in Ashtanga Hridaya, which is neither too short nor too elaborate.

Ashtanga Ayurveda – Eight branches of Ayurveda:

कायबालग्रहोर्ध्वाङ्गशल्यदंष्ट्राजरावृषान्||५||
अष्टावङ्गानि तस्याहुश्चिकित्सा येषु संश्रिता|

1. Kaya Chikitsa – General medicine
2. Bala Chikitsa – Paediatrics
3. Graha Chikitsa – Psychiatry
4. Urdhvanga Chikitsa – Diseases and treatment of ear, nose, throat, eyes and head (neck and above region)
5. Shalya Chikitsa – Surgery
6. Damshrta Chikitsa – Toxicology
7. Jara Chikitsa – Geriatrics

8. VrushyaChikitsa – Aphrodisiac therapy.
These are the eight branches of Ayurveda.

Tridosha and their distribution:

वायुः पित्तं कफश्चेति त्रयो दोषाः समासतः||६||
विकृताविकृता देहं घ्नन्ति ते वर्तयन्ति च||
ते व्यापिनोऽपि हृन्नाभ्योरधोमध्योर्ध्वसंश्रयाः||७||

Vayu (Vata), Pitta and Kapha are the three Doshas of the body.
A perfect balance of three Doshas leads to health and their imbalance leads to diseases.
The Tridosha are present all over the body, but their presence is especially seen in particular parts.
If you divide the body into three parts,
The upper part up to the chest is dominated by Kapha Dosha,
The part between the chest and umbilicus is dominated by Pitta,
The part below the umbilicus is dominated by Vata.

Dosha predominance in the body according to Age, Time of the day and Stage of digestion:

वयोहोरात्रिभुक्तानां तेऽन्तमध्यादिगाः क्रमात्|

In a person's life,
Childhood is dominated by Kapha,
Middle age is dominated by Pitta,
Old age is dominated by Vata.
During the day and night (separately),
First part is dominated by Kapha,
Second part is dominated by Pitta and
Third part is dominated by Vata.
While eating and during digestion,
First part (gastric phase) is dominated by Kapha,
Second part (intestinal phase) is dominated by Pitta and
Third part (colonic phase) is dominated by Vata.

Agni Bheda – Types of Digestive fire:

तैर्भवेद्विषमस्तीक्ष्णो मन्दश्चाग्निः समैः समः||८||

There are four types of Digestive fires (Agni)
1. Vishama Agni – A person with Vishama Agni will sometimes have high

appetite, and sometimes, low appetite.

2. Teekshna Agni -A person with Teeksna Agni will have high digestion power and appetite.

3. Manda Agni -A person with Manda Agni will have low digestion power and appetite.

4. Sama Agni –A person with Sama Agni will have proper appetite and digestion power. Here, digestion occurs at an appropriate time.

Koshta Bheda – Types of digestive tract:

कोष्ठः क्रूरो मृदुर्मध्यो मध्यः स्यातैः समैरपि|

There are three types of digestive tracts (Koshta):

1. Kroora Koshta – hard bowels
2. Mrudu Koshta – soft bowels
3. Madhyama Koshta –normal bowels.

Deha Prakriti – Body type:

शुक्रार्तवस्थैर्जन्मादौ विषेणेव विषक्रिमे:||९||

तैश्च तिस्रः प्रकृतयो हीनमध्योतमाः पृथक्|

समधातुः समस्तासु श्रेष्ठा निन्द्या द्विदोषजाः||१०||

Like the Visha (poison) is natural and inherent to poisonous insects, similarly, the Prakruti (body type) is inherent to humans. The body type is decided during conception, based on qualities of shukra (sperm) and arthava (ovum).

Vata prakruti – Vata body type is considered as low quality

Pitta Prakruti – Pitta body type is considered as moderate quality

Kapha Prakruti – Kapha body type is considered good quality.

Tridosha Prakruti – Body type influenced equally by Vata, Pitta and Kapha is considered the best quality.

Dual body types, like Vata-Pitta, Pitta-Kapha, Vata-Kapha body types are not considered good.

Vata Dosha Lakshana – Characteristics of Vata Dosha:

तत्र रूक्षो लघुः शीतः खरः सूक्ष्मश्चलोऽनिलः|

Rooksha – dryness,

Laghu – lightness,

Sheeta – coldness,

Khara – roughness,
Sookshma – minuteness,
Chala – movement are the qualities of Vata.

Pitta Dosha Lakshana – Characteristics of Pitta Dosha:

पित्तं सस्नेहतीक्ष्णोष्णं लघु विस्रं सरं द्रवम्||११||

Sasneha – slightly oily, unctuous,
Teekshna – piercing, entering into deep tissues,
Ushna – hotness,
Laghu – lightness,
Visram – having bad smell,
Sara – having fluidity, movement,
Drava – liquidity are the qualities of Pitta.

Kapha Dosha Lakshana – Characteristics of Kapha Dosha:

स्निग्धः शीतो गुरुर्मन्दः श्लक्ष्णो मृत्स्नः स्थिरः कफः|

Snigdha – oily, unctuous,
Sheeta – cold,
Guru – heavy,
Manda – mild, viscous,
Shlakshna – smooth, clear,
Mrutsna – slimy, jelly-like,
Sthira – stability, immobility are the qualities of Kapha.

Samsarga and Sannipata:

संसर्गः सन्निपातश्च तद्द्विद्वत्रिक्षयकोपतः||१२||

The increase, decrease or imbalance of two Doshas together is called Samsarga. Imbalance of all the three Doshas together is called Sannipata.

Dhatu and Mala – Body tissues and excretory products:

रसासृङ्मांसमेदोऽस्थिमज्जशुक्राणि धातवः|

सप्त दूष्याः मला मूत्रशकृत्स्वेदादयोऽपि च||१३||

Body tissues and waste products are called Dushyas (Those that are influenced and affected by Doshas).

Sapta Dhatu - Seven body tissues

· Rasa - Lymph or plasma

· Rakta -Blood
· Mamsa -Muscle
· Meda -Fat tissue
· Asthi -Bones and cartilages
· Majja -Bone marrow
· Shukra -Semen / Ovum or entire male and female genital tract and its secretions

Tri Mala – Three waste products of the body

Shakrut / Pureesha (faeces),
Sweda (sweat) and
Mootra (urine) constitutes the Tri Mala (three waste products of the body).

Status of Tridosha and health

वृद्धिः समानैः सर्वेषां विपरीतैर्विपर्ययः|

Samana means similar or equal; Viparita means opposite.
Equal qualities lead to increase, and opposing qualities lead to decrease.

Shad Rasa – Six Tastes:

रसाः स्वाद्वम्ललवणतिक्तोषणकषायकाः||१४||
षड् द्रव्यमाश्रितास्ते च यथापूर्वंबलावहाः|

There are 6 types of tastes (Rasa) mentioned -
Svadu / Madhura – sweet,
Amla – Sour,
Lavana – Salt,
Tikta – Bitter,
Ushna / Katu – Pungent,
Kashaya – Astringent.
They are successively lower in energy. It means sweet taste imparts maximum energy to the body and astringent, the least.

Alleviation of Dosha According to Taste:

तत्रद्या मारुतं घ्नन्ति त्रयस्तिक्तादयः कफम्||१५||
कषायतिक्तमधुराः पित्तमन्ये तु कुर्वते|
शमनं कोपनं स्वस्थहितं द्रव्यमिति त्रिधा||१६||

In the list of tastes, the first three, i.e.Madhura (sweet), Amla (sour) and Lavana (salt) mitigates Vata and increases Kapha.

The last three, i.e.Tikta (bitter), Katu (pungent) and Kashaya (astringent) tastes mitigate Kapha and increase Vata.

Kashaya (astringent), Tikta (bitter) and Madhura (sweet) tastes mitigate Pitta.

Amla (sour), Lavana (salt) and Katu (pungent) tastes increase Pitta.

Dravya Bheda - Types of Substance:

Shamana – that which decreases –A substance that brings down the increased Dosha to normalcy

Kopana – that which increases -A substance that increases the lowered Dosha to normalcy

Swasthahita – 'Swasta' means 'health', 'Hita' means 'good for' - A substance that maintains the normalcy of Tridosha and health.

Two types of Virya (Potency):

उष्णशीतगुणोत्कर्षात्तत्र वीर्यं द्विधा स्मृतम्‌|

Ushna veerya – Foods that are hot in potency

Sheeta veerya – Foods that are cold in potency.

Three types of Vipaka (Taste conversion after digestion):

त्रिधा विपाको द्रव्यस्य स्वाद्वम्लकटुकात्मकः||१७||

Swadu (Madhura) Vipaka - Sweet taste conversion after digestion

Amla Vipaka– Sour taste conversion after digestion

Katu Vipaka – Pungent taste conversion after digestion.

Gurvadi Guna – Attributes or Qualities:

गुरुमन्दहिमस्निग्धश्लक्ष्णसान्द्रमृदुस्थिराः|

गुणाः ससूक्ष्मविशदा विंशतिः सविपर्ययाः||१८||

The twenty types of gunas (qualities) -

Guru(heavy) X laghu (light)

Manda(slow) X tiksna(quick,fast)

Hima (cold) X ushna (hot)

Snigdha (unctuous) X ruksa (dry)

Slaksna (smooth) X khara (rough)

Sandra (solid) X drava (liquid)

Mrdu (soft) X kathina (hard)

Sthira (stable) X cala (moving, unstable)
Suksma (stable, small) X sthula (big, gross)
Vishada (non slimy) X picchila (slimy)

Roga Arogya Karana – Cause of Disease and Health:

कालार्थकर्मणां योगो हीनमिथ्यातिमात्रकः|
सम्यग्योगश्च विज्ञेयो रोगारोग्यैककारणम्||१९||

Hina (less), ati (more) or mithya (wrong) unison of Kala(time), Artha (senses) and Karma(functions)is the reason for diseases and the right unison of these three factors is the reason for health.

Disease and health:

रोगास्तु दोषवैषम्यं, दोषसाम्यमरोगता|

Imbalance in Tridosha leads to Roga (disease).
Samya (perfect balance) of Dosha is health.

Roga Bheda – Types of Disease:

निजागन्तुविभागेन तत्र रोगा द्विधा स्मृताः||२०||

The two types of diseases:
Nija roga – Disease caused due to imbalance in internal factors.|
Agantu Roga -Disease caused due to external factors.

Roga Bheda According to Adhishtana(Disease classification according to location):

तेषां कायमनोभेदादधिष्ठानमपि द्विधा|

Based on Adhishtana (location), the doshas are of two types i.e.,
Kaya / sharirika dosha (Vata, Pitta and Kapha)
Mano dosha (psychic doshas)

Types of Mano (psychic) Doshas:

रजस्तमश्च मनसो द्वौ च दोषावुदाहृतौ||२१||

There are two types of Mano Doshas -
Rajas – quality of mind that drives us to take actions,
Tamas – that leads to inaction and lethargy.

Rogi and Roga Pariksha:

दर्शनस्पर्शनप्रश्नैः परीक्षेत च रोगिणम्|

रोगं निदानप्रागूपलक्षणोपशयाप्तिभिः||२२||

Methods of Rogi Pariksha (Examination of patient) -

Darshana –by means of inspection, observation

Sparshana - by means of touching

Prashna –by means of asking

Methods of Roga Pariksha (Examination of the disease) -

Disease should be examined by its -

Nidana - causes, etiology

Pragrupa – Purvarupa – prodromal symptoms, premonitory symptoms

Lakshana – Specific signs and symptoms, clinical features

Upashaya – diagnostic tests

Apti – Samprapti – Pathogenesis of the disease.

Desha Bheda - Types of Habitat:

भूमिदेहप्रभेदेन देशमाहुरिह द्विवधा|

जाङ्गलं वातभूयिष्ठमनूपं तु कफोल्बणम्||२३||

साधारणं सममलं त्रिधा भूदेशमादिशेत्|

In the context of medicine, Desha is said to be of two kinds -

Bhumi desha– region of land and

Dehadesha – the body.

Bhumi desha (land region) is of three kinds -

Jangala (arid or desert-like land) - which is predominant of Vata

Anupa (marshy land with more of water)- which is predominant of Kapha

Sadharana(land with moderate water, vegetation, sunlight) - which has all Tridosha in balance.

Kala Bheda – Types of time:

क्षणादिव्र्याध्यवस्था च कालो भेषजयोगकृत्||२४||

Two kinds are considered -

Kshanadi kala - One is normal time, beginning with seconds.

Vyadhi Avastha Kala - Stages of disease.

Aushadha Bheda – Classification of Medicine:

शोधनं शमनं चेति समासादौषधं द्विवधा |

There are two types of medicines -

Shamana - Palliative treatment – which brings the Dosha to normalcy, useful in initial stages of diseases

Shodhana – Purification treatment – which expels imbalanced Dosha out of body – Useful in aggravated stages of the disease.

Main therapies and ingredient for Doshas:

शरीरजानां दोषाणां क्रमेण परमौषधम्||२५||

बस्तिर्विरेको वमनं तथा तैलं घृतं मधु|

For diseases of the body, under Shodhana (purification) regimen,

For Vata – Basti(enema)

For Pitta – Virechana (Purgation)

For Kapha – Vamana (emesis).

For diseases of the body, under Shamana (palliative) regimen,

For Vata – Taila (oil)

For Pitta – Grita (ghee)

For Kapha – Madhu (honey).

Treatment for Mano Dosha (Dosha pertaining to the psyche):

धीधैर्यात्मादिविज्ञानं मनोदोषौषधं परम्||२६||

Dhee – improving intelligence

Dhairya – improving courage and

Atmavijnana – Self realization - are the means to treat mental imbalance.

Chikitsa Chatushpada – Four factors in treatment:

भिषक् द्रव्याण्युपस्थाता रोगी पादचतुष्टयम्|

चिकित्सितस्य निर्दिष्टं, प्रत्येकं तच्चतुर्गुणम्||२७||

Bhishak (Doctor), Dravya (medicine), Upasthata (Nurse) and Rogi (patient) are the four factors in treatment. Each of these four factors have four qualities each.

Qualities of Bhishak (doctor):

दक्षस्तीर्थातशास्त्रार्थो दृष्टकर्मा शुचिर्भिषक्|

Daksha – Alert, disciplined

Tirthathashastrarhta – Having detailed knowledge about diseases and treatment

Drushtakarma – Having practical experience

Shuchi – Cleanliness

Qualities of Dravya / Aushada (medicine):

बहुकल्पं बहुगुणं सम्पन्नं योग्यमौषधम्||२८||

Bahukalpa – Ability to formulate into different dosage forms, like decoction, powder, herbal oil etc.

Bahuguna – Having enormous qualities

Sampanna – Endowed with virtues

Yogya – Suitable and appropriate for specific diseases.

Qualities of Upasthata / Paricharaka (nurse):

अनुरक्तः शुचिर्दक्षो बुद्धिमान् परिचारकः|

Anurakta – Compassion towards patients

Shuchi – Cleanliness

Daksha – Alert, active

Buddhiman – Intelligence

Qualities of Rogi (patient):

आढ्यो रोगी भिषग्वश्यो ज्ञापकः सत्त्ववानपि||२९||

Adhya - Rich

Bhishagvashya – Obedience towards doctor

Jnapaka – Having good memory

Satvavaan – Having good strength to tolerate disease and treatment.

Vyadhi Bheda based on Sadhyasadhyata (Disease classification based on prognosis):

साध्योऽसाध्य इति व्याधिर्द्विधा, तौ तु पुनर्द्विधा|

सुसाध्यः कृच्छ्रसाध्यश्च, याप्यो यश्चानुपक्रमः ||२९+(१) ||

There are two types of diseases, which are further divided into two each -

1.Sadhya - Thatwhich can be cured.

It is of two types –

Sukha Sadhya (Easily curable),

Krichra Sadhya (Cured with difficulty)

2.Asadhya – That which cannot be cured.

It is of two types –

Yapya (which cannot be cured but can be managed),

Anupakrama (Incurable).

Qualities of Sukha Sadhya Vyadhi – easily curable disease:

सर्वौषधक्षमे देहे यूनः पुंसो जितात्मनः।
अमर्मगोऽल्पहेत्वग्ररूपरूपोऽनुपद्रवः।।३०।।
अतुल्यदूष्यदेशर्तुप्रकृतिः पादसम्पदि।
ग्रहेष्वनुगुणेष्वेकदोषमार्गो नवः सुखः।।३१।।

Qualities of Sukha Sadhya Vyadhi – easily curable disease:

Sarvaushadhakshame dehe – The body of the patient is able to tolerate all types of medicines

Yunaha – Young patient

Pumsa – Male patient

Jitatmanaha – Patient having good control over sense organs, who follows abstinence

Amarmaga – If the disease has not affected sensitive areas like brain, heart, kidney

Alpahetu – If the cause for disease is mild

Alparoopa – Mild symptoms

Anupadrava – no complications

Atulya dushya desha rutu prakruti – If the Dosha and Dhatu (body tissue) involved, Desha (place), Rutu (season) and Prakruti (body type) are not influenced by one particular Dosha,

Pada sampadi - If all the sixteen qualities of the doctor, patient etc. explained above are present

Graha anuguna - If astrology is in favour of the patient

Eka Doshaja - Disease due to only one Dosha

Eka Marga - If only one body channel is affected

Nava - Disease of recent origin / onset.

Qualities of Krichra Sadhya Vyadhi – Diseases which are cured with difficulty:

शस्त्रादिसाधनः कृच्छ्रः सङ्करे च ततो गदः।
Diseases which require the use of surgical instruments etc. in treatment and also those which have a mixture of factors enumerated in previous verses are krichra sadhya (curable with difficulty).

Qualities of Yapya Vyadhi – Diseases which are manageable:

शेषत्वादायुषो याप्यः पथ्याभ्यासादिविपर्यये।।३२।।

A disease is Yapya (manageable) if, although its presentation is opposite to Sukha Sadhya lakshanas,the patient can be managed with Pathya - diet, activities and medicine.

Qualities of Anupakrama Vyadhi – Diseases which are not curable:

अनुपक्रम एव स्यात्स्थितोऽत्यन्तविपर्यये।
औत्सुक्यमोहारतिकृद् दृष्टरिष्टोऽक्षनाशनः॥३३॥

Diseases which have features entirely opposite to those of curable diseases, which have stayed for long periods of time, involving all the important tissues and vital organs, which have produced anxiety (fear of death), delusion and restlessness; which are presenting with fatal signs and which causes damage to sense organs are impossible to cure.

Patient worth rejection:

त्यजेदार्तं भिषग्भूपैर्द्विष्टं तेषां द्विषं द्विषम्।
हीनोपकरणं व्यग्रमविधेयं गतायुषम्॥३४॥
चण्डं शोकातुरं भीरुं कृतघ्नं वैद्यमानिनम्।

The physician should reject the patient -
who is hated by the physician and the king and who hates them;
who hates himself (dejected in life), who is not having the equipments and other facilities required for treatment,
who is busy with other activities,
who is not having the required attention etc. towards the treatment,
who is disobedient (to the physician),
whose life is coming to an end,
who has an evil mindset (violent, destructive),
who is afflicted with great grief,
who is full of fear,
who is ungrateful and
who thinks himself to be a physician (in respect of deciding drugs, therapies, food, activities etc.)

Adhyaya Sangraha – List of Chapters:

तन्त्रस्यास्य परं चातो वक्ष्यतेऽध्यायसङ्ग्रहः॥३५॥

The list of other Adhyayas (chapters) explained in Ashtanga Hridaya are

Sutra Sthana:

आयुष्कामादिनर्त्वीहारोगानुत्पादनद्रवाः| अन्नज्ञानान्नसंरक्षामात्राद्रव्यरसाश्रयाः||३६||
दोषादिज्ञानतद्भेदतच्चिकित्साद्युपक्रमाः|
शुद्ध्यादिस्नेहनस्वेदरेकास्थापननावनम्||३७||
धूमगण्डूषदृक्सेकतृप्तियन्त्रकशस्त्रकम्| शिराविधिः   शल्यविधिः
शस्त्रक्षाराग्निकर्मिकौ||३८||
सूत्रस्थानमिमेऽध्यायास्त्रिंशत्शारीरमुच्यते|

The list of chapters explained in Sutra Sthana -

1. Ayuskamiyaadhyaya (desire for long life). 2. Dinacaryaadhyaya (daily regimen).

3. Rtucaryaadhyaya (seasonal regimen). 4. Roganutpadaniyaadhyaya (prevention of diseases).

5. Dravadravyavijnaniyaadhyaya (knowledge of liquid materials).

6. Annasvarupavijnaniyaadhyaya (nature of food materials).

7. Annaraksadhyaya (Protection of foods). 8. Matrasitiyadhyaya (Proper quantity of food).

9. Dravyadivijnaniyaadhyaya (Knowledge of substances etc.).

10. Rasabhediyaadhyaya (classification of tastes).

11. Dosadivijnaniyaadhyaya (Knowledge of dosas etc.).

12. Dosabhediyaadhyaya (classification of dosas).

13. Dosopakramaniyaadhyaya (treatment of the dosas).

14. Dvividhopakramaniyaadhyaya (two kinds of treatments).

15. Sodhanadiganasangrahaadhyaya (groups of drugs for purificatory therapies etc.).

16. Sneha vidhiadhyaya (oleation therapy). 17. Svedavidhiadhyaya (sudation therapy).

18. Vamana virecanavidhiadhyaya (emesis and purgation therapies).

19. Basti vidhiadhyaya (enema therapy). 20. Nasya vidhiadhyaya (nasal medication).

21. Dhumapanavidhiadhyaya (inhalation of smoke therapy).

22. Gandusadividhiadhyaya (mouth gargles and other therapies).

23. Ascyotana-anjanavidhiadhyaya (eye drops, collyrium therapies).

24. Tarpana-putapakavidhiadhyaya (satiating the eye and other therapies).

25. Yantra vidhiadhyaya (use of blunt instruments).

26. Sastra vidhiadhyaya (use of sharp instruments).

27. Siravyadhavidhiadhyaya (venesection).

28. Salyaharanavidhiadhyaya (removal of foreign bodies).

29. Sastrakarmavidhiadhyaya (surgical operation).

30. Ksaragnikarmavidhiadhyaya (alkaline and thermal cautery)

Sharira Sthana:

गर्भावक्रान्तितद्व्यापदङ्गमर्मविभागिकम्||३९|| विकृतिर्दूतजं षष्ठम्

The list of chapters explained in Sharira Sthana –

1. Garbhavakrantisarira (embryology). 2. Garbhavyapadsarira (disorders of pregnancy).

3. Anga vibhaga sarira (different parts of the body). 4. Marma vibhaga sarira (classification of vital spots). 5. Vikruti vijnaniyasarira (knowledge of bad prognosis).

6. Dutadivijnaniyasarira (knowledge of messenger etc.)

Nidana Sthana:

निदानं सार्वरोगिकम्| ज्वरासृक्श्वासयक्ष्मादिमदाद्यर्शोतिसारिणाम्||४०||

मूत्राघातप्रमेहाणां विद्रध्याद्युदरस्य च| पाण्डुकुष्ठानिलार्तानां वातास्रस्य च षोडश||४१||

The list of chapters explained in Nidana Sthana–

1. Sarvroganidanam (diagnosis of diseases in general).

2. Jvaranidanam (diagnosis of fever).

3. Raktapitta, Kasa nidanam (diagnosis of bleeding disease and cough).

4. Svasa-Hidhmanidanam (diagnosis of dyspnoea and hiccup).

5. Rajayaksmadinidanam (diagnosis of pulmonary tuberculosis etc.).

6. Madatyayanidanam (diagnosis of alcoholic intoxication).

7. Arsasnidanam (diagnosis of haemorrhoids).

8. Atisara-Grahani nidanam (diagnosis of diarrhoea and duodenal disorders).

9. Mutraghatanidanam (diagnosis of retention of urine).

10. Prameha nidanam (diagnosis of diabetes).

11. Vidradhi-Vrddhi-Gulma nidanam (diagnosis of abscess, enlargement of the scrotum and abdominal

tumour).

12. Udara nidanam (diagnosis of enlargement of the abdomen).

13. Panduroga-sopha-visarpa nidanam (diagnosis of anaemia, dropsy and herpes).

14. Kustha-svitra-kriminidanam (diagnosis of leprosy, leucoderma and parasites).

15. Vata vyadhi nidanam (diagnosis of diseases of the nervous system).

16. Vatasonitanidanam (diagnosis of gout).

Chikitsa Sthana:

चिकित्सितं ज्वरे रक्ते कासे श्वासे च यक्ष्मणि| वमौ मदात्ययेऽर्शःसु, विशि द्वौ, द्वौ च मूत्रिते||४२||

विद्रधौ गुल्मजठरपाण्डुशोफविसर्पिषु| कुष्ठश्वित्रानिलव्याधिवातास्रेषु चिकित्सितम्||४३|| द्वाविंशतिरिमेऽध्यायाः

The list of chapters explained in Chikitsa Sthana –

1. Jvara cikitsita (treatment of fevers). 2. Raktapitta cikitsita (treatment of bleeding disease).

3. Kasa cikitsita (treatment of cough). 4. Svasa-Hidhma cikitsita (treatment of dyspnoea and hiccup).

5. Rajayaksmadi cikitsita (treatment of pulmonary tuberculosis, etc.).

6. Chardi-Hrdroga-Trsna cikitsita (treatment of vomiting, heart disease and thirst).

7. Madatyaya cikitsita (treatment of alcoholic intoxication). 8. Arsascikitsita (treatment of haemorrhoids). 9. Atisara cikitsita (treatment of diarrhoea).

10. Grahani dosa cikitsita (treatment of duodenal disorder). 11. Mutraghata cikitsita (treatment of retention of urine). 12. Prameha cikitsita (treatment of diabetes). 13. Vidradhi-vrddhi cikitsita (treatment of abscess, enlargement of the scrotum). 14. Gulma cikitsita (treatment of abdominal tumour). 15. Udara cikitsita (treatment of enlargement of the abdomen). 16. Pandu roga cikitsita (treatment of anaemia). 17. Svayathu (sopha) cikitsita (treatment of dropsy). 18. Visarpa cikitsita (treatment of herpes). 19. Kustha cikitsita (treatment of leprosy). 20. Svitra-krimicikitsita (treatment of leucoderma and parasites). 21. Vata vyadhi cikitsita (treatment of diseases of the nervous system). 22. Vatasonita cikitsita (treatment of gout).

KalpaSiddhi Sthana:

कल्पसिद्धिरतः परम्| कल्पो वमेर्विरेकस्य तत्सिद्धिर्बस्तिकल्पना||४४|| सिद्धिर्बस्त्यापदां षष्ठो द्रव्यकल्पोऽत|

The list of chapters explained in Kalpa - Siddhi Sthana -

1. Vamana kalpa (emetic recipes). 2. Virecanakalpa (purgative recipes).

3. Vamana virecana vyapat siddhi (management of complications of emesis and purgation therapies). 4. Basti kalpa (enema recipes). 5. Basti vyapat siddhi (management of complications of enema therapy). 6. Dravya-kalpa

(pharmaceutics).

Uttara Sthana:
उत्तरम्| बालोपचारे तद्व्याधौ तद्ग्रहे, द्वौ च भूतगे||४५|| जन्मादेऽथ स्मृतिभ्रंशे, द्वौ द्वौ वर्त्मसु सन्धिषु|
दृक्तमोलिङ्गनाशेषु त्रयो, द्वौ द्वौ च सर्वगे||४६|| कर्णनासामुखशिरोव्रणे, भङ्गे भगन्दरे|
ग्रन्थ्यादौ क्षुद्ररोगेषु गुह्यरोगे पृथग्द्वयम्||४७|| विषे भुजङ्गे कीटेषु मूषकेषु रसायने|
चत्वारिंशोऽनपत्यानामध्यायो बीजपोषणः||४८||

The list of chapters explained in Uttara Sthana –
1. Balopacaraniyaadhyaya (care of the new born baby). 2. Balamayapratisedha (treatment of diseases of children). 3. Balagrahapratisedha (treatment of evil spirits). 4. Bhuta vijnaniya (knowledge of demons). 5. Bhuta pratisedha (treatment of demons). 6. Unmada pratisedha (treatment of insanity).

7. Apasmara pratisedha (treatment of epilepsy). 8. Vartma roga vijnaniya (knowledge of diseases of eyelids). 9. Vartma roga pratsedha (treatment of diseases of eyelids). 10. Sandhisitasita roga vijnaniya (knowledge of diseases of fornices, sclera and cornea). 11. Sandhisitasita roga pratisedha (treatment of diseases of fornices, sclera and cornea). 12. Drsti roga vijnaniya (knowledge of diseases of vision). 13. Timira pratisedha (treatment of blindness). 14. Linganasa pratisedha (treatment of blindness). 15. Sarvaksi roga vijnaniya (knowledge of diseases of the whole eye).

16. Sarvaksi roga pratisedha (treatment of diseases of the whole eye). 17. Karna roga vijnaniya (knowledge of diseases of the ear). 18. Karna roga pratisedha (treatment of diseases of the ear).

19. Nasa roga vijnaniya (knowledge of diseases of the nose). 20. Nasa roga pratisedha (treatment of diseases of the nose). 21. Mukha roga vijnaniya (knowledge of the diseases of the mouth). 22. Mukha roga pratisedha (treatment of diseases of the mouth). 23. Siro roga vijnaniya (knowledge of the diseases of the head). 24. Siro roga pratisedha (treatment of diseases of the head). 25. Vrana pratisedha (treatment of ulcers). 26. Sadyovrana pratisedha (treatment of traumatic wounds). 27. Bhanga pratisedha (treatment of fractures). 28. Bhagandara pratisedha (treatment of rectal fistula).

29. Granthi-arbuda-slipada-apaci-nadi vijnaniya (knowledge of tumours, cancers, filariasis, scrofula and sinus ulcer). 30. Granthyadipratisedha

(treatment of tumours etc.). 31. Kshudra roga vijnaniya (knowledge of minor diseases). 32. Kshudra roga pratisedha (treatment of minor diseases). 33. Guhya roga vijnaniya (knowledge of diseases of genital organs). 34. Guhya roga pratisedha (treatment of diseases of genital organs). 35. Visa pratisedha (treatment of poisoning). 36. Sarpa visa pratisedha (treatment of snake bite poison). 37. Kitalutadi visa pratisedha (treatment of poison of insects, spiders etc.). 38. Musika-alarka visa pratisedha (treatment of mouse poison, rabid dog etc.). 39. Rasayana vidhi (rejuvenation therapy). 40. Vajikarana vidhi (aphrodisiac therapy).

इत्यध्यायशतं विंशं षड्भिः स्थानैरुदीरितम् ॥४८॥

Thus enlisted are the 120 chapters under 6 titles.

इति श्रीवैद्यपतिसिंहगुप्तसूनुवाग्भटविरचितायामष्टाङ्गहृदयसंहितायां सूत्रस्थाने आयुष्कामीयो नाम प्रथमोऽध्यायः॥१॥

Thus ends the chapter called Ayushkamiyam, the first in Sutrasthana of Astanga Hrudaya composed by SrimadVaghata, son of Sri Vaidyapati Simhagupta.

2

दिनचर्याध्यायम्
(dinacharya adhyayam)

This is the second Chapter of Ahstanga Hrudaya Sutrasthana called Dinacharya – Ayurvedic daily routine. Dina means daily, Charya means regimen/routine. This chapter covers mental, speech and physical aspects of well being, that you should follow every day.

अथातो दिनचर्याध्यायं व्याख्यास्यामः| इति ह स्माहुरात्रेयादयो महर्षयः| (गद्यसूत्रे)||२||

As advised by Maharshi Atreya, henceforth is described the chapter named 'Dinacharya Adhyaya'.

This chapter covers the daily routine which is to be followed by a healthy person.

Ideal time to wake up:

ब्राह्मे मुहूर्त उत्तिष्ठेत्स्वस्थो रक्षार्थमायुषः|

For living a wholesome life, a healthy person should get up from bed at Brahmi Muhurtha. That is, before dawn, or around 1 and 1/2 hours before sunrise (i.e. around 4:30 – 5:30 AM/14th muhurtha of night).

Danta dhavana - Brushing of the teeth:

शरीरचिन्तां निर्वर्त्य कृतशौचविधिस्ततः||१||

अर्कन्यग्रोधखदिरकरञ्जककुभादिजम्|

प्रातर्भुक्त्वा च मृद्वग्रं कषायकटुतिक्तकम्||२||

कनीन्यग्रसमस्थौल्यं प्रगुणं द्वादशाङ्गुलम्|

भक्षयेद्दन्तपवनं दन्तमांसान्यबाधयन्||३||

After analyzing for a while about the condition of his body, the individual should pass urine and faeces, then clean his teeth with any of the twigs of following herbs -

Arka (Calotropis procera),

Nyagrodha/Vata (Ficus benghalensis),

Khadira (Acacia catechu),

Karanja (Pongamia pinnata),

Kakubha (Terminalia arjuna).

The sharp edges of the twig should be chewed and made soft before use. The twig should be Kashaya (astringent), Katu (pungent) or Tikta (bitter) in taste. To use the twig as a toothbrush, the thickness of the twig should be approximately equal to the tip of one's little finger and its length should be 12 Angula. The teeth should be brushed after every meal, and care should be taken not to hurt the gums (danta mamsa).

Contra-indications for brushing of teeth:

नाद्यादजीर्णवमथुश्वासकासज्वरादिती।

तृष्णास्यपाकहृन्नेत्रशिरःकर्णामयी च तत्॥४॥

People suffering from the following conditions are contra-indicated for brushing of teeth:

Ajeerna - indigestion,

Vamathu - vomiting,

Swasa - dyspnoea,

Kasa - cough,

Jwara - fever,

Arditha - facial paralysis,

Trishna - excessive thirst,

Asyapaka - ulceration of mouth,

Hridroga - heart disease,

Netraroga - diseases of eyes,

Shiroroga - diseases of head,

Karnaroga - diseases of ears.

Sauviramanjanam – Daily collyrium application:

सौवीरमञ्जनं नित्यं हितमक्ष्णोस्ततो भजेत्।

चक्षुस्तेजोमयं तस्य विशेषात् श्लेष्मतो भयम्॥५॥

योजयेत्सप्तरात्रेऽस्मात्स्रावणार्थं रसाञ्जनम्।

Sauvira anjanam is considered Hita (good) for the eyes and hence can be used daily.

The use of Sauvira anjana makes the Pakshma (eyelashes) snigdha (unctuous, shining) and ghana (thick). The eyes with well defined tricolours (black, white and red in appropriate areas), becomes Vimala (clean), Manojna (beautiful) and Sookshma darshana (vision becomes sharp).

Rasanjanam – Weekly collyrium application:
चक्षुस्तेजोमयं तस्य विशेषात् श्लेष्मतो भयम्||५||
योजयेत्सप्तरात्रेऽस्मात्स्रावणार्थं रसाञ्जनम्|

Vision is a function of Agni/Tejo Mahabhuta, and hence the eye is especially prone to diseases caused by Kapha dosha. To prevent this, Rasanjana (aqueous extract of Berberis aristata), should be applied once in a week, to drain out Kapha (secretions) from the eyes.

Procedures done following Anjana (collyrium) application:
ततो नावनगण्डूषधूमताम्बूलभाग्भवेत्||६||
Thereafter,
Navana (Nasya) – Nasal instillation of medicine,
Gandusha – holding of liquid medicine orally,
Dhuma – inhalation of herbal smoke,
Tambula sevana – chewing betel leaves with condiments should be done.

Contra-indications of Tambula Sevana (Chewing betel leaves):
ताम्बूलं क्षतपित्तास्ररूक्षोत्कुपितचक्षुषाम्| विषमूर्च्छामदार्तानामपथ्यं शोषिणामपि||७||
Chewing of betel leaves is contraindicated in those suffering from
Kshata - wounds,
Pittasra - bleeding diseases,
Roukshya - dryness,
Utkupita chakshu - inflammation of eye,
Visha - poisoning,
Murcha - unconsciousness,
Mada - intoxication and
Shosha – emaciation.

Abhyanga – Oil Massage:

अभ्यङ्गमाचरेन्नित्यं,   स   जराश्रमवातहा|

दृष्टिप्रसादपुष्ट्यायुःस्वप्नसुत्वक्त्वदार्ढ्यकृत्||८||

शिरःश्रवणपादेषु तं विशेषेण शीलयेत्|

Abhyanga means oil massage.

It should be done daily (Nitya).

Benefits of Abhyanga:

It delays Jara (aging),

Relieves Srama (tiredness),

Relieves excess of Vata (aches and pains).

Drishti Prasada - It improves vision,

Pushti - nourishes body tissues,

Ayu - prolongs lifespan,

Swapna - induces good sleep,

Sutvaktva - improves skin tone and complexion and

Dardyakrit – helps maintain a good physique.

Massage should be specially done on shira (head), sravana (ears) and pada (legs).

Abhyanga Conta-indications:

वर्ज्योऽभ्यङ्गः कफग्रस्तकृतसंशुद्ध्यजीर्णिभिः||९||

Massage should be avoided when -

- There is increase of Kapha in the body,
- Soon after Shodhana (Panchakarma procedure) and
- During Ajeerna (indigestion).

Vyayama – Physical exercise:

लाघवं कर्मसामर्थ्यं दीप्तोऽग्निर्मेदसः क्षयः|

विभक्तघनगात्रत्वं व्यायामादुपजायते||१०||

Exercise brings about

Laghavam – lightness of the body,

Karma Samarthyam - it improves work capacity,

Deepto Agni - increases digestion power,

Medasa Kshaya – wanes obesity,

Vibhakta Ghana Gatra – Renders a consistent body structure.

Vyayama Conrta-indications:

वातपित्तामयी बालो वृद्धोऽजीर्णो च तं त्यजेत्|

Vata Pitta Amayi - People with diseases originating from Vata and Pitta,

Bala - Children,

Vriddha - Elders,

Ajeerna - People suffering from indigestion,

should not do exercise.

Strength upto which exercise should be done:

अर्धशक्त्या निषेव्यस्तु बलिभिः स्निग्धभोजिभिः||११||

शीतकाले वसन्ते च, मन्दमेव ततोऽन्यदा|

तं कृत्वाऽनुसुखं देहं मर्दयेच्च समन्ततः||१२||

Strong individuals, who consume fat rich diet, should regularly practice exercise in winter and spring, using only half the strength one can gather.

In other seasons, exercise should be done using lesser strength.

At the end of the exercise, one should undergo mild massage (pressing the body parts with mild to moderate pressure).

Complications due to Ati Vyayama (excessive exercise):

तृष्णा क्षयः प्रतमको रक्तपित्तं श्रमः क्लमः| अतिव्यायामतः कासो ज्वरश्छर्दिश्च जायते||१३||

Trishna - excessive thirst,

Kshaya - emaciation,

Pratamaka - severe dyspnoea (difficulty in breathing),

Raktapitta - bleeding disorders,

Srama - exhaustion,

Klama - feeling of debility (even without any work),

Kasa - cough,

Jwara - fever and

Chardi - vomiting

are caused as a result of excessive exercise.

Ill effects of excessive indulgence:

व्यायामजागराध्वस्त्रीहास्यभाष्यादि साहसम्| गजं सिंह इवाकर्षन् भजन्नति विनश्यति||१४||

If indulged in excess in -

Vyayama - exercise,

Jagara - keeping awake at night,

Adhva - walking,

Stri - sexual activities,

Hasya - laughter and

Bhashya - talk

would destroy an individual like a lion perishing while attacking an elephant.

Udvartana – Dry powder Massage:

उद्वर्तनं कफहरं मेदसः प्रविलायनम्‌|

स्थिरीकरणमङ्गानां त्वक्प्रसादकरं परम्‌||१५||

Udvartana is a method of using medicated powders for massage.

Benefits of Udvartana -

- Kaphahara - It helps to calm down aggravated Kapha,
- Medasa pravilayanam - helps to dissolve fat,
- Sthirikaranam Anganam - brings about stability to body parts and
- Twak prasadakaram param - improves skin complexion.

Benefits of Snana (Bathing):

दीपनं वृष्यमायुष्यं स्नानमूर्जाबलप्रदम्‌|

कण्डूमलश्रमस्वेदतन्द्रातृइदाहपाप्मजित्‌||१६||

Bathing has the following benefits -

Deepana - improves digestion,

Vrishyam - acts as aphrodisiac,

Ayushyam - prolongs life,

Urja - increases enthusiasm,

Balapradam – improves strength.

It helps to get rid of -

Kandu - dirt,

Mala - waste products,

Srama - tiredness,

Sweda - sweat,

Tandra – lethargy,

Trit - excessive thirst,

Daha - burning sensation,

Papma – ill feeling.

Use of Hot water for bath:

उष्णाम्बुनाऽधःकायस्य परिषेको बलावहः|

तेनैव तूत्तमाङ्गस्य बलहृत्केशचक्षुषाम्||१७||

Pouring warm (hot) water below the neck bestows strength, but the same over the head, results in loss of strength of Kesha (hair) and Chakshu (eyes).

Snana (bath) contra-indications:

स्नानमर्दितनेत्रास्यकर्णरोगातिसारिषु|

आध्मानपीनसाजीर्णभुक्तवत्सु च गर्हितम्||१८||

Bathing is contra- indicated in those suffering from -

Arditha - facial paralysis,

Netra, Asya, Karna roga - diseases of the eyes, mouth and ears,

Atisara - diarrhoea,

Adhmana - flatulence,

Pinasa - rhinitis,

Ajeerna - indigestion and

Bhuktavat - who has just taken food.

Sadvritta - Code of right conduct:

जीर्णे हितं मितं चाद्यान्न वेगानीरयेद्बलात्|

न वेगितोऽन्यकार्यः स्यान्नाजित्वा साध्यमामयम्||१९||

Jeerne hitam mitam chaadyat – One should always eat, only after digestion of previous food, in limited quantity,

Na vegan neerayet – one should not induce natural urges forcefully,

Na Vegito anya kaaryaha – one should immediately attend to natural urges, whenever they occur, prior to

other involvements.

Na ajitva sadhyam amayam – A curable disease should be treated before anything else.

सुखार्थाः सर्वभूतानां मताः सर्वाः प्रवृत्तयः|

सुखं च न विना धर्मात्तस्माद्धर्मपरो भवेत्||२०||

भक्त्या कल्याणमित्राणि सेवेतेतरदूरगः|

Sukhartha sarvabhutanam - All the creatures in the universe aim towards comfort.

Mataha sarva pravrittaya – All their activities are also aimed at happiness and comforts.

Sukham ca na vina dharmat - There is no happiness, without Dharma (righteousness).

Tasmat dharmaparo bhavet - Hence all should follow the path of Dharma (righteousness).

Bhaktya kalyana mitrani seveta – Good friends shall be served with affection,

Itara dooragaha - Whereas the others (wicked) should be kept at a distance.

Dasha Vidha Paapa Karma (Ten Sins):

हिंसास्तेयान्यथाकामं पैशुन्यं परुषानृते ॥२१॥ सम्भिन्नालापं व्यापादमभिध्यां दृग्विपर्ययम्‌।

पापं कर्मेति दशधा कायवाङ्मनसैस्त्यजेत्‌ ॥२२॥

The following are the ten sins that should not be committed by the body, speech or the mind -

1. Himsa – violence, injury, torture etc.
2. Steya - theft,
3. Anyathakama - unlawful sexual activity, infidelity,
4. Paisunya - abusive, false speech,
5. Parusha vachana - harsh speech,
6. Anruta vacana - speaking untruth,
7. Sambhinna alapa - speech causing separation, breaking of company,
8. Vyapada - quarrel, intention of harming,
9. Abhidya - jealousy, longing for others belongings
10. Drgviparyaya - finding fault, misunderstanding, faithlessness etc. with scriptures, elders etc.

These ten sins pertaining to the body, speech and mind should be avoided.Of these ten,

The first three - are related to the body,

The next four- are related to speech and

The last three – are related to the mind.

People who should be helped:

अवृत्तिव्याधिशोकार्ताननुवर्तेत शक्तितः।

आत्मवत्सततं पश्येदपि कीटपिपीलिकम्||२३||

One should lend as much help to

Avritti - those who have no means of livelihood,

Vyadhi - who are suffering from diseases and

Shoka - who are afflicted with grief.

Even the keeta (insects) and pipilika (ants) should be seen with respect.

Respected persons:

अर्चयेद्देवगोविप्रवृद्धवैद्यनृपातिथीन्|

One should worship -

Deva – God, Go – Cow,

Vipra – Scholars, Vaidya – Physicians,

Vridha – Old people, Nripa – Rulers and

Atithi - Guests.

विमुखान्नार्थिनः कुर्यान्नावमन्येत नाक्षिपेत्||२४||

A wealthy person should not send back someone who approached for help, empty handed, insulted or abused.

उपकारप्रधानः स्यादपकारपरेऽप्यरौ|

One should be willing to help even his foes, even though they are not helpful.

One should maintain Eka Mana (balanced mind) both during calamity and prosperity.

One should not be jealous of other's wealth and happiness.

सम्पदिविपत्स्वेकमना, हेतावीर्ष्येत्फले न तु||२५||

काले हितं मितं ब्रूयादविसंवादि पेशलम्|

पूर्वाभिभाषी, सुमुखः सुशीलः करुणामृदुः||२६|||

नैकः सुखी, न सर्वत्र विश्रब्धो, न च शङ्कितः|

Kale bruyat – speak only on the right occasion.

Hitam bruyat – speak good words, be pleasant.

Mitam bruyat – speak little, as per necessity.

Avisamvadi peshalam – speak without giving a chance for arguments.

Purva abhibhashi - be the first to greet, to start a conversation.

Sumukhaha – have a smiling face.

Susheelaha – have a good character.

Karuna – be courteous.

Mrudu - be soft in speech and activity.

Na Eka sukhee – Do not be a person who likes to be alone always.

Na sarvatah vishrabdo – do not believe everything around you.

Na shankhitaha – do not suspect everything around you.

न कञ्चिदात्मनः शत्रुं नात्मानं कस्यचिद्रिपुम्||२७|| प्रकाशयेन्नापमानं न च निःस्नेहतां प्रभोः|

Na kanchit atmanaha shatrum - Do not instantly consider someone as your foe.

Na aatmanam kasyachit ripum - Do not consider anybody's hostility toward self.

Prakashayet na apamanam - Do not publicly talk about insults that you faced.

Na cha nisnehata prabho - Do not publicly talk about disaffection towards your king.

जनस्याशयमालक्ष्य यो यथा परितुष्यति||२८|| तं तथैवानुवर्तेत पराराधनपण्डितः|

One who is skilled in pleasing others, should keep in mind the nature of people, should deal with them in a manner best pleasing to them, and become well-versed in the art ofadoring others.

न पीडयेदिन्द्रियाणि न चैतान्यति लालयेत् ॥ २९ ॥
त्रिवर्गशून्यं नारम्भं भजेतं चाविरोधयन्|

Na peedayet indriyani – Never induce much strain over the Indriyas (sense organs).

Na chaythanyatilalayet – Never let the Indriyas (sense organs) remain inert. Do not engage yourself in deeds that are devoid of Trivarga (The three objects of worldly existence) -

Dharma (righteousness),

Artha (wealth) and

Kama (desire)

One should carry out his deeds without going contrary to the Trivargas.

अनुयायात्प्रतिपदं सर्वधर्मेषु मध्यमाम्||३०||

In Sarva Dharma (all dealings/activities) one should adopt the Madhyama (middle) Pratipadam (means) only.

Personal hygiene:

नीचरोमनखश्मश्रुनिर्मलाङ्घ्रिमलायनः| स्नानशीलः सुसुरभिः

सुवेषोऽनुल्बणोज्ज्वलः||३१||

धारयेत्सततं रत्नसिद्धमन्त्रमहौषधीः|

One should cut his Roma (hair), Nakha (nails), and Smashru (moustache/ beard) regularly.

Keep the feet and excretory orifices (ears, nose, eyes, urethra and anus) clean.

Snatha sheela - One should take bath regularly,

Susurabhi - use substances with pleasant fragrance,

Suvesha - be well dressed,

Anuthbanojwala – dress should not be superfluous but should be pleasant to look at.

Dharayet ratna - wear precious stones,

Siddha mantra and oushadhi – wear potent hymns and herbs (kept inside amulets) on the body.

सातपत्रपदत्राणो विचरेद्युगमात्रदृक्||३२|| निशि चात्ययिके कार्ये दण्डी मौली सहायवान्|

Walk holding an umbrella, putting on foot wear and looking straight to a distance of 3 yuga (i.e. four arms length) in front of you while walking.

In case of urgent travel at nights, one should go equipped with a danda (baton), mouli (head-dress) and sahayavan (an assistant).

Places that should not be trespassed:

चैत्यपूज्यध्वजाशस्तच्छायाभस्मतुषाशुचीन्||३३||

नाक्रामेच्छर्कगलोष्टबलिस्नानभुवो न च|

One should not trespass the shadows of

Chaitya - a holy tree on which deities reside (or a Buddhist shrine),

Pujya - materials (or men) of worship,

Dvaja – flag posts,

Ashasta - unholy things,

One should not tread upon

Bhasma - heap of ash,

Tusha – husk,

Ashuchi - dirt,

Sarkara - sand dunes,

Loshta – lumps of earth,

Places of Bali (offering sacrifices to Gods, demons etc.) and Snana (bathing).

नदीं तरेन्न बाहुभ्यां, नाग्निस्कन्धमभिव्रजेत्||३४||
सन्दिग्धनावं वृक्षं च नारोहेद्दुष्टयानवत्|

Nadi taret na bahubyam - One should not swim across rivers using arms,
Na agni skandham abhivrajet – One should not walk facing a huge fire,
One should not travel in a risky boat (Navam), not climb a tree (vriksham) doubtful of strength; or ride on a vehicle (yana), which is in bad condition (dushta).

नासंवृतमुखः कुर्यात्क्षुतिहास्यविजृम्भणम्||३५||
नासिकां न विकुष्णीयान्नाकस्मादिवलिखेद्भुवम्|
नाङ्गैश्चेष्टेत विगुणं, नासीतोत्कटकश्चिरम्||३६||

Without covering the mouth, one should not sneeze (kshuti), laugh (hasya) or yawn (vijrimbanam).
One should not blow his nose (nasika), except for forcing out the excretions,
One should not dig the ground (bhumi) without any reason,
One should not move the body parts (anga) in an awkward manner (vigunam),
Sitting on one's own heels (utkutika) for a long time should be avoided.

देहवाक्चेतसां चेष्टाः प्राक् श्रमादिवनिवर्तयेत्|
नोर्ध्वजानुश्चिरं तिष्ठेत् नक्तं सेवेत न द्रुमम्||३७||
तथा चत्वरचैत्यान्तश्चतुष्पथसुरालयान्|
सूनाटवीशून्यगृहश्मशानानि दिवाऽपि न||३८||

One should stop the activities of the body (deha), speech (vak) and the mind (chetas) before getting exhausted;
One should not keep his knees (janu) raised (urdhva) or flexed for a long period.
One should not reside at night (nakta) -
On trees – druma,
At the meeting place of three roads - chatvara,
Chaityanta - vicinity of a holy tree (or a Buddhist shrine),
Chatushpada - meeting place of four roads and
Suralaya – temple (house of God).

One should not reside even during daytime in -
Suna - a place of slaughter,
Atavi – lonely places,
Shunya griha - a haunted house and
Shmashaana - burial grounds.

सर्वथेक्षेत नादित्यं, न भारं शिरसा वहेत्‌।
नेक्षेत प्रततं सूक्ष्मं दीप्तामेध्याप्रियाणि च||३९||
मद्यविक्रयसन्धानदानादानानि नाचरेत्‌।

Sarvatha iksheta na adityam - Never gaze at the sun (aditya) for a long time,
Na bharam shirasa vahet - One should not carry heavy weight (bhara) on his head (shiras), One should not see continuously, objects which are minute (sukshma), shining (deepta), dirty (amedhya) or unpleasant (apriya).
One should not engage in selling (vikriya), brewing (sandhana), free distributing (daana), or receiving (paana) of wine (madya).

The following should be avoided:
पुरोवातातपरजस्तुषारपरुषानिलान्‌||४०||

Exposure to the following should be avoided -
Purovata – eastern wind,
Atapa – heat,
Raja – dust,
Tushara – frost,
Parusha anila – storm.
अनृजुः क्षवथूद्गारकासस्वप्नान्नमैथुनम्‌।

Indulgence in the following while adopting an awkward posture should be avoided -
Kshavathu – sneezing, Udgara – belching,
Kasa – cough, Swapna – sleep,
Anna – taking food and Maithunam – Sexual intercourse.

The following are to be avoided -
कूलछायां नृपद्विष्टं व्यालदंष्ट्रिविषाणिनः||४१||
Koola chaya – shadows of a barricade, Nripa dvishta – adversaries of rulers,
Vyala – wild animals, Damshtri – venomous animals,

Vishani – animals with horns.

हीनानार्यातिनिपुणसेवां विग्रहमुत्तमैः।
सन्ध्यास्वभ्यवहारस्त्रीस्वप्नाध्ययनचिन्तनम्॥४२॥

Dependence on those who are socially inferior (heena) and crooked should be avoided.

Quarrel with people of excellent (uttama) conduct should be avoided.

The following activities should be avoided at the time of meeting of night and sunrise -

Abhyavahara – intake of food,

Stri – sexual intercourse,

Swapna – sleep,

Adhyayana – learning,

Chintanam – thinking.

Foods to be avoided:

शत्रुसत्रगणाकीर्णगणिकापणिकाशनम्।

Food of the following types should be avoided -

Shatru – offered by enemies,

Satra – served during sacrificial ceremony, or food served to a gathering,

Ganika – offered by merchants,

Panika – offered by prostitutes.

गात्रवक्त्रनखैर्वाद्यं हस्तकेशावधूननम्॥४३॥

One should not make sound with the body parts (gatra), mouth (vaktra) and nails (nakha).

One should not flicker his hands (hastha) or hair (kesha).

तोयाग्निपूज्यमध्येन यानं धूमं शवाश्रयम्।
मद्यातिसक्तिं विश्रम्भस्वातन्त्र्ये स्त्रीषु च त्यजेत्॥४४॥

The following should be avoided -

Toya madhyena yanam – Walking amidst water,

Agni madhyena yanam – Walking amidst fire,

Poojya madhyena yanam – Walking between respectable personalities,

Dhumam shavashrayam – Inhalation of smoke of funeral pyre,

Madya atisaktim – Alcohol addiction,

Strishu visrambha – Over trust in (wicked) females,

Strishu svathantrye – Freedom in (wicked) females.

The world as a teacher:

आचार्यः सर्वचेष्टासु लोक एव हि धीमतः।
अनुकुर्यात्तमेवातो लौकिकेऽर्थे परीक्षकः॥४५॥

For an intelligent person the world (loka) is a teacher, hence one should imitate the world after carefully considering their meaning and effects of such actions.

Ethics to follow:

आर्द्रसन्तानता त्यागः कायवाक्चेतसां दमः।
स्वार्थबुद्धिः परार्थेषु पर्याप्तमिति सद्व्रतम्॥४६॥

Ardrasanthanata - Compassion towards all living beings,

Tyaga - charity,

Kaya, vak, chetasam damaha - controlling the activities of the body, speech and mind,

Parartheshu svarthabuddhi – showing selfless devotion to the cause of others (looking after their interests as if it is his own).

These are sufficient rules of good conduct.

नक्तंदिनानि मे यान्ति कथम्भूतस्य सम्प्रति।
दुःखभाङ्न भवत्येवं नित्यं सन्निहितस्मृतिः॥४७॥

He, who is constantly involved in how his nights (nakta) and days (dina) are passing and adopts the right way, will never become a victim of sorrow (dukha).

इत्याचारः समासेन, यं प्राप्नोति समाचरन्।
आयुरारोग्यमैश्वर्यं यशो लोकांश्च शाश्वतान्॥४८॥

Thus was enumerated, in brief the rules of good conduct; he who adopts it will attain

Ayu – A long life, Arogya – Health,

Aishwaryam – Wealth, Yashaha – Reputation, fame and

Shaashvata loka – The eternal world.

इति श्रीवैद्यपतिसिंहगुप्तसूनु श्रीमद्वाग्भटविरचितायामष्टाङ्गहृदयसंहितायां सूत्रस्थाने दिनचर्या नाम द्विवतीयोऽध्यायः॥२॥

Thus ends the chapter called Dinacarya, the second in Sutrasthana of Astanga Hrudaya composed by Srimad Vaghata, son of Sri Vaidyapati Simhagupta.

3

ऋतुचर्याध्यायम्
(ritucharya adhyayam)

The word Ritucharya is made of two words – Rutu means seasons, Charya means regimen. This chapter discusses in detail regarding different seasons and the specific regimen to be followed.

अथातो ऋतुचर्याध्यायं व्याख्यास्यामः । इति ह स्माहुरात्रेयादयो महर्षयः ॥

Maharshi Atreya and other sages pledge that they will henceforth be explaining the chapter named Ritucharya.

Shad Ritu – Six seasons:

मासैर्द्विवसंख्यैर्माघाद्यैः क्रमात् षड्ऋतवः स्मृताः।
शिशिरोऽथ वसन्तश्च ग्रीष्मो वर्षाशरदि्धमाः॥१॥

A season (Ritu) is comprised of two months (two Masa) to constitute a seasonal cycle.

- **Shishira Ritu** (winter, dewy season) – Magha and Phalguna (Mid January – Mid March)
- **Vasanta Ritu** (Spring season) – Chaitra and Vaishakha (Mid March – Mid May)
- **Greeshma Ritu** (Summer season) – Jyeshta and Ashadha (Mid May to Mid July)
- **Varsha Ritu** (Rainy Season) – Shravana and Bhadrapada (Mid July – mid September)

- **Sharat Ritu** (Autumn season) – Ashvayuja and Karthika – (Mid September to Mid November)
- **Hemantha Ritu** (Winter season) – Margashira and Pushya - (Mid November to Mid January).

Uttarayana – Adana kala – Northern Solstice – mid January to mid July:

शिशिराद्यैस्त्रिभिस्तैस्तु विद्यादयनमुत्तरम् ।
आदानं च तदादत्ते नृणां प्रतिदिनं बलम् ॥ २ ॥

The three consecutive Ritus of Shishira (winter), Vasanta (spring) and Grishma (summer) comprise Uttarayana (Northern solstice). It is also called Adana Kala (period of extraction), wherein the human strength relatively reduces day by day.

तस्मिन् ह्यत्यर्थतीक्ष्णोष्णरूक्षा मार्गस्वभावतः ।
आदित्यपवनाः सौम्यान् क्षपयन्ति गुणान् भुवः ॥ ३ ॥
तिक्तः कषायः कटुको बलिनोऽत्र रसाः क्रमात् ।
तस्मादादानमाग्नेयं

Because of the nature of the path (marga svabhava), both the Sun (aditya) and wind (pavana) become very sharp (tikshna), hot (ushna) and dry (ruksha).
It takes away all the cooling qualities (soumya) of the Earth.
Bitter (Tikta), Astringent (Kashaya), and Pungent (Katu) Rasa will be more powerful, respectively, in the successive Ritus.
Hence Adana Kala is dominated by fire (agneyam).

Dakshinayana – Visarga Kala – Southern Solstice – mid July to mid January:

ऋतवो दक्षिणायनम् ॥ ४ ॥
वर्षादयो विसर्गश्च यद्बलं विसृजत्ययम् ।

The seasons of Varsha (rainy season), Sharat (autumn) and Hemanta (early winter) comprise Dakshinayana (Southern Solstice).
This period is also called Visarga Kala (period of discharge) as the body gains strength during this season.

Dakshinayana:
सौम्यत्वादत्र सोमो हि बलवान् हीयते रविः ॥ ५ ॥

मेघवृष्ट्यनिलैः शीतैः शान्ततापे महीतले ।
स्निग्धाश्चेहाम्ललवणमधुरा बलिनो रसाः ॥ ६ ॥

During this period, due to the predominance of Somabhava (gentleness), the moon (Soma) becomes more powerful, weakening the properties of the Sun (Ravi). The Earth is cooled down due to clouds (megha), rain (varsha) and cold wind (sheeta anila).

Sour (amla), salt (lavana) and sweet (madhura) tastes which have snigdha (unctuous) properties, gain strength during the three seasons of this period.

Variation in body strength as per season:

शीतेऽग्र्यं वृष्टिघर्मेऽल्पं बलं मध्यं तु शेषयोः ।

Winter – Hemantha and Shishira – mid November to mid March – Highest strength.

Summer and rainy seasons – Grishma and Varsha - mid May to mid September – Lowest strength.

Spring and Autumn – Vasanta and Sharat - Medium strength.

Hemanta Ritucharya – Ayurveda winter regimen: Mid November – Mid January:

बलिनः शीतसंरोधाद्धेमन्ते प्रबलोऽनलः ॥ ७ ॥
भवत्यल्पेन्धनो धातून् स पचेद्वायुनेरितः ।
अतो हिमेऽस्मिन् सेवेत स्वाद्वम्ललवणान् रसान् ॥ ८ ॥

During Hemantha, the body is strong, digestive fire becomes powerful, because it gets obstructed from flowing outwards due to the external cold atmosphere. Like fire consumes the things that it comes in contact with, the digestive fire may digest the body tissues and cause emaciation. Hence, in this period, one should consume food predominantly of sweet (madhura), sour (amla) and salt (lavana) tastes.

Regime to be followed:

दैर्घ्यान् निशानामेतर्हि प्रातरेव बुभुक्षितः ।
अवश्यकार्यं सम्भाव्य यथोक्तं शीलयेदनु ॥ ९ ॥
वातघ्नतैलैरभ्यङ्गं मूर्ध्नि तैलं विमर्दनम्।
नियुद्धं कुशलैः सार्धं पादाघातं च युक्ततः ॥१०॥

As the nights (nisha) are longer (deerga), a person feels hungry (bubhukshita) early in the morning (prataha). So, after attending to ablution (avashyakaaryam sambhavya),

one should resort to the following -
Abhyanga (oil massage) - with oils that have Vata balancing properties,
Murdha taila – Oil application on scalp and forehead,
Vimardana - Mild massaging,
Niyudha - wrestling till one's half strength and
Padaghata – body massage with feet.

Snana (bath):

कषायापहृतस्नेहस्ततः स्नातो यथाविधि ।
कुङ्कुमेन सदर्पेण प्रदिग्धोऽगुरुधूपितः ॥ ११ ॥

Thereafter, one should take bath using astringent (kashaya rasa) drugs to wash off the oil. Then fine powders of Kumkuma (Saffron) and Darpa (kasthuri / musk) are applied over the body.
Then, Dhupana (exposure to fumes) of the body is done using Aguru (Aquilaria agallocha).

Foods to be consumed:

रसान् स्निग्धान् पलं पुष्टं गौडमच्छसुरां सुराम् ।
गोधूमपिष्टमाषेक्षुक्षीरोत्थविकृतीः शुभाः ॥ १२ ॥
नवमन्नं वसां तैलं शौचकार्ये सुखोदकम् ।

The following are the recommended foods during Hemanta Ritu -
Rasan snigdhan - meat soup mixed with fats,
Palam pushtam - meat of well nourished animals,
Gouda - wine prepared with jaggery,
Acha sura - supernatant part of wine (Sura),
Food prepared with
Godhuma - wheat flour,
Masha - black gram,
Ikshu vikriti - products of sugarcane,
Kshirotha vikriti – products prepared using milk,
Navam annam - food prepared from freshly harvested paddy,
Vasa - muscle fat and
Taila - edible oils.
Shouryakaryam sukhodakam - Warm water (sukhodaka) should be used for ablutions.

प्रावाराजिनकौशेयप्रवेणीकौचवास्तृतम् ॥ १३ ॥

उष्णस्वभावैर्लघुभिः प्रावृतः शयनं भजेत् ।
युक्त्यार्ककिरणान्स्वेदं पादत्राणं च सर्वदा ॥ १४ ॥

Thick sheets made of Pravara (cotton), Ajina (leather), Kausheya (silk), Praveni (wool) Kauchava (woollen blanket) which are warm and light in weight should be used during sleep.

Exposure to Arka kirana (sunlight) and Sweda (sudation) should be resorted to, judiciously. Padatrana (foot wear) should be worn always.

पीवरोरुस्तनश्रोण्यः समदाः प्रमदाः प्रियाः ।
हरन्ति शीतमुष्णाङ्ग्यो धूपकुङ्कुमयौवनैः ॥ १५ ॥

The embrace of loving young women, who are passionate and warm, having applied saffron all over and have fumigated, will keep out cold.

Ideal place to reside:

अङ्गारतापसन्तप्तगर्भभूवेश्मचारिणः ।
शीतपारुष्यजनितो न दोषो जातु जायते ॥ १६ ॥

One who resides in underground chambers (garbha bhuveshma), warmed with burning charcoal (angara), will not be affected by diseases due to Sheeta (cold) and Parushya (dryness).

Shishira Rutu charya – Ayurveda winter regimen – Mid January to Mid March:

अयमेव विधिः कार्यः शिशिरेऽपि विशेषतः ।
तदा हि शीतमधिकं रौक्ष्यं चादानकालजम् ॥ १७ ॥

Even in Shishira Ritu, the same regimen, as described above should be adopted with more intensity. During this period Sheeta (cold) and Roukshya (dryness), which is characteristic of Adana Kala is present.

Vasanta Rutucharya - Ayurveda Spring regimen – Mid March to Mid May:

कफश्चितो हि शिशिरे वसन्तेऽर्कांशुतापितः ।
हत्वाग्निं कुरुते रोगानतस्तं त्वरया जयेत् ॥ १८ ॥

Kapha which has undergone increase in Shishira (cold season) becomes liquefied by the heat of the Arka (Sun) in Vasanta (spring).

It diminishes the digestive fire (Hatva Agni) and gives rise to many Roga (diseases).

Methods to pacify aggravated Kapha:

तीक्ष्णैर्वमननस्याद्यैर्लघुरूक्षैश्च भोजनैः ।
व्यायामोद्वर्तनाघातैर्जित्वा श्लेष्माणमुल्बणम् ॥ १९ ॥
स्नातोऽनुलिप्तः कर्पूरचन्दनागुरुकुङ्कुमैः ।

The aggravated Kapha should be controlled quickly, by resorting to

Tikshna vamana - strong emesis therapy,

Nasya - nasal medication etc.,

Laghu, ruksha bhojana - Foods that are easily digestible and dry,

Vyayama - Physical exercises,

Udvartana - dry massage and

Aghata – Massage using more pressure.

Having thus mitigated the Kapha, the person should take bath and then anoint the body with pastes of -

Karpura (camphor), Candana (sandalwood), Aguru (Aquilaria agallocha) and Kumkuma (saffron).

Foods to be consumed:

पुराणयवगोधूमक्षौद्रजाङ्गलशूल्यभुक् ॥ २० ॥
सहकाररसोन्मिश्रानास्वाद्य प्रिययार्पितान् ।
प्रियास्यसङ्गसुरभीन् प्रियानेत्रोत्पलाङ्कितान् ॥ २१ ॥
सौमनस्यकृतो हृद्यान् वयस्यैः सहितः पिबेत् ।

Purana yava - old barley,

Godhuma – wheat,

Madhu - honey,

Jangala - meat of animals of desert-like land, and

Shulya - meat roasted over fire

Drink the juice of mango fruit mixed with fragrant substances, in the company of friends, getting it served by the beloved; the drink, thereby producing satisfaction.

निर्गदानासवारिष्टसीधुमाद्वीकमाधवान् ॥ २२ ॥
शृङ्गवेराम्बु साराम्बु मध्वम्बु जलदाम्बु वा।

Beverages such as

Asava - fermented infusion, Arista - fermented decoction,

Sidhu - fermented infusion, Mardvika - fermented grape juice, or

Sringavera ambu – water boiled with ginger (Zingiber officinalis),

Sara ambu – water boiled with extract of asana, chandana etc.

Madhvambu - water mixed with honey, Jaladambu - water boiled with jalada

(Musta – Cyperus rotundus).

Ways to spend the mid-day hours:

दक्षिणानिलशीतेषु परितो जलवाहिषु ॥ २३ ॥
अदृष्टनष्टसूर्येषु मणिकुट्टिटमकान्तिषु ।
परपुष्टविघुष्टेषु कामकर्मान्तभूमिषु ॥ २४ ॥
विचित्रपुष्पवृक्षेषु काननेषु सुगन्धिषु ।
गोष्ठीकथाभिश्चित्राभिर्मध्याह्नं गमयेत्सुखी ॥ २५ ॥

Dakshina anila sheeteshu - In the gardens cooled by the breeze from south direction,

Paritaha jalavahishu - with plenty of reservoirs of water all around,

Adrishta nashta suryeshu – Half hidden sun among the clouds,

Mani kuttima kanthishu - the land covered with shining crystals,

Parapushta vigushteshu kamakarmantha - with the cuckoo everywhere making pleasant sounds and engaged in love-play,

Vichitra pushpa vriksheshu – amongst trees with exotic blooms,

the person should spend his mid-day hours (madhyahnam) in the company of friends engaged in pleasant games, pastimes, storytelling etc., in forests (or gardens).

The following are to be avoided:

गुरुशीतदिवास्वप्नस्निग्धाम्लमधुरांस्त्यजेत् ।

Guru, sheeta ahara - hard to-digest and cold foods,

Divaswapna - sleeping at day time,

Snigdha ahara - foods which are fatty,

Amla - sour and

Madhura - sweet.

Greeshma Ritucharya (Ayurveda Summer Regimen) Mid May – Mid July:

तीक्ष्णांशुरतितीक्ष्णांशुर्ग्रीष्मे सङ्क्षिपतीव यत् ॥ २६ ॥
प्रत्यहं क्षीयते श्लेष्मा तेन वायुश्च वर्धते ।

In Greeshma (summer) the sun rays become powerful (tikshnaamshu) and appear to be destructive.

Kapha decreases (ksheeyate) day by day (pratyaham) and Vata increases consequently (vateshu vardhate).

The following are to be avoided:

अतोऽस्मिन् पटुकट्वम्ल व्यायामार्ककरांस्त्यजेत् ॥ २७ ॥

Hence, in Greeshma, the following are to be avoided -

Patu (lavana) – salty,

Katu – pungent,

Amla – sour tastes,

Vyayama – exercise,

Arka – exposure to sun.

Foods that are recommended:

भजेन्मधुरमेवान्नं लघु स्निग्धं हिमं द्रवम् ।

सुशीततोयसिक्ताङ्गो लिह्यात् सक्तून् सशर्करान् ॥ २८ ॥

The anna (food) recommended shall be of -

Madhura rasa – sweet,

Laghu – light,

Snigdha – unctuous,

Hima – cool,

Drava – in liquid form.

After taking bath in Susheeta toya (cool water), Saktu (powder of parched paddy) mixed with sharkara (sugar) is licked.

Limited use of wine during summer:

मद्यं न पेयं पेयं वा स्वल्पं सुबहुवारि वा ।

अन्यथा शोफशैथिल्यदाहमोहान् करोति तत् ॥ २९ ॥

Madyam na peyam – Alcoholic beverages are forbidden,

Peyam va svalpam – If very necessary, taken in very small quantity,

Subahuvari va – or consumed by mixing it with a lot of water.

Otherwise it may lead to -

Shopha – inflammatory conditions,

Shaithilya – generalised debility,

Daha – burning sensation and

Moha - fainting.

Foods indicated:

कुन्देन्दुधवलं शालिमश्नीयाज्जाङ्गलैः पलैः ।

पिबेद्रसं नातिघनं रसालं रागखाण्डवौ ॥ ३० ॥

पानकं पञ्चसारं वा नवमृद्भाजने स्थितम् ।

मोचचोचदलैर्युक्तं साम्लं मृन्मयशुक्तिभिः ॥ ३१ ॥

पाटलावासितं चाम्भः सकर्पूरं सुशीतलम् ।

Shali (rice) as white as kunda (jasmine flower) or indu (moon) is consumed along with the meat of Jangala animals (animals residing in arid regions).

The following can be used as a drink -

Rasa (meat soup), which is not very ghana (thick),

Rasala - curds churned and mixed with pepper powder and sugar,

Raga - syrup which is sweet, sour and salty,

Khandava - syrup which has all the tastes, prepared with many substances,

Panaka panchasara - syrup prepared with raisins (draksha), madhuka, dates (karjura), kasmarya, and parushaka fruits all in equal quantities, cooled and added with powder of cinnamon leaves, cinnamon and cardamom etc. and kept inside a fresh mud pot (nava mrit bhajana), along with leaves of plantain (mocha) and jackfruit (chocha dala), and made sour / fermented (sa amlam), should be drunk in mugs made of mud (mrinmaya) or shell (shukti).

Very cool water kept in mud pots along with flowers of patala and karpura (camphor) should be used for drinking.

शशाङ्ककिरणान् भक्ष्यान् रजन्यां भक्षयन् पिबेत् ॥ ३२ ॥
सासितं माहिषं क्षीरं चन्द्रनक्षत्रशीतलम् ।

Food articles like shashanka kirana (hollow, finger-like, fried pastry made of corn flour) should be taken at night.

Mahisha kshira (Buffalo milk) mixed with Sita (sugar) and cooled by Chandra (moonlight) and the Nakshatra (stars) should be used for drinking.

अभ्रङ्कषमहाशालतालरुद्धोष्णरश्मिषु ॥ ३३ ॥ वनेषु माधवीश्लिष्टद्राक्षास्तबकशालिषु ।
सुगन्धिहिमपानीयसिच्यमानपटालिके ॥ ३४ ॥ कायमाने चिते चूतप्रवालफललुम्बिभिः ।
कदलीदलकल्हारमृणालकमलोत्पलैः ॥ ३५ ॥ कोमलैः कल्पिते तल्पे हसत्कुसुमपल्लवे ।
मध्यन्दिनेऽर्कतापार्तः स्वप्यादुधारागृहेऽथवा ॥ ३६ ॥
पुस्तस्त्रीस्तनहस्तास्यप्रवृत्तोशीरवारिणि ।

Day time should be spent in forests having tall trees which seem to touch the sky (abhra), such as shala (Shorea robusta), Tala (Borassus flabellifera) etc., which obstruct the hot rays of the sun (ruddha ushna rashmi), or in houses around which bunches of flowers and grapes (draksha) are hanging from their creepers.

Sheets of cloth dribbling with sweet scented water are arranged all around. The person should sleep on a soft bed prepared with Kadali dala (banana leaves), kalhara (soughandika – a water plant), mrinala (lotus stalk), kamala (lotus flower), utpala (water lily) etc. with fully blossomed flowers placed all over.

Spend the remaining day inside the house cooled by water fountains, water being scented with Ushira (vetiver grass), and thereby relieving oneself from the heat of the sun.

Ratricharya (Night regimen):

निशाकरकराकीर्ण सौधपृष्ठे निशासु च ॥ ३७ ॥
आसना स्वस्थचित्तस्य चन्दनार्द्रस्य मालिनः ।
निवृत्तकामतन्त्रस्य सुसूक्ष्मतनुवाससः ॥ ३८ ॥
जलार्द्रस्तालवृन्तानि विस्तृताः पद्मिनीपुटाः ।
उत्क्षेपाश्च मृदूत्क्षेपा जलवर्षिहिमानिलाः ॥ ३९ ॥
कर्पूरमल्लिकामाला हाराः सहरिचन्दनाः ।
मनोहरकलालापाः शिशवः सारिकाः शुकाः ॥ ४० ॥
मृणालवलयाः कान्ताः प्रोत्फुल्लकमलोज्ज्वलाः ।
जङ्गमा इव पद्मिन्यो हरन्ति दयिताः क्लमम् ॥ ४१ ॥

At night, one should sleep on the terrace, under the moonlight.

Exhaustion due to heat of the day is relieved by -

Anointing the body with moist paste of chandana (sandalwood),

Wearing garlands (mala),

Nivritta kama tantrasya - avoidance of sexual activities,

Sukshma tanu vasa - wearing of very light and thin dresses,

Fanning with fans made of Tala vrinta – ornamental fans made of peacock feathers, or large leaves of Padmini (lily) made wet,

Jala varsha hima anila - cool breeze sprinkling water droplets,

Garlands of flowers of camphor, jasmine and of pearls and beads of sandalwood,

Sweet coquetry of children,

Sarika (mynah bird) and Shuka (parrot) talking pleasantly;

Beautiful woman wearing bangles of soft lotus stalk, blossoms of lotus in their hair, moving about nearby.

Varsha Ritu carya- Ayurveda seasonal regimen for rainy season – Mid July – Mid September

आदानग्लानवपुषामग्निः सन्नोऽपि सीदति ।
वर्षासु दोषैर्दुष्यन्ति तेऽम्बुलम्बाम्बुदेऽम्बरे ॥ ४२ ॥

सतुषारेण मरुता सहसा शीतलेन च ।
भूबाष्पेणाम्लपाकेन मलिनेन च वारिणा ॥ ४३ ॥
वह्निनैव च मन्देन तेष्वित्यन्योऽन्यदूषिषु ।
भजेत्साधारणं सर्वमूष्मणस्तेजनं च यत् ॥ ४४ ॥

The weak digestive fire of Adanakala is further deteriorated by doshas in Varsha ritu (rainy season). Thick clouds full of water spread and the cold wind blows with water droplets, causing the warmth of the earth to generate amla vipaka.

This amla vipaka thus generated, the turbid water (due to rain) and the manda vahni (weak digestive fire) are responsible for the vitiation of the doshas.

Thus it is advisable to adopt a seasonal regimen that does not vitiate doshas and increases the digestive fire (ushmana tejanam).

Recommended diet:

आस्थापनं शुद्धतनुर्जीर्णं धान्यं रसान् कृतान् ।
जाङ्गलं पिशितं यूषान् मध्वरिष्टं चिरन्तनम् ॥ ४५ ॥
मस्तु सौवर्चलाढ्यं वा पञ्चकोलावचूर्णितम् ।
दिव्यं कौपं शृतं चाम्भो भोजनं त्वतिदुर्दिने ॥ ४६ ॥
व्यक्ताम्ललवणस्नेहं संशुष्कं क्षौद्रवल्लघु ।

After cleansing the body (Shuddha tanu) by emesis and purgation,
The person should be administered asthapana basti (decoction enema therapy).
He should consume -
Jeerna dhanya - old grains,
Krita rasa - meat juice processed with spices etc.,
Jangalam pishitam - Meat of animals of desert-like lands,
Yusha - soup of pulses,
Chirantam madhu arishtam - wine prepared from grapes and fermented decoctions, which are old
Mastu (whey, thin water or curds) processed with more of sauvarchala (Sochal salt) and powder of Panchakola.
Well boiled rain or well water should be used for drinking.
On days of no sunlight at all (durdina), the food should be -
predominantly of Amla (sour), Lavana (salty) rasa
Added with sufficient Sneha dravyas (unctuous substances),
Samshushka (dry),

Kshoudravat (mixed with honey) and
Laghu (easily digestible).

Regime to be followed:
अपादचारी सुरभिः सततं धूपिताम्बरः ॥ ४७ ॥
हर्म्यपृष्ठे वसेद्बाष्पशीतसीकरवर्जिते ।
Apadachari – walking without footwear – is not recommended,
Surabhi – Body shall be scented with perfumes,
Satatam dhupita ambara – Clothes worn should be fumigated,
Harmyaprishte vaset – dwell in upper storeys of the house,
Bashpa sheeta shikara varjite – Which is devoid of moisture, cold and mist.

The following has to be avoided -
नदीजलोदमन्थाहः स्वप्नायासातपांस्त्यजेत् ॥ ४८ ॥
Nadi jala – river water,
Udamantha - beverage prepared with flour of corns mixed with ghee,
Aaha swapna – sleeping during daytime,
Aayasa – exertion and
Tapta – exposure to sun.

Sharat Ritucharya – Ayurveda autumn regimen – Mid September – Mid November:
वर्षाशीतोचिताङ्गानां सहसैवार्करश्मिभिः ।
तप्तानां सञ्चितं वृष्टौ पित्तं शरदि कुप्यति ॥ ४९ ॥
During Varsha ritu, the person becomes accustomed to the cold atmosphere. When he suddenly gets exposed to the warm rays of Sun, the Pitta, which has undergone increase in Varsha (rainy season) becomes greatly aggravated during Sharat ritu (autumn).

Methods to pacify aggravated Pitta:
तज्जयाय घृतं तिक्तं विरेको रक्तमोक्षणम् ।
तिक्तं स्वादु कषायं च क्षुधितोऽन्नं भजेल्लघु ॥ ५० ॥
शालिमुद्गसिताधात्रीपटोलमधुजाङ्गलम् ।
To pacify Pitta aggravation,
Tikta grita - medicated ghee recipe prepared with tikta (bitter) dravyas,
Virechana - purgation therapy and
Raktamokshana - bloodletting should be resorted to.

When hungry, the person should take foods
Which are of Tikta (bitter), Madhura (sweet) and Kashaya (astringent)
tastes,
Laghu - easily digestible such as
Shali (rice), Mudga (green gram),
Sita (sugar), Dhatri / Amla (Indian gooseberry),
Patola (snake gourd), Madhu (honey) and
Jangala mamsa (meat of animals of desert-like lands).

Hamsodaka:

तप्तं तप्तांशुकिरणैः शीतं शीतांशुरश्मिभिः ॥ ५१ ॥
समन्तादप्यहोरात्रमगस्त्योदयनिर्विषम् ।
शुचि हंसोदकं नाम निर्मलं मलजिज्जलम् ॥ ५२ ॥
नाभिष्यन्दि न वा रूक्षं पानादिष्वमृतोपमम् ।

The water heated by the hot rays of the sun during day time and cooled by
the rays of the moon at night,
Which has been de-poisoned (detoxified) by the rise of the star Agastya,
Which is pure,
Uncontaminated and capable of mitigating the malas (dosas) is known as
Hamsodaka.
It is neither abhisyandi (does not produce more secretion or moisture inside
the minute channels so as to block them) nor ruksha (dry),
such water is like Amrita (nectar) for drinking and other purposes.

चन्दनोशीरकर्पूरमुक्तास्रग्वसनोज्ज्वलः ॥ ५३ ॥
सौधेषु सौधधवलां चन्द्रिकां रजनीमुखे ।

Evenings should be spent on the terrace of houses which are painted white,
after anointing the body with the paste of Chandana (Sandalwood), Ushira
(Cus Cus grass), Karpura (Camphor), wearing garlands of Mukta (pearls)
and brilliant clothes and enjoying the moonlight.

The following are to be avoided:

तुषारक्षारसौहित्यदधितैलवसातपान् ॥ ५४ ॥ तीक्ष्णमद्यदिवास्वप्नपुरोवातान् परित्यजेत्
।

The following should be avoided -
Tushara – Exposure to fog,
Kshara – Alkalis,

Souhitya – Heavy food,
Dadhi – Curd,
Taila – Oil,
Vasa – Muscle fat,
Atapa – Exposure to sun,
Tikshna madya – Strong alcoholic beverages,
Divaswapna – Sleeping during daytime,
Puro vata – Eastern wind.

Use of taste as per season:

शीते वर्षासु चाद्यांस्त्रीन् वसन्तेऽन्त्यान् रसान्भजेत् स्वादुं निदाघे, शरदि स्वादुतिक्तकषायकान्|

During Hemanta, Shishira (winter season) and Varsha (rainy season) – Madhura (Sweet), Amla (Sour) and Lavana (salt) tastes should be especially used.

During Vasanta (spring season) – Tikta (Bitter), Katu (pungent) and Kashaya (astringent) tastes should be used more.

Madhura (sweet) taste should be used more during Nidagha (summer) and Svadu (Sweet), Tikta (bitter) and Kashaya (astringent) tastes should be used during Sharat (autumn season).

Qualities of food as per season:

शरद्वसन्तयो रूक्षं शीतं घर्मघनान्तयोः ॥ ५६ ॥ अन्नपानं समासेन विपरीतमतोऽन्यदा ।

During Sharat and Vasanta (autumn and spring) - the foods and drinks should be Ruksha (dry, moisture less, fat-less).

During Gharma (summer) and Ghananta (end of rainy season) - food should be Sheeta (cool).

During the other four Ritus (Sisira, Vasanta, Varsha, Hemanta), hot foods are preferred.

नित्यं सर्वरसाभ्यासः स्वस्वाधिक्यामृतावृतौ ॥ ५७ ॥

The habit of using all the six tastes every day is ideal for maintenance of health. However, during particular seasons, the tastes that are particularly indicated should be given special emphasis.

तत्र पूर्वो विधिस्त्याज्यः सेवनीयोऽपरः क्रमात् ॥ ५८ ॥

असात्म्यजा हि रोगाः स्युः सहसा त्यागशीलनात् ॥ ५८ ॥

The last seven days of a season and the first seven days of the next season is known as Ritusandhi (inter seasonal period).

During this period, the regimen of the preceding season should be discontinued gradually and that of the succeeding season should be gradually adopted.

Sudden discontinuance or sudden adoption gives rise to diseases caused by asatmya (non-habituation).

इति श्रीवैद्यपतिसिंहगुप्तसूनुश्रीमद्वाग्भटविरचितायामष्टाङ्गहृदयसंहितायां सूत्रस्थाने ऋतुचर्या नाम तृतीयोऽध्यायः॥३॥

Thus ends the chapter named Ritucharya, the third of Sutrasthana of Astanga Hridaya Samhita composed by Srimad Vagbhata, Son of Sri Vaidyapati Simhagupta.

4

रोगानुत्पादनीयमध्यायम् (roganutpadaniyam adhyayam)

The fourth chapter of Astanga Hridaya is called Roganutpadaniya Adhyaya, which means - preventive healthcare. It explains the method of adjusting the body according to natural signs so as to avoid toxic material accumulation and onset of disease process.

Roganutpadaneeya is made up of two words - Roga and Anutpadaneeya.

Roga means disease. Utpadana means production. Anutpadana means prevention of production.

So, Roga Anutpadaneeya means prevention of onset of disease. This chapter deals with preventive healthcare.

अथातो रोगानुत्पादनीयमध्यायं व्याख्यास्यामः । इति ह स्माहुरात्रेयादयो महर्षयः ॥

Maharshi Atreya and other sages pledge that henceforth they will be explaining the chapter named Roganutpadaniyam.

Adharaneeya Vega – Natural urges that should not be suppressed:

वेगान्न धारयेद्वातविण्मूत्रक्षवतृट्क्षुधाम् । निद्राकासश्रमश्वासजृम्भाश्रुच्छर्दिरेतसाम् ॥ १ ॥

One should not suppress these natural urges by force -

1. Vata – flatus

2. Vit – faeces

3. Mutra – urine

4. Kshavatu – sneeze

5. Trut – thirst

6. Kshudha – hunger

7. Nidra – sleep

8. Kasa – cough

9. Shramashvasa – panting

10. Jrumbha – yawning

11. Ashru – tears, weeping

12. Chardi – vomiting

13. Retas – semen ejaculation

Adhovata vega rodha – Suppression of the urge of flatus:

अधोवातस्य रोधेन गुल्मोदावर्तरुक्क्लमाः ।

वातमूत्रशकृत्सङ्ग दृष्ट्यग्निवधहृद्गदाः ॥ २ ॥

Suppression of the urge of flatus causes -

- Gulma - abdominal bloating, tumour,
- Udavarta – retrograde movement of Vata,
- Ruk – abdominal pain,
- Klama – fatigue,
- Vata mutra shakrut sanga – Obstruction to passage of flatus, urine and stools,
- Drishti vadha - loss of vision,
- Agni vadha - loss of digestive power,
- Hrid gada - diseases related to epigastric region and heart.

Methods to induce proper Vata anulomana (Downward movement of Vata):

स्नेहस्वेदविधिस्तत्र वर्तयो भोजनानि च ।

पानानि वस्तयश्चैव शस्तं वातानुलोमनम् ॥ २+१ ॥

Snehana – oleation,

Svedana – sudation,

Varti - Phala varti – rectal suppositories,

Bhojana – Vatahara bhojana – foods that alleviate Vata,

Pana – Sukhoshna udaka pana – drinking lukewarm water,

Vasti - enema

Shakrut Nirodhaja Roga – Diseases caused by suppressing the urge to defecate:

शकृतः पिण्डिकोद्वेष्टप्रतिश्यायशिरोरुजः ।
ऊर्ध्ववायुः परीकर्तो हृदयस्योपरोधनम् ॥ ३ ॥
मुखेन विट्प्रवृत्तिश्च पूर्वोक्ताश्चामयाः स्मृताः ।

Shakrut vega rodha (suppressing the urge to defecate) leads to the following -

Pindikodveshta – twisting pain of calf muscles,

Pratishyaya – running nose,

Shiroruja – headache,

Urdhvavayu – upward movement of Vata,

Parikarta – fissure-in-ano,

Hrudayasya Uparodhana – tightness in the chest region,

Mukhena Vit pravrutti – foul breath, faecal vomiting,

and other diseases which manifest due to Adhovata vega rodha (suppression of flatus), mentioned above.

Mutra vega rodha - Suppression of the urge for urination:

अङ्गभङ्गाश्मरीवस्तिमेढ्रवङ्क्षणवेदनाः ॥ ४ ॥
मूत्रस्य रोधात्पूर्वे च प्रायो रोगास्तदौषधम् ।

Suppression of micturition reflex leads to -

Angabhanga – body pain,

Ashmari – Urinary calculi,

Vasti vedana - Pain in the urinary bladder,

Medra vedana – Pain in the penis,

Vankshana vedana – Pain in the inguinal region.

Diseases that are mentioned under suppression of flatus and defecation reflexes may also occur in this condition.

Management of diseases due to suppression of Vata, Shakrut and Mutra:

वर्त्यभ्यङ्गावगाहाश्च स्वेदनं बस्तिकर्म च ॥ ५ ॥

The recommended treatment includes -

Varti – Rectal and urethral suppositories,

Abhyanga – Oil massage,

Avagaha – tub bath, sitz bath,

Svedana – sweating therapy, sudation therapy,
Bastikarma – rectal enema.

Treatment of diseases due to suppression of the urge to defecate:
अन्नपानं च विड्भेदि विड्रोधोत्थेषु यक्ष्मसु ।
In diseases due to suppression of defecation reflex (Vit rodha),
Annapaanam ca vidbhedi – all food that helps to induce purgation should
be administered.

Treatment of diseases due to suppression of the urge of micturition:
मूत्रजेषु तु पाने च प्राग्भक्तं शस्यते घृतम् ॥ ६ ॥
जीर्णान्तिकं चोत्तमया मात्रया योजनाद्वयम् ।
अवपीडकमेतच्च सञ्ज्ञितं धारणात्पुनः ॥७॥
In diseases caused by suppression of urination reflex, drinking of grita
(ghee) before food is ideal. Administration of Uttama matra (maximum
dose) of ghee in two divided doses, before and after food is called
Avapidaka Sneha.
(One part of ghee is administered before food; and its complete digestion is
awaited. Food is administered and after its proper and complete digestion,
the second part of ghee is given.)

Udgara vega dharana - Suppression of belching:
उद्गारस्यारुचिः कम्पो विबन्धो हृदयोरसोः ।
आध्मानकासहिध्माश्च हिध्मावत्तत्र भेषजम् ॥ ८ ॥
Suppression of belching may cause -
Aruchi – Anorexia, lack of interest in taking food,
Kampa – tremors,
Vibhando hrudaya uraso – feeling of obstruction in hridaya (heart) and uras
(chest) regions,
Adhmana – bloating, gaseous distension of abdomen,
Kasa – cough,
Hidhma – hiccups.
The treatment for this is similar to the treatment for suppression of hiccups.

Kshavathu vega dharana - Suppression of sneezing:
शिरोऽर्तीन्द्रियदौर्बल्य मन्यास्तम्भार्दितं क्षुतेः ।
Suppression of sneezing may cause –

Shiro Arti – headache,
Indriya Daurbalya – weakness of sense organs,
Manyasthamba – neck stiffness,
Ardita – facial palsy.

Treatment for diseases due to Kshavathu vega dharana:
तीक्ष्णधूमाञ्जनाघ्राणनावनार्कविलोकनैः ॥ ९ ॥
प्रवर्तयेत् क्षुतिं सक्तां स्नेहस्वेदौ च शीलयेत् ।
Treatment measures include -
Teekshna Dhooma – strong herbal smoking,
Teekshna Anjana – strong collyrium,
Teekshna Grana – snuffing with powder of herbs like maricha (black pepper),
Teekshna Navana – instillation of strong nasal medication,
Arkavilokana – watching the sun directly for a few seconds,
Sneha – oleation, oil massage,
Sveda - sudation therapies.

Trit vega dharana - Suppression of thirst:
शोषाङ्गसादबाधिर्यसम्मोहभ्रमहृद्गदाः ॥ १० ॥
तृष्णाया निग्रहात्तत्र शीतः सर्वो विधिर्हितः ।
Suppression of thirst causes -
Shosha – Emaciation,
Angasada – debility, weakness,
Badhirya – deafness,
Sammoha – loss of consciousness,
Bhrama – giddiness,
Hrut Gada – cardiac disorders.
Treatment:
Sheeta sarva vidhi hita - All procedures that are cooling in nature are recommended.

Kshut vega dharana - Suppression of hunger:
अङ्गभङ्गारुचिग्लानिकार्श्यशूलभ्रमाः क्षुधः ॥ ११ ॥

The symptoms that occur due to suppression of hunger reflex:
Angabhanga – body ache, myalgia,
Aruchi – Anorexia, lack of interest in taking food,

Glani – debility,
Karshya – emaciation, weight loss,
Shoola – abdominal colic pain,
Bhrama – giddiness.

Treatment:
तत्र योज्यं लघु स्निग्धमुष्णमल्पं च भोजनम् ।
Treatment measures include -
Laghu - Light meals,
Snigdha - with oily substance (such as ghee),
Ushna - which is hot in nature,
Alpa – in limited quantities should be given.

Nidra vega dharana - Suppression of sleep:
निद्राया मोहमूर्धाक्षिगौरवालस्यजृम्भिकाः ॥ १२ ॥
अङ्गमर्दश्च तत्रेष्टः स्वप्नः संवाहनानि च ।
Suppression of sleep causes -
Moha – delusion,
Murdha Gourava – heaviness of head,
Akshi Gourava – heaviness of eyes,
Alasya – laziness, lassitude,
Jrumbhika – yawning,
Angabhanga – body ache, myalgia.
Treatment:
Swapna – sleep,
Samvahana - mild massage.

Kasa vega dharana - Suppression of cough:
कासस्य रोधात्तद्वृद्धिः श्वासारुचिहृदामयाः ॥ १३ ॥
शोषो हिध्मा च कार्योऽत्र कासहा सुतरां विधिः ।
Kasasya rodhat vridhi - By suppressing cough, it further increases.
It leads to -
Shvasa – Asthma, COPD, wheezing, dyspnoea,
Aruchi – Anorexia, lack of interest in taking food,
Hrudamaya – cardiac disorders,
Shosha – Emaciation,
Hidhma – hiccup.
Treatment:

Regular treatment for Kasa (cough) should be given.

Srama swasa vega dharana – Suppression of urge for panting:

गुल्महृद्रोगसम्मोहाः श्रमश्वासादिवधारितात् ॥ १४ ॥
हितं विश्रमणं तत्र वातघ्नश्च क्रियाक्रमः ।

Suppression of the urge to breathe heavily after heavy work may lead to
Gulma – Abdominal tumour, bloating,
Hrudroga - Cardiac disorders,
Sammoha – loss of consciousness.
Treatment:
Vishrama – rest
Vataghna kriya - Vata balancing treatment.

Jrmbha vega dharana -Suppression of yawning:

जृम्भायाः क्षववद्रोगाः सर्वश्चानिलजिद्विधिः ॥ १५ ॥

Suppression of yawning produces similar symptoms to that of suppression
of sneezing. Here, Vata balancing activities should be taken up.

Bashpa vega dharana -Suppression of tears:

पीनसाक्षिशिरोहृद्रुङ्मन्यास्तम्भारुचिभ्रमाः ।
सगुल्मा बाष्पतस्तत्र स्वप्नो मद्यं प्रियाः कथाः ॥ १६ ॥

Suppression of tear causes -
Peenasa – running nose, rhinitis,
Akshi roga – eye disorders,
Shiro roga – disorders of the head,
Hridruk – heart diseases associated with pain,
Manyasthamba – Neck stiffness,
Aruchi – Anorexia, lack of interest in taking food,
Bhrama – giddiness,
Gulma – Abdominal tumour, bloating.
Treatment:
Swapna -sleep,
Madya - alcohol and
Priya katha - sweet talk with friends and family.

Vami vega dharana - Suppression of vomiting reflex:

विसर्पकोठकुष्ठाक्षिकण्डूपाण्डुवामयज्वराः ।

सकासश्वासहृल्लासव्यङ्गश्वयथवो वमेः ॥ १७ ॥

Suppression of vomiting causes -

Visarpa – Herpes, spreading skin diseases,

Kotha – allergic skin rashes,

Kushta – skin diseases,

Akshi Roga – eye disorders,

Kandu – itching sensation,

Pandu – Anaemia,

Jvara – fever,

Kasa – cough,

Shwasa – Asthma, COPD, wheezing, breathing difficulty,

Hrullasa – nausea,

Vyanga – Hyper pigmented patches on face,

Shvayathu – oedema, inflammation.

Treatment:

गण्डूष धूमानाहारारूक्षं भुक्त्वा तदुद्वमः।

व्यायामः सुतिरसस्य शस्तं चात्र विरेचनम् ॥ १८ ॥

सक्षारलवणं तैलमभ्यङ्गार्थे च शस्यते ।

Treatment for suppression of vomiting reflex includes -

Gandusha – gargling,

Dhumapana – herbal smoke inhalation,

Anahara – fasting,

Rooksha aahara vamana – eating dry food and inducing vomiting,

Vyayama – exercise,

Asra sruti – Bloodletting,

Virechana – purgation type of Panchakarma treatment.

Sakshara lavana taila abhyanga – Massage using oils processed with Kshara (alkalis) and Lavana (salt).

Shukra vega dharana -Suppression of Semen ejaculation:

शुक्रात्तत्स्रवणं गुह्यवेदनाश्वयथुज्वराः ॥ १९ ॥

हृद्व्यथामूत्रसङ्गाङ्गभङ्गवृद्ध्यश्मषण्ढताः ।

Suppression of ejaculation causes -

Sravana – seminal exudation,

Guhya Vedana – pain in perineal region,

Shvayathu – oedema, inflammation,

Jvara – fever,

Hrid Vyatha – cardiac pain, cardiac distress,

Mutrasanga – obstruction to the flow of urine,

Angabhanga – body ache, myalgia,

Vruddhi – hernia,

Ashma – stone formation,

Shandata – impotency.

Treatment:

ताम्रचूडसुराशालिवस्त्यभ्यङ्गावगाहनम् ॥ २० ॥
बस्तिशुद्धिकरैः सिद्धं भजेत्क्षीरं प्रियाः स्त्रियः ।

Treatment measures include:

Tamrachuda – chicken,

Sura – beer, alcohol,

Shali – rice,

Basti – medicated enema,

Abhyanga – oil massage,

Avagaha – immersion bath with oil,

Basti shuddhi – cleansing of urinary bladder with enema,

Ksheera – treatment with milk processed with herbs,

Priya Striyaha – copulation.

Persons contra-indicated for treatment:

तृट्शूलार्तं त्यजेत् क्षीणं विड्वमं वेगरोधिनम् ॥ २१ ॥

Those who are habituated to the suppression of urges and who presents with

Trit - intense thirst,

Shula - intense pain,

Ksheena – who are severely emaciated,

Vit vamam - those who vomit faeces.

Such patients are not to be treated.

Root cause for all diseases:

रोगाः सर्वेऽपि जायन्ते वेगोदीरणधारणैः ।
निर्दिष्टं साधनं तत्र भूयिष्ठं ये तु तान् प्रति ॥ २२ ॥
ततश्चानेकधा प्रायः पवनो यत्प्रकुप्यति ।
अन्नपानौषधं तस्य युञ्जीतातोऽनुलोमनम् ॥ २३ ॥

All diseases are caused due to -

Vegodeerana – initiation of urges forcefully and

Vegadhaarana – Suppression of naturally initiated urges.

For those common diseases arising from these acts, specific treatments have been counted so far. By disturbing the nature, it is Vata that is mainly vitiated.

Hence the symptoms arising from suppression of natural urges should be treated with food and treatments which clear the passages of Vata and help in restoring Vata's natural downward movement.

Dharaneeya vega - Urges that should be suppressed:

धारयेत्तु सदा वेगान् हितैषी प्रेत्य चेह च ।

लोभेर्ष्याद्वेषमात्सर्यरागादीनां जितेन्द्रियः ॥ २४ ॥

The one who wishes to live an auspicious life should suppress the following vegas -

Lobha – greed

Irshya – envy

Dvesha – hatred

Matsarya – jealousy

Raga – unlawful, excessive attraction,

while having perfect control over his senses (indriya).

Importance of timely Shodhana (purification procedure):

यतेत च यथाकालं मलानां शोधनं प्रति ।

अत्यर्थसञ्चितास्ते हि क्रुद्धाः स्युर्जीवितच्छिदः ॥ २५ ॥

One must exercise precaution to clear out Doshas and waste products at suitable times. Accumulation of such toxins could lead to their aggravation and subsequently even death may occur due to this.

Effectiveness of shodhana (purification procedure):

दोषाः कदाचित् कुप्यन्ति जिता लङ्घनपाचनैः ।

ये तु संशोधनैः शुद्धा न तेषां पुनरुद्भवः ॥ २६ ॥

The Doshas that are pacified by Langhana (fasting etc.) and Pachana (digestives) therapies may aggravate later.

However, Doshas that have been eliminated by Shodhana therapy will never recur again.

यथाक्रमं यथायोगमत ऊर्ध्वं प्रयोजयेत् ।

रसायनानि सिद्धानि वृष्ययोगांश्च कालवित् ॥ २७ ॥

After proper Shodhana procedures at suitable times, timely administration of Rasayana (rejuvenation) and Vajikarana (aphrodisiac) formulations should be taken up.

Treatment for those who are exhausted due to Panchakarma treatment:

भेषजक्षपिते पथ्यमाहारैर्बृंहणं क्रमात् ।
शालिषष्टिकगोधूममुद्गमांसघृतादिभिः ॥ २८ ॥
हृद्यदीपनभैषज्यसंयोगादुचिपक्तिदैः ।
साभ्यङ्गोद्वर्तनस्नाननिरूहस्नेहवस्तिभिः ॥ २९ ॥
तथा स लभते शर्म सर्वपावकपाटवम् ।
धीवर्णेन्द्रियवैमल्यं वृषतां दैर्घ्यमायुषः॥ ३० ॥

It is desirable for those exhausted by various therapeutic procedures to resort to the following:

Bruhmana Ahara – nourishing eatables such as

Shashtika Shali – rice that matures in 60 days,

Godhuma – wheat, Mudga – green gram,

Mamsa – meat, Ghrita – ghee.

Medicine with Hrudya (cardiac tonic) and Deepana (digestive, carminative) qualities should be mixed with food and consumed.

Abhyanga – oil massage,

Udvartana – powder massage,Snana – herbal bath,

Niruha Basti – enema treatment, Snehabasti – oil / ghee enema treatment.

All these help to restore the health of the debilitated. By these measures, one could gain -

Sharma - health, happiness,

Sarva pavaka patavam – digestive power,

Dhi - intelligence,

Varna – good complexion,

Indriya vaimalyam - clarity of vision,

Vrishata - sexual vigour and

Ayusha dairghyam - longevity.

Agantu Roga - Exogenous diseases:

ये भूतविषवाय्वग्निक्षतभङ्गादिसम्भवाः ।
रागद्वेषभयाद्याश्च ते स्युरागन्तवो गदाः ॥ ३१ ॥

Those diseases produced by

Bhuta (evil spirits, bacteria, parasites, insects and such microbes),

Visha (poisons),

Vayu (air, hurricane, cyclone),

Agni (fire, electricity, radiation etc.),

Kshata (injury, wounds etc.),

Bhanga (fracture of bones) etc.,

and also those due to

Raga (desire, lust),

Dvesha (hatred),

Bhaya (fear) etc.

are known as Agantu rogas (diseases arising from external causes).

Sarvaroga samanya chikitsa- (General treatment for all diseases):

त्यागः प्रज्ञापराधानामिन्द्रियोपशमःस्मृतिः ।

देशकालात्मविज्ञानं सद्वृत्तस्यानुवर्तनम् ॥ ३२ ॥

अथर्वविहिता शान्तिः प्रतिकूलग्रहार्चनम् ।

भूताद्यस्पर्शनोपायो निर्दिष्टश्च पृथक् पृथक् ॥ ३३ ॥

अनुत्पत्यै समासेन विधिरेष प्रदर्शितः ।

निजागन्तुविकाराणामुत्पन्नानां च शान्तये ॥ ३४ ॥

Tyagaha pranjaparadhanam - Avoidance of improper activities of body, mind and speech by wilful transgression of rules,

Indriyopashama smriti - Control of the senses, remembering previous experiences and acting rightly,

Desha kala atma vijnanam - good knowledge of the habitat, season and the self,

Sadvrittasya anuvartanam - adherence to rules of good conduct and rituals,

Atharva vihita shanti - Peaceful procedures as mentioned in Atharva Veda,

Pratikoola graham archanam - Worship of celestial powers – Grahashanti (astronomical palliative

procedures),

Bhutadi asparshana upaya - Staying away from Bhuta (evil spirits, microbes).

Respective treatment followed as per the principles explained above, are the general guidelines to prevent the origin of both Nija (endogenous) and Agantu (exogenous) diseases and to cure those diseases which are already manifested.

Seasons for Panchakarma treatment:

शीतोद्भवं दोषचयं वसन्ते विशोधयन् ग्रीष्मजमभ्रकाले ।

घनात्यये वार्षिकमाशुसम्यक् प्राप्नोति रोगान् ऋतुजान् न जातु ॥ ३५ ॥

Doshas which attain the state of chaya (accumulation) during the Sheeta Ritu (cold season) of Hemanta (early winter) and Sisira (winter), are evacuated in Vasanta Ritu (spring).

Doshas which undergo chaya (accumulation) in Greeshma (summer), are eliminated in Varsha Ritu (rainy season).

Doshas which undergo chaya (accumulation) in Varsha (rainy season), are eliminated in Sharat Ritu (autumn).

By this, a person will not become a victim of diseases arising out of seasonal variations.

Secret to Arogya (good health):

नित्यं हिताहारविहारसेवी समीक्ष्यकारी विषयेष्वसक्तः ।

दाता समः सत्यपरः क्षमावान् आप्तोपसेवी च भवत्यरोगः ॥ ३६ ॥

Nityam hita ahara vihara sevi - He who indulges daily in healthy foods and activities,

Sameekshyakari - who discriminates between the good and bad of all aspects and then acts wisely,

Vishayeshu asakta - who is not too much attached to the objects of the senses,

Daata - who develops the habit of charity,

Sama - considers all as equal,

Satyapara – is truthful,

Kshamavan – pardons,

Aptopasevi - and keeping company of good persons only,

becomes free from all diseases.

इति श्रीवैद्यपति सिंहगुप्तसूनु श्रीमद्वाग्भटविरचितायामष्टाङ्गहृदय संहितायां सूत्रस्थाने रोगानुत्पादनीयो नाम चतुर्थोऽध्यायः ॥४॥

Thus ends the chapter called Roganutpadaniyam, the fourth in Sutrasthana of Astangahrdaya Samhita of Srimad Vagbhata, son of Sri Vaidyapati Simhagupta.

5

द्रवद्रव्यविज्ञानीयमध्यायम् (dravadravya vijnaniyam adhyayam)

The 5th chapter of Sutrasthana is known as Dravadravya Vijnaneeya Adhyaya.

Drava means liquid; dravya means substance. This chapter deals with the types and health benefits of all liquid foods. It explains in detail the types and benefits of water, milks, dairy products, sugarcane juices, honey, oils, wines and urine.

अथातो द्रवद्रव्यविज्ञानीयमध्यायं व्याख्यास्याम: इति ह स्माहुरात्रेयादयोमहर्षय: ॥

Maharshi Atreya and other sages pledge that they would henceforth be explaining the chapter named Dravadravyavijnaniyam.

Toya varga – Group of waters:
Gangambu – Rain water – Benefits:
जीवनं तर्पणं हृद्यं ह्लादि बुद्धिप्रबोधनम्।
तन्वव्यक्तरसं मृष्टं शीतं लघ्वमृतोपमम्॥१॥
गङ्गाम्बु नभसो भ्रष्टं स्पृष्टं त्वर्कन्दुमारुतैः।
हिताहितत्वे तद्भूयो देशकालावपेक्षते॥२॥

Rain water, which has come into contact with sunlight (arka), moon light (indu) and wind (maruta) is

Jeevana – enlivening, improves quality of life,

Tarpana – satiating,
Hrudya – good for heart,
Hladi – calming and soothing to the mind and stomach,
Buddhi prabodhanam – Stimulates intellect,
Tanu – thin,
Avyaktarasa – imperceptible taste,
Mrshta – purifactory,
Sheeta – cold,
Laghu – light to digest,
Amrutopama – similar to nectar.
Whether rain water is good or bad depends on the place (desha) and season (kala) where it rains.

Gangambu – Test for quality:

येनाभिवृष्टममलं शाल्यन्नं राजते स्थितम्।
अक्लिन्नमविवर्णं च तत्पेयं गाङ्गमन्यथा॥३॥

Water that does not cause decomposition (aklinnam) or change in colour (avivarnam) of cooked Shaali (rice) kept in silver (rajata) vessel can be considered as Gangambu and can be used for drinking.

Samudrambu (Seawater) qualities:

सामुद्रं, तन्न पातव्यं मासादाश्वयुजादिवना।

Water having properties opposite to those described above is Samudrambu (sea water) and is not suitable for drinking (napatavyam) except in the month of Ashvayuja (the month of September – October, characterised by the appearance of Agastya nakshatra – the star Canopus).

Water to be used for drinking:

ऐन्द्रमम्बु सुपात्रस्थमविपन्नं सदा पिबेत्॥४॥
तदभावे च भूयिष्ठमान्तरिक्षानुकारि यत्।
शुचिपृथ्व्यासितश्वेते देशेऽर्कपवनाहतम्॥५॥

Rain water, which is
Supatrastham – collected in a clean vessel,
Avipannam – which has not changed in colour, taste and odour,
should always be used for drinking.
In its absence, the water from the earth, which resembles rainwater in all its qualities, is collected from a clean vast place that has black or white soil and

which is exposed to sunlight and breeze.

Dushtajala – Contaminated water:

न पिबेत्पङ्कशैवालतृणपर्णाविलास्तृतम्। सूर्येन्दुपवनादृष्टमभिवृष्टं घनं गुरु॥६॥

फेनिलं जन्तुमत्तप्तं दन्तग्राह्यतिशैत्यतः। अनार्तवं च यदिदव्यमार्तवं प्रथमं च यत्॥७॥

लूतादितन्तुविण्मूत्रविषसंश्लेषदूषितम्।

Water that is unfit for drinking:

Water that is contaminated by

Panka – dirt, mixed with mud,

Shaivala – algae,

Trina – weeds,

Parna – leaves,

Surya indupavanaadrishta – which is not exposed to sunlight, moonlight and wind,

Abhivrishta – which is a mixture of old and freshwater,

Gana – which is thick,

Guru – not easily digestible,

Phenilam – frothy,

Jantumat – containing worms,

Taptam – hot in nature,

Dantagrahiatishaityataha – causes tingling sensation of teeth by being very cold,

Anarthavam – that rainwater which is non–seasonal,

Arthavamprathamam – though seasonal, that of the first rain,

Water contaminated by

Tantu – webs,

Vit – faeces,

Mutra – urine,

Visha – poison of

Luta adi – spider etc., should not be used for drinking.

Diseases caused due to usage of Dushtajala:

तत्कुर्यात्स्नानपानाभ्यां तृष्णानाहोदरज्वरान्।

Using Dushtajala (polluted water) for Snana (bath) and Paana (drinking) will lead to

Trishna – thirst,

Anaha – abdominal distension,

Udara – ascites,

Jwara – Fever.

Nadijala – River water:

पश्चिमोदधिगाः शीघ्रवहा याश्चामलोदकाः ॥८॥

पथ्याः समासाता नद्यो विपरीतास्त्वतोऽन्यथा।

Water of the rivers which is suitable for use:

Paschimodadhiga – that which flows into the west sea,

Shigravaha – with high speed,

Amala udaka – which is pure (uncontaminated) is good for health.

Water of a river flowing in the opposite (viparita) direction, i.e. eastern sea is not ideal for consumption.

Water of rivers arising from Himalaya and Malaya mountains:

उपलास्फालनाक्षेपविच्छेदैः खेदितोदकाः ॥९॥

हिमवन्मलयोद्भूताः पथ्यास्ता एव च स्थिराः।

कृमिश्लीपदहृत्कण्ठशिरोरोगान् प्रकुर्वते ॥१०॥

The water of rivers arising from Himalaya and Malaya mountains, and which gets churned up well by dashing against rocks is considered Pathya (suitable for use and good for health).

The same water if stagnated (sthira) gives rise to

Krimi – worms (intestinal parasites),

Shlipada – filariasis,

Hridroga – diseases of the heart,

Kantaroga – diseases of the throat and

Shiro roga – diseases of the head.

Diseases caused by water of rivers originating from various regions:

प्राच्यावन्त्यपरान्तोत्था दुर्नामानि महेन्द्रजाः।

उदरश्लीपदातङ्कान् सह्यविन्ध्योद्भवाः पुनः ॥११॥

कुष्ठपाण्डुशिरोरोगान् दोषघ्न्यः पारियात्रजाः।

बलपौरुषकारिण्यः सागराम्भस्त्रिदोषकृत् ॥१२॥

Water of rivers of the Prachya (gauda), Avanti (malwa) and Aparanta (konkana) countries causes Arshas (haemorrhoids);

Water of rivers arising from Mahendra mountains causesUdara (enlargement of the abdomen) and Shlipada (filariasis);

Those arising from Sahya and Vindhya mountains causes Kushta (skin

diseases), Pandu (anaemia) and Shiroroga (diseases of the head);
Those arising from Pariyatrais doshagna (mitigates the aggravated dosas), bestows bala (strength) andpourusha (sexual vigour);
The Sagaraambu (sea water) is tridoshakrit (causes vitiation of all the three dosas).

Qualities of water in wells and ponds:

विद्यात्कूपतडागादीन् जाङ्गलानूपशैलतः।

The water in kupa (deep wells), tadaga (artificial ponds) etc., should be considered to be similar (in qualities and properties) to the corresponding desha (place) in which they are located and the hills situated nearby.

Jalapanavarjya– contra–indications for drinking water:

नाम्बु पेयमशक्त्या वा स्वल्पमल्पाग्निगुल्मिभिः ॥१३॥
पाण्डूदरातिसारार्शोग्रहणीशोषशोथिभिः।

Water should not be consumed (naambupeyam) or consumed in very little quantity (swalpam), by those suffering from
Alpaagni – poor digestive function,
Gulma – tumours of the abdomen,
Pandu – anaemia,
Udara – enlargement of the abdomen,
Atisara – diarrhoea,
Arshas – haemorrhoids,
Grahani dosha – diseases of the duodenum,
Shotha – oedema.

Consumption of water based on seasons:

ऋते शरन्निदाघाभ्यां पिबेत्स्वस्थोऽपि चाल्पशः ॥१४॥

Even a healthy person is recommended to drink only small quantities of water in all other seasons except Sharad (autumn) and Nidagha (summer).

Effects of drinking water with respect to meals:

समस्थूलकृशा भुक्तमध्यान्तप्रथमाम्बुपाः।

Drinking water in between meals is considered healthy, such a person will neither be too thin nor too fat.
Drinking water after meals causes obesity,
Drinking water before meals causes emaciation, weakness.

Sheetajala – cold water:

शीतं मदात्ययग्लानिमूर्छाछर्दिश्रमभ्रमान्॥१५॥ तृष्णोष्णदाहपित्तास्रविषाण्यम्बु नियच्छति।

Cold water relieves

Madatyaya – alcoholic intoxication,

Glani – exhaustion,

Murcha – fainting,

Chardi – vomiting,

Shrama – debility (fatigue),

Bhrama – giddiness,

Trushna – thirst,

Ushna – heat (of the sun),

Daha – burning sensation,

Pittasra – bleeding conditions and Pitta dominant conditions and

Visha – poison / toxins.

Ushnajala– Hot water:

दीपनं पाचनं कण्ठ्यं लघूष्णं बस्तिशोधनम्॥१६॥ हिध्माध्मानानिलश्लेष्मसद्यःशुद्धिनवज्वरे। कासामपीनसश्वासपार्श्वरुक्षु च शस्यते॥१७॥

Hot water is

Deepana – stimulates hunger,

Pachana – helps in digestion,

Kantya – good for the throat,

Laghu – easily to digest,

Ushna – hot in potency,

Basti shodhana – cleanses the urinary bladder,

It relieves

Hidhma –hiccup,

Adhmana – abdominal distension,

Anila – aggravation of Vata,

Shleshma – aggravation of Kapha,

Sadhyashudhi – ideal soon after Shodana therapy,

Navajvara – fever of recent origin,

Kasa – cough,

Ama – accumulation of undigested materials,

Peenasa – rhinitis (running nose),
Shwasa – dyspnoea and
Parshvaruja – pain in the flanks.

Kvathitha sheetala jala – Boiled and cooled water:

अनभिष्यन्दि लघु च तोयं क्वथितशीतलम्।
पित्तयुक्ते हितं दोषे द्युषितं तत्त्रिदोषकृत्॥१८॥

Water which is boiled and then cooled is

Anabhishyandi – does not increase moisture or stickiness in the body,

Laghu – light to digest.

Useful in conditions associated with Pitta dosha.

Water which is kept overnight is not ideal for consumption. It increases Tridosha.

पानीयं न तु पानीयं पानीयेऽन्यप्रदेशजे।

It is not desirable to drink water before the digestion of water of anyapradesha (another region) is completed.

अजीर्णे क्वथितं चामे पक्वे जीर्णेऽपि नेतरम्॥

Drinking boiled water (kwathita jala) before the digestion of unboiled water (ama jala), and unboiled water soon after the digestion of boiled water is not recommended.

शीते विधिरयं तप्ते त्वजीर्णे शिशिरं त्यजेत्॥

Cold water (sheetajala) should not be consumed before hot water (taptajala) undergoes digestion.

Effects of excessive consumption of water:

अतियोगेन सलिलं तृष्यतोऽपि प्रयोजितम्।
प्रयाति श्लेष्मपित्तत्वं ज्वरितस्य विशेषतः॥

Water taken in excess (atiyoga), even in trishna (thirst), gets transformed into Kapha and Pitta, especially in Jwara (fever).

पानीयं प्राणिनां प्राणाः विश्वमेवचतन्मयम्।
अतोत्यन्त निषेधेन नक्वचिद्धारिवर्यते॥

Water (paniyam) is the life (prana) for living beings (prani), and they are made up of water. Hence there is no instance where water is totally restricted.

Effects of unavailability of water:

आस्यशोषाङ्गसादाद्यामृत्युर्वातदलाभतः।

नहितोयादि्वनावृतिस्स्वस्थस्यव्याधितस्यवा॥
Unavailability of drinking water causes
Asyashosha – dryness of mouth,
Angasada – debility and
Mrityu – death.
Hence, life without water is equally impossible for the healthy (swastha) and the diseased (vyadhita).

Narikelodaka– Coconut water benefits:
नारिकेलोदकं स्निग्धं स्वादुं वृष्यं हिमं लघु। तृष्णापितानिलहरं दीपनं वस्तिशोधनम्॥१९॥
Tender coconut water is
Snigdha – unctuous, oily,
Swadu – sweet,
Vrushya – aphrodisiac,
Hima – coolant,
Laghu – easy to digest.
It relieves
Trushna – thirst,
Pitta hara – balances Pitta,
Anila hara – balances Vata,
Deepana – increases hunger and
Bastishodhana – cleanses urinary bladder.
वर्षासु दिव्यनादेये परं तोये वरावरे।
During varsa (rainy season) rain water is the best and river water is least suitable for consumption.

Ksheeravarga – Group of milk and milk products:
अथ क्षीरवर्गः ।
स्वादुपाकरसं स्निग्धमोजस्यं धातुवर्धनम्॥२०॥ वातपितहरं वृष्यं श्लेष्मलं गुरु शीतलम्।
प्रायः पयोऽत्र गव्यं तु जीवनीयंरसायनम्॥२१॥
Generally milk is
Svadupakarasa – sweet in taste (rasa) and also at the end of digestion (vipaka),
Snigdha – unctuous,
Ojovardhana – increases Ojas (essence of body tissues),
Dhatuvardhana – nourishes and increases body tissues,
Vata Pittahara – mitigates Vata and Pitta,

Vrushya – aphrodisiac,
Shleshmala – increases Kapha,
Guru – heavy to digest,
Sheetala – coolant.
Cow's milk is
Jeevaneeya – promotes long life,
Rasayana – anti aging, rejuvenating.

Cow milk benefits:
क्षतक्षीणहितं मेध्यं बल्यं स्तन्यकरं सरम्। श्रमभ्रममदालक्ष्मीश्वासकासातितृट्क्षुधः॥२२॥
जीर्णज्वरं मूत्रकृच्छ्रं रक्तपित्तं च नाशयेत्।
Cow's milk is
Kshataksheenahita – good to relieve weakness due to injury,
Medhya – increases intelligence,
Balya – strengthening,
Stanyakara – promotes breast milk production,
Sara – helps in easy movement of the bowels,
It relieves
Shrama – exhaustion,
Bhrama – dizziness,
Mada – intoxication,
Alakshmi – inauspiciousness,
Shwasa – dyspnoea,
Kasa – cough,
Atitrut Kshudha – severe thirst and hunger,
Jeernajvara – chronic fevers,
Mutrakrichra – dysuria and
Raktapitta – bleeding diseases.

Mahisha Kshira – Buffalo milk:
हितमत्यग्न्यनिद्रेभ्यो गरीयो माहिषं हिममम्॥२३॥
Buffalo milk is good for those affected with
Atyagni – very strong digestion power,
Anidra – insomnia.
It is
Guru – heavy and
Sheeta – cool.

Aja ksheera – Goat milk:

अल्पाम्बुपानव्यायामकटुतिक्ताशनैर्लघु।
आजं शोषज्वरश्वासरक्तपित्तातिसारजित्॥२४॥

Goats drink less water (alpaambupana) and do a lot of walking (vyayama). It eats pungent (katu) and bitter (tikta) grass and vegetables that are light to digest (laghu). Hence goat's milk also carries these qualities.

Goat's milk is useful in

Shosha – emaciation,

Jvara – fever,

Shwasa – dyspnoea, asthma, chronic bronchial disorders,

Raktapitta – bleeding disorders of Pitta origin,

Atisara – diarrhoea, dysentery.

Ustraksheera–Camel's milk:

ईषद्रूक्षोष्णलवणमौष्ट्रकं दीपनं लघु। शस्तं वातकफानाहकृमिशोफोदरार्शसाम्॥२५॥

Ushtraksheera (camel's milk) is

Ishatruksha – slightly dry,

Ushna – hot,

Lavana – salty taste,

Deepana – increases digestion strength,

Laghu – easy to digest,

Vatakaphanshastam – useful in Vata and Kapha disorders,

Anaha – abdominal distension,

Krumi –worm infestation,

Shopha – oedema,

Udara –ascites and

Arshas – haemorrhoids.

Manushapaya – Breast milk:

मानुषं वातपित्तासृग्‌अभिघाताक्षिरोगजित्। तर्पणाश्चोतनै: नस्यै:

Breast milk is useful in

Vata and Pitta imbalance disorders,

Asruk – blood vitiation disorders,

Abhighata –injuries,

Akshiroga – diseases of the eye.

It is used in Tarpana (retention of medicine in the eye) and Ashchotana (eye drops) types of eye treatments. It is also used in Nasya (instillation of nasal drops) treatment.

Avikaksheera – Ewe's milk:
अहृद्यं तृष्णमाविकम्॥२६॥ वातव्याधिहरं हिध्माश्वासपित्तकफप्रदम्।
Ewe's milk is
Ahridyam – not good for the heart,
Ushna – hot in nature,
Vata vyadhi hara – alleviates Vata disorders,
It causes
Hidhma – hiccup,
Swasa – dyspnoea,
Pitta Kaphapradam – vitiates Pitta and Kapha.

Hastiksheera (Elephant milk), Ekashaphaksheera (milk of single hoofed animals):
हस्तिन्याःस्थैर्यकृद् बाढमुष्णं त्वैकशफं लघु॥२७॥ शाखावातहरं साम्ललवणं जडताकरम्।
Hastiksheera (Elephant milk) is
Sthairyakrit – strengthening in nature.
Ekashaphaksheera– milk of single hoofed animals like horse, donkey, etc. is
Badamushnam – very hot in potency,
Laghu – light for digestion,
Vataharam – useful in vata disorders,
Sa amla lavanam– slightly sour and salty, and
Jadathakaram – causes lassitude.

Qualities of different types of milk based on processing:
पयोऽभिष्यन्दि गुर्वामं युक्त्या शृतमतोऽन्यथा॥२८॥
भवेद्गरीयोऽतिशृतं धारोष्णममृतोपमम्।
Ama ksheera (unboiled milk) is
Abhisyandi – causes excess secretion in the tissue pores, causing their blockage,
Guru – heavy to digest,
Amakara – causes Ama, indigestion.
Sruthaksheera (boiled milk) has opposite properties.
Atishrutaksheera – condensed milk – is guru (heavy).
Dharoshnaksheera– Milk that is freshly drawn from the udder (nipple)

is similar to nectar (provided, the cow is perfectly healthy without any infection).

Dadhi (curds/soured milk/coagulated milk) benefits:
अम्लपाकरसं ग्राहि गुरूष्णं दधि वातजित्॥२९॥ मेदःशुक्रबलश्लेष्मपित्तरक्ताग्निशोफकृत्।
रोचिष्णु शस्तमरुचौ शीतके विषमज्वरे॥३०॥ पीनसे मूत्रकृच्छ्रे चरूक्षंतुग्रहणीगदे।
Curd has the following properties –
Amlapaka rasa – sour taste and sour taste conversion after digestion,
Grahi – absorbent, constipative,
Guru – heavy to digest,
Ushna – hot in nature,
Vatajit – balances Vata.
It increases
Meda – fat,
Shukra – semen,
Bala – strength,
Increases Sleshma (Kapha), Pitta, Rakta,
Agni (digestion strength) and
Shotha (inflammation).
It is Rochishnu – increases taste
Curd is indicated in –
Aruchi –anorexia,
Sheetajwara – fever with chills,
Vishamajwara – chronic, recurrent fever,
Peenasa – rhinitis,
Mutrakruchra – dysuria,
Grahani – malabsorption syndrome, after making it ruksha – dry (by removing the cream).

Rules for curd consumption:
नैवाद्यान्निशि नैवोष्णं वसन्तोष्णशरत्सुन॥३१॥
नामुद्गसूपं नाक्षौद्रं नाघृतं नासितोपलम्।
न चानामलकं नापि नित्यं नो मन्दमन्यथा॥३२॥
ज्वरासृक्पित्तवीसर्पकुष्ठपाण्डुभ्रमप्रदम्।
Curd should not be eaten at nishi (night),
It should not be made hot,
It is contra–indicated in Vasanta (spring), Ushna (summer) and Sharat

(autumn).
Curd can taken along with mudga supa (green gram soup),
It can taken along with kshoudra (honey), grita (ghee), sitopalam (rock sugar) and amla (Indian gooseberry).
Curd should not be too thick, half prepared (manda).
It should not be taken daily.
If used daily, it may cause / worsen
Jwara – fever,
Asrukpitta – bleeding disorders,
Visarpa – spreading skin diseases, herpes,
Kushta – skin disorders,
Pandu – anaemia and
Bhrama – dizziness.

Takra – buttermilk:
तक्रं लघु कषायाम्लं दीपनं कफवातजित्॥३३॥ शोफोदराश्शोग्रहणीदोषमूत्रग्रहारुची:।
गुल्मप्लीहघृतव्यापद्गरपाण्डुवामया न् जयेत् ॥३४॥
Takra (buttermilk) is –
Laghu – easy to digest,
Kashaya, amla – sour, astringent in taste,
Deepana – improves digestion strength,
Kaphavatajit – balances Kapha and Vata,
It is indicated in –
Shopha – inflammatory conditions,
Udara – ascites,
Arsha – haemorrhoids,
Grahanidosha – malabsorption syndrome,
Mutragraha – dysuria,
Aruchi – anorexia,
Gulma – abdominal distension,
Pleeha – splenomegaly,
Ghritavyapat –indigestion caused by excess consumption of ghee,
Garavisha – chronic intoxication and
Pandu – anaemia.

Mastu – Supernatant liquid of curds (whey/watery part of curds):
तद्वन्मस्तु सरं स्रोत:शोधि विष्टम्भजिल्लघु।

Mastu is similar to buttermilk. It is

Sara – promotes movement of fluids inside body channels,

Srotahshodhi – cleanses body channels,

Vishtambhajit – relieves constipation,

Laghu – easy to digest.

Navanita (Butter):

नवनीतं नवं वृष्यं शीतं वर्णबलाग्निकृत्॥३५॥ सङ्ग्राहि
वातपित्तासृक्क्षयार्शोऽदितकासजित्।
क्षीरोद्भवं तु सङ्ग्राहि रक्तपित्ताक्षिरोगजित्॥३६॥

Fresh Navanita (butter) is

Vrushya – aphrodisiac,

Sheeta – coolant,

Varnakrit – improves skin complexion,

Balakrit – improves strength,

Agnikrut – improves digestion strength,

Sangrahi – absorbent, useful in diarrhoea,

Vatapittasrukjit – balances Vata, Pitta and detoxifies blood

Useful in

Kshaya – emaciation,

Arsha – haemorrhoids,

Ardita– paralysis,

Kasa – cough.

The butter made directly from milk is

Sangrahi – absorbent,

Raktapittajit – useful in bleeding disorders,

Akshirogajit – useful in eye diseases.

Ghrita – (ghee/clarified butter):

शस्तं धीधृतिमेधाग्निबलायुःशुक्रचक्षुषाम्।
बालवृद्धप्रजाकान्तिसौकुमार्यस्वरार्थिनाम्॥३७॥
क्षतक्षीणपरीसर्पशस्त्राग्निग्लपितात्मनाम्। वातपित्तविषोन्मादशोषालक्ष्मीज्वरापहम्॥३८॥
स्नेहानामुत्तमं शीतं वयसः स्थापनं परम्। सहस्रवीर्यं विधिभिर्घृतं कर्मसहस्रकृत्॥३९॥

Ghee is ideal for improving

Dhi–intelligence,

Smriti – memory,

Medha – discriminative ability,

Agni – digestion,

Bala – strength,

Ayu – long life,

Shukra – semen (sexual vigour) and

Chakshu – eye sight.

Ghee is good for

Bala – children,

Vridha – the aged,

Praja – those who desire more children,

Kanti – to enhance complexion,

Soukumarya – tenderness of the body and

Swara – pleasant voice.

Ghee is indicated in those suffering from

Kshataksheena – emaciation as a result of injury,

Parisarpa – herpes,

Shastragata – injury from weapons,

Agnidaha – injury by fire,

Disorders of Vata and Pitta origin,

Visha – poison,

Unmada – insanity,

Shosha – pulmonary tuberculosis,

Alakshmi – inauspicious activities (witchcraft, etc.) and

Jwara – fevers.

Snehanamuttamam – Of all the fatty materials, ghee is the best.

It is

Sheeta– coolant,

Vayasthapanam – best for retaining of youth,

It is capable of giving a thousand good effects by a thousand kinds of processing.

Purana Ghrita – Old ghee:

मदापस्मारमूर्च्छायशिरःकर्णाक्षियोनिजान्। पुराणं जयति व्याधीन् व्रणशोधनरोपणम्॥४०॥

Purana Ghrita (at least one year old ghee) is used in the treatment of

Mada – intoxication,

Apasmara – epilepsy,

Murcha – fainting,

Shiro roga – diseases of the head,

Karnaroga – diseases of the ear,

Akshiroga – diseases of the eye,

Yoni roga – diseases of the vagina,

Vranashodhana – cleanses wounds,

Vranaropana – heals wounds.

Milk preparations, fatty dairy products:

बल्या: कीलाटपीयूषकूर्चिकामोरटादय: । शुक्रनिद्राकफकरा विष्टम्भिगुरुदोषला: ॥४१॥

Kilata, Piyusa, Kurcika, Morata (various dairy products), etc. are

Balya – strengthening,

Shukrakara – increase the semen,

Nidrakara – induces sleep,

Kaphakara – increases Kapha,

Vishtambhi – causes constipation,

Guru – heavy to digest and

Doshala – aggravates the Doshas.

Best and worst qualities of milk and ghee:

गव्ये क्षीरघृते श्रेष्ठे निन्दिते चाविसम्भवे। इति क्षीरवर्ग:

Milk and ghee obtained from the cow (gavya) is the best and those obtained from ewe (avi), the least.

IksuVarga – Group of sugarcane juice and its products:

इक्षो: सरो गुरु: स्निग्धो बृंहण: कफमूत्रकृत्॥४२॥

वृष्य: शीतोऽस्रपित्तघ्न: स्वादुपाकरसो सर: ।

Iksurasa Guna – Properties of sugarcane juice:

Juice of sugar cane is

Sara – laxative,

Guru – heavy for digestion,

Snigdha – unctuous,

Brihmana – nutritive, improves weight,

Kaphakrut – increases Kapha,

Mutrakrut – increases urine volume,

Vrushya – aphrodisiac,

Sheeta – coolant,

Asrapittaghna – useful in bleeding disorders,

Swadupaka rasa – sweet in rasa and vipaka.

सोऽग्रे सलवणो दन्तपीडितः शर्करासमः ॥४३॥

The tips of shoots of sugarcane have a salty taste. Its juice obtained when chewed has properties similar to sugar (sharkara).

मूलाग्रजन्तुजग्धादिपीडनान्मलसङ्करात्।

किञ्चित्कालं विधृत्या च विकृतिं याति यान्त्रिकः ॥४४॥

विदाही गुरुविष्टम्भी तेनासौ तत्र पौण्ड्रकः।

शैत्यप्रसादमाधुर्यैर्वरस्तमनु वांशिकः ॥४५॥

If the roots, shoots and worm infested parts of the cane are crushed together, the juice gets mixed with dirty materials. Hence it becomes guru (heavy) and causes

Vidaha – burning sensation,

Vishtambha – constipation.

The Poundraka variety of cane is superior in view of its sheetaguna (coolant property), prasada (clarity) and madhurya (sweetness) of its juice; next to it is the Vamsika variety.

Sataparvaka, Kantara, Naipala varieties of sugarcane:

शातपर्वककान्तारनैपालाद्यास्ततः क्रमात्।

सक्षाराः सकषायाश्च सोष्णाः किञ्चिद्विदाहिनः ॥४६॥

Varieties of sugarcane such as Sataparvaka, Kantara, Naipala etc., in respective order are qualitatively inferior. This means Sataparvaka is the best and Naipala the worst among the three. They are slightly Kshara (alkaline) and Kashaya (astringent) in taste, hot in potency and cause slight burning sensation (vidaha).

Phanita – Half – cooked molasses, unrefined treacle:

फाणितं गुर्वभिष्यन्दि चयकृन्मूत्रशोधनम्।

Phanita (half – cooked molasses) is

Guru – heavy to digest,

Abhisyandi – increases the secretions in the tissues pores and blocks them,

Chayakrit – causes accumulation of Tridosha and

Mutra shodanam – cleanses the urine.

Guda – Jaggery:

नातिश्लेष्मकरो धौतः सृष्टमूत्रशकृद्गुडः ॥४७॥

प्रभूतकृमिमज्जासृङ्मेदोमांसकफोऽपरः।

हृद्यः पुराणः पथ्यश्च नवः श्लेष्माग्निसादकृत् ॥४८॥

Guda (jaggery, molasses), washed well, made white and purified is–
Natishleshmakara – does not increase Kapha to a large extent,
Srishtamutrashakrit – increases volume of urine and faeces.
If it is not purified properly, it causes
Krimi – intestinal worms,
Increases chances of Kapha disorders in majja (marrow), asruk (blood),
medas (fat tissue) and mamsa (muscles).
Purana guda (old jaggery) is –
Hridya – good for heart,
Pathya – wholesome.
Nava guda (freshly prepared jaggery) is
Sleshmakrut – increases Kapha,
Agnisadakrut – weakens digestive fire.

Sugarcane preparations – Matsyandika, Khanda, Sita:
वृष्या: क्षीणक्षतहिता रक्तपित्तानिलापहा: ।
मत्स्यण्डिकाखण्डसिता: क्रमेण गुणवत्तमा: ॥४९॥
Matsyandika (brown sugar), Khanda (sugar candy) and Sita (white
crystalline sugar) in their succeeding order are better. This means, Sita is
the best and Matsyandika is the least beneficial.
They are
Vrishya – aphrodisiac,
Kshataksheenahita – good for those emaciated due to injuries,
Raktapittapaha – useful in bleeding diseases,
Anilapaha – useful in aggravation of Vata.

Yasa Sarkara :
तद्गुणा तिक्तमधुरा कषाया यासशर्करा।
YasaSarkara (sugar prepared from Yavasaka – a resinous plant) is similar
in properties to sugar (sharkara) but is tikta (bitter), madhura (sweet) and
kashaya (astringent) in taste.

Indications of Sharkara (sugar):
दाहतृट्छर्दिमूर्छासृक्पित्तघ्न्य: सर्वशर्करा: ॥५०॥
All types of sugars are useful in
Daha – burning sensation,
Trit – thirst,

Chardi – vomiting,
Murcha – fainting and
Asrukpitta – bleeding diseases.

Best and worst
शर्करेक्षुविकाराणां फाणितं च वरावरे।
Among the products of sugarcane, Sharkara (sugar) is the best and Phanita
(half cooked molasses) is the worst.

Madhu (Honey) properties:
चक्षुष्यं छेदि तृट्श्लेष्मविषहिध्मास्रपित्तनुत्॥५१॥
मेहकुष्ठकृमिच्छर्दिश्वासकासातिसारजित्।
व्रणशोधनसन्धानरोपणं वातलं मधु॥५२॥
रूक्षं कषायमधुरं तत्तुल्या मधुशर्करा।
Madhu (honey) is
Chakshushya – good for the eyes (vision),
Chedi – breaks up hard masses,
Trut – relieves thirst,
Sleshmahara – balances Kapha.
It is indicated in –
Visha – toxicity,
Hidhma – hiccup,
Asrapitta – bleeding conditions,
Kushta – skin diseases,
Meha – diabetes, urinary tract diseases,
Krumi – worm infestation,
Chardi – vomiting,
Shwasa – dyspnoea, chronic respiratory diseases,
Kasa – cough,
Atisara – diarrhoea,
Vranashodhana – wound cleansing,
Vranasandhana – wound abridgement,
Vranaropana – heals wounds quickly,
Vatala – increases Vata,
Ruksha – dry,
Kashaya, Madhura – astringent and sweet in taste.
Crystallized honey (Madhu Sarkara) is similar to honey in properties.

यक्ष्मार्शोऽर्दितपित्तासृइग्नाशनं ग्राहिदीपनम्॥५३ a॥

Madhu (honey) is indicated in the following conditions –

Yakshma – tuberculosis,

Arshas – haemorrhoids,

Ardita – facial palsy,

Pittasruk – bleeding disorders of Pitta origin.

It is

Grahi – constipative,

Deepana – increases appetite.

Rules for usage of Madhu (honey):
उष्णमुष्णार्तमुष्णे च युक्तं चोष्णैर्निहन्ति तत्॥५३॥
प्रच्छर्दने निरूहे च मधूष्णं न निवार्यते।
अलब्धपाकमाश्वेव तयोर्यस्मान्निवर्तते॥५४॥

Taking honey that is hot, during hot season, mixed with hot dishes or by a person afflicted by heat is destructive.
But honey does not cause any harm when used warm in medicines for Prachardana (vomiting) or for administration of Niruha Basti (decoction enema) because it comes out of the body before it undergoes digestion.

Taila Varga – Group of oils and other fats:
तैलं स्वयोनिवत्तत्र मुख्यं तीक्ष्णं व्यवायि च।
त्वग्दोषकृदचक्षुष्यं सूक्ष्मोष्णं कफकृन्न च॥५५॥
कृशानां बृंहणायालं स्थूलानां कर्शनाय च।
बद्धविट्कं कृमिघ्नं च संस्कारात्सर्वरोगजित्॥५६॥

Oils are generally similar to their source (oil seeds).
Sesame oil (Tilataila) is the most important among all oils.
Sesame oil is
Tikshna – sharp in action,

Vyavayi – quickly spreading,

Tvakdoshakrut – causes skin disorders,

Chakshushya – good for the eyes,

Sukshma – subtle, penetrates deep into the tissues,

Ushna – hot,

Na kaphakrit – does not increaseKapha,

Krushanambrumhanaya – nourishes the lean,

Sthulanamkarshanaya – emaciates the obese,

Badhavitkam – Useful to relieve constipation,

Krimignam – relieves worm infestation.

Samskaratsarvarogajit – When it is processed (samskara) with other herbs, it is capable of curing various diseases.

Eranda Taila – Castor oil Benefits:

सतिक्तोषणमैरण्ड तैलं स्वादु सरं गुरु। वर्धमगुल्मानिलकफानुदरं विषमज्वरम्॥५७॥
रुक्शोफौ च कटीगुह्यकोष्ठपृष्ठाश्रयौ जयेत्। तीक्ष्णोष्णं पिच्छिलं विस्रं रक्तैरण्डोद्भवं
त्वति॥५८॥

Castor oil is tikta (bitter), ushana/katu (pungent) and swadu (sweet) in taste,

Sara – promotes natural movement of body fluids (laxative),

Guru – hard to digest,

It pacifies

Vardhma – enlargement of the scrotum (hernia),

Gulma – abdominal tumours,

Anilakaphahara – alleviates Vata and Kapha,

Udara – ascites,

Vishamajwara – chronic intermittent fevers,

Ruk (pain) and shopha (swellings) of the kati (waist), guhya (genitals), koshta (abdomen) and prishta (back),

Tikshna – is capable of penetrating deep,

Ushna – hot in potency and

Visra – odourous.

Oil of red variety of castor seeds (raktaeranda) is

Atitikshna – still more penetrating,

Atiushna – very hot in potency,

Pichila – slimy and

Visra – odourous.

Sarshapa Taila – Mustard oil:

कटूष्णं सार्षपं तीक्ष्णं कफशुक्रानिलापहम्। लघु पित्तास्रकृत्
कोठकुष्ठार्शोव्रणजन्तुजित्॥५९॥

SarsapaTaila (mustard oil) is

Katu – pungent in taste,

Ushna – hot in potency,

Tikshna – penetrates deep,
Kaphapaham – mitigates Kapha,
Shukrapaham – reduces semen,
Anilapaham – mitigates Anila (Vata),
Laghu – easy to digest,
Pittasrakrit – causes bleeding diseases.
It relieves the following conditions –
Kota – rashes on the skin,
Kushta – skin diseases,
Arshas – haemorrhoids,
Vrana – ulcers,
Jantu – worms (bacteria etc).

AkshaTaila – Oil of Vibhitaka (Terminalia bellirica):
आक्षं स्वादु हिमं केश्यं गुरु पित्तानिलापहम्।
Aksa Taila – oil obtained from seeds of Vibhitaka is
Swadu – sweet,
Hima – cold in potency,
Keshya – good for the hair,
Guru – hard to digest,
Pitta anilapaha – mitigates Pitta and Vata.

Nimba Taila – Neem oil:
नात्युष्णं निम्बजं तिक्तं कृमिकुष्ठकफप्रणुत्॥६०॥
Neem oil is
Na atiushna – not very hot (slightly hot) in potency,
Tiktam – bitter,
Krimipranut – antimicrobial,
Kushtanut – cures skin diseases,
Kaphanut – mitigates Kapha.

Uma–Kusumbha Taila – Linseed oil and Safflower oil:
उमाकुसुम्भजं चोष्णं त्वग्दोषकफपित्तकृत्।
Taila of Uma (linseed) and Kusumbha is
Ushnam – hot in potency,
Twakdoshakrit – produces skin diseases,
Kaphapittakrit – aggravates Kapha and Pitta.

Properties of animal fats (Vasa) and bone marrow (Majja):

वसा मज्जा च वातघ्नौ बलपित्तकफप्रदौ॥६१॥

मांसानुगस्वरूपौ च विद्यान्मेदोऽपि ताविव।

Vasa (muscle–fat) and Majja (bone–marrow) is

Vatagna – mitigates Vata,

Balaprada – increases strength,

Pitta kaphaprada – increases Pitta and Kapha.

They are similar in properties as the meat of animals from which they are obtained.

Karanja taila – Karanja seed oil:

कषायतिक्तकटुकं कारञ्जं व्रणशोधनम्॥६११+१॥

Oil obtained from Karanja seed (Pongamia pinnata) is –

Kashaya tiktakatu – Astringent, bitter, pungent in taste,

VranaShodhana – It cleanses the wounds.

Madya Varga – Alcoholic beverages:

दीपनं रोचनं मद्यं तीक्ष्णोष्णं तुष्टिपुष्टिदम्॥६२॥ सस्वादुतिक्तकटुकम्अम्लपाकरसं सरम्।

सकषायं स्वरारोग्यप्रतिभावर्णकृल्लघु॥६३॥ नष्टनिद्रातिनिद्रेभ्यो हितं पित्तास्रदूषणम्।

कृशस्थूलहितं रूक्षं सूक्ष्मं स्रोतोविशोधनम्॥६४॥ वातश्लेष्महरं युक्त्या पीतं विषवदन्यथा।

गुरु त्रिदोषजननं नवं जीर्णमतोऽन्यथा॥६५॥

Madya (alcoholic beverages) in general is –

Deepana – stimulates digestion,

Rochana – helps improve taste,

Teekshna – penetrates deep,

Ushna – hot in potency,

Tushtipushtida – give satisfaction and nourishment,

Sasvadutiktakatukam – slightly sweet, bitter and pungent in taste,

Amlapaka rasa – sour in taste and sour taste conversion at the end of digestion,

Sara – laxative,

Sakashaya – slightly astringent,

Svara – confers good voice,

Arogya – improves health,

Pratibha – intellect,

Varnakrit – improves colour and complexion,
Laghu – easy to digest.
It is indicated in the following conditions –
Nashtanidra – loss of sleep,
Atinidra – excessive sleep.
Pitta asra dushanam – it vitiates pitta and asra (rakta).
Krisha sthula hitam – beneficial for both lean and stout persons,
Ruksham – is non–viscid,
Sukshmam – capable of entering minute pores,
Srotovishodhanam – cleanses the metabolic pathways,
Vata sleshma hara – mitigates Vata and Kapha.
These benefits are obtained if used judiciously.
If taken in a non–recommended form, they act like poison.

Nava madya (freshly prepared alcoholic beverages) is
Guru – hard to digest,
Tridoshajanana – increases all the three Doshas.
Seasoned beverages have opposite qualities.

Best ingredient to prepare madya (alcohol)
द्राक्षेक्षवः सखर्जूराः शालिपिष्टंयवस्यच। पञ्चमद्याकाराः श्रेष्ठा द्राक्षा तेषां विशिष्यते ॥६५१+१॥
Draksha – grapes,
Ikshu – sugarcane,
Karjura – dates,
Shalipishtam – ground cereals,
Yava – barley,
Among these five substances used in the preparation of Madya (fermented beverages), Draksha (grapes) is considered sreshta (superior).

Contra indication for wine intake:
पेयं नोष्णोपचारेण न विरिक्तक्षुधातुरैः। नात्यर्थतीक्ष्णमृद्वल्पसम्भारं कलुषं न च ॥६६॥
Na ushnopacharena – wine should not be consumed hot.
Na virikta – It should not be consumed by a person who has undergone Virechana (purgation) panchakarma therapy.
Na kshudathura – It should be avoided by a person who is hungry.
Na atitikshnamridu – wines which are very strong or very weak should not

be consumed,

Na alpasambhara – wine which is prepared using insufficient quantity of ingredients,

Na kalusham – very turbid and those which are spoiled, should not be used for drinking.

Sura – Alcoholic drink

गुल्मोदरार्शोग्रहणीशोषहृत् स्नेहनी गुरुः। सुरानिलघ्नी मेदोऽसृक्स्तन्यमूत्रकफावहा॥६७॥

Sura is indicated in

Gulma – abdominal tumours,

Udara – enlargement of the abdomen,

Arshas – haemorrhoids,

Grahani – duodenal diseases,

Shosha – emaciation.

It is

Snehani – lubricating,

Guru – hard to digest,

Anilagna – mitigates Vata,

Medoasrukstanya mutra kaphavaha – causes increase of fat, blood, breast milk, urine and Kapha.

Varuni – Toddy:

तद्गुणा वारुणी हृद्या लघुस्तीक्ष्णा निहन्ति च। शूलकासवमिश्वासविबन्धाध्मानपीनसान्॥६८॥

The properties of Varuni are similar to that of Sura.

It is

Hrudya – good for heart,

Laghu – light for digestion,

Tikshna – sharp in action,

It cures

Shula – colic,

Kasa – cough,

Vami – vomiting,

Swasa – dyspnoea,

Vibandha – constipation,

Adhmana – abdominal distension,

Pinasa – running nose.

Vibhitaka Sura – Alcoholic drink prepared using Vibhitaki:
नातितीव्रमदा लघ्वी पथ्या वैभीतकी सुरा। व्रणे पाण्डुवामये कुष्ठे न चात्यर्थं विरुध्यते॥६९॥
Sura prepared from Vibhitaka (Terminalia bellirica) is

Na atiteevramada – not very intoxicating,

Laghu – easy to digest,

Pathya – good for health,

It is not totally contra–indicated (as other wines) in Vrana (wounds), Pandu (anaemia), and Kushta (skin disorders).

Yava Sura – Alcoholic drink prepared using Barley:
विष्टम्भिनी यवसुरा गुर्वी रूक्षा त्रिदोषला।
Sura prepared from Yava (Barley – Hordeum vulgare) is

Vishtambi – causes constipation,

Guru – heavy to digest,

Ruksha – non–unctous and

Tridoshala – aggravates all the three Doshas.

Arista – Fermented decoctions:
यथाद्रव्यगुणोऽरिष्टः सर्वमद्यगुणाधिकः ॥७०॥ ग्रहणीपाण्डुकुष्ठार्शःशोफशोषोदरज्वरान्।
हन्ति गुल्मकृमिप्लीहनः कषायकटुवातलः ॥७१॥
Arista (fermented decoction) possesses properties of the materials from which it is prepared, and is the most intoxicating of all alcoholic beverages.
It is useful in

Grahani – disease of the duodenum,

Pandu – anaemia,

Kushta – skin diseases,

Arsha – haemorrhoids,

Shopha – oedema,

Shosha – emaciation,

Udara – enlargement of the abdomen,

Jwara – fever,

Gulma – abdominal tumours,

Krimi – worms (intestinal parasites) and

Pleeha – disorders of the spleen.

It is Kashaya (astringent), Katu (pungent) and Vatala (aggravates Vata).

Mardvika – Wine prepared from grapes:

माद्वीकं लेखनं हृद्यं नात्युष्णं मधुरं सरम्। अल्पपित्तानिलं
पाण्डुमेहार्शःकृमिनाशनम्॥७२॥

Mardvika (wine prepared from grapes) is

Lekhana – scraping,

Hridyam – good to the heart,

Na atiushnam – not very hot in potency,

Madhuram – sweet,

Sara – laxative,

Alpa pitta anilam – causes slight increase of Pitta and Anila (Vata),

Indicated in

Pandu – anaemia,

Meha – diabetes, urinary disorders,

Arshas – haemorrhoids and

Krimi – worms (intestinal parasites).

Kharjura – Wine prepared from dates:

अस्मादल्पान्तरगुणं खार्जूरं वातलं गुरु।

Wine prepared from dates (kharjura) is inferior in properties to that prepared from grapes, vatala (aggravates Vata) and is guru (heavy to digest).

Sarkara – Wine prepared using sugar:

शार्करः सुरभिःस्वादुहृद्यो नातिमदो लघुः॥७३॥

Wine prepared using sugar is

Surabhi – sweet smelling,

Swadu – sweet in taste,

Hridya – good for the heart,

Na atimada – not very intoxicating and

Laghu – easy to digest.

Gouda – Beverage prepared by using molasses/treacle:

सृष्टमूत्रशकृद्वातो गौडस्तर्पणदीपनः।

Gouda increases volume of mutra (urine), shakrut (faeces) and vata (flatus), is tarpana (nourishing) and deepana (increases hunger).

Sidhu – Wine prepared from sugarcane juice:

वातपित्तकरः सीधुः स्नेहश्लेष्मविकारहा॥७४॥

मेदःशोफोदरार्शोघ्नस्तत्र पक्वरसो वरः।

Sidhu (prepared from fermenting sugarcane juice) is

Vata pittakara – aggravates Vata and Pitta,

Decreases sneha (lubrication) and

Sleshmavikaraha – mitigates diseases due toKapha.

It is indicated in

Medoroga – obesity,

Shopha – oedema,

Udara – enlargement of the abdomen and

Arsha – haemorrhoids,

Sidhu madya prepared by boiling sugarcane juice is excellent when compared to the non–boiled variety.

Madhvasava – Wine prepared from honey:

छेदी मध्वासवस्तीक्ष्णो मेहपीनसकासजित्॥७५॥

Madhvasava (wine prepared from honey) is

Chedi – breaks up hard masses,

Tikshna – penetrates deep,

Indicated in

Meha – diabetes, urinary disorders,

Pinasa – chronic nasal catarrh and

Kasa – cough.

Sukta – Wine prepared from roots and tubers:

रक्तपित्तकफोत्क्लेदि शुक्तं वातानुलोमनम्।

भृशोष्णतीक्ष्णरूक्षाम्ल हृद्यं रुचिकरं सरम्॥७६॥

दीपनं शिशिरस्पर्श पाण्डुहृत्कृमिनाशनम्।

Sukta (wine prepared from roots and tubers) is

Rakta pitta kaphautkledi – increases the moisture of blood, Pitta and Kapha,

Vatanulomanam – expels Vata in downward direction,

Brishaushna – very hot in potency,

Tikshna – is penetrating,

Ruksha – causes dryness,

Amla – sour,

Hridyam – good for the heart,

Ruchikara – increases taste (appetite),

Sara – promotes bowel movements (laxative),

Deepanam – enhances digestive fire,
Shishirasparsham – is cold to touch,
Indicated in
Pandu – anaemia,
Drik – diseases of the eye and
Krimi–worms (intestinal parasites).

गुडेक्षुमद्यमाद्वींकशुक्तं लघु यथोत्तरम्॥७७॥

Sukta prepared from guda (jaggery), ikshu (sugarcane), madya (alcohol) and mardvika (grapes) are successively laghu (light to digest). This means, sukta prepared from mardvika (grapes) is the lightest to digest and that prepared from guda (jaggery) is the heaviest.

Asava –Fermented infusion:

कन्दमूलफलाद्यं च तद्वद्विद्यात्तदासुतम्।

kandamūlaphalādyaṃ ca tadvadvidyāttadāsutam |

Asava prepared by using kanda (tubers), moola (roots), phala (fruits) etc, is similar to shukta.

Asava prepared using Sandaki:

शाण्डाकी चासुतं चान्यत्कालाम्लं रोचनं लघु॥७८॥

Asava prepared by using Sandaki (balls of fried paddy mixed with spices, dried in sun and then deep fried in oil) and other materials (such as oil–cakes etc) which have turned sour (amla) by lapse of time are rochana (appetizers) and laghu (easy to digest).

Dhanyamla (prepared using rice and such other grains):

धान्याम्लं भेदि तीक्ष्णोष्णं पित्तकृत्स्पर्शशीतलम्

श्रमक्लमहरं रुच्यं दीपनं बस्तिशूलनुत्॥७९॥

शस्तमास्थापने हृद्यं लघु वातकफापहम्।

एभिरेव गुणैर्युक्ते सौवीरकतुषोदके॥८०॥

कृमिहृद्रोगगुल्मार्शःपाण्डुरोगनिबर्हणे।

ते क्रमादिवतुषैर्विद्यात्सतुषैश्च यवैः कृते॥८१॥

Dhanyamla (liquor prepared by fermenting the water in which rice and such other grains, pulses etc. have been slightly cooked or merely washed) is
Bhedi – purgative,
Tikshna – penetrating,

Ushna – hot in potency,

Pittakrit – aggravates Pitta,

Sparshasheetalam – cold to touch,

Shramaklama hara – relieves fatigue and exhaustion,

Ruchyam – increases appetite,

Deepanam – increases digestive strength,

Vastishoolanut – relieves pain in the urinary bladder,

Ideal for use as Asthapana (decoction enema),

Hridyam – good to the heart,

Laghu – easy to digest,

Vata kaphapaham – balances Vata and Kapha.

Sauviraka and Tushodaka also possess similar properties and areuseful in

Krimi – worms,

Hridroga – heart disease,

Gulma – abdominal tumour,

Arsha – haemorrhoids and

Pandu roga – anaemia.

These are prepared from dehusked (vitusha) barley and barley–with–husk (satusha).

गण्डूष धारणाद्वक्त्रमलदौर्गन्ध्यशोषजित्॥८०१+१॥

Dhanyamla is used for –

Gandusha – oral retention of medication,

It alleviates mala (dirt), dourgandya (odour) and shosha (dryness) of the vaktra (oral cavity).

Mutra Varga – Group of urine:

मूत्रं गोऽजाविमहिषीगजाश्वोष्ट्रखरोद्भवम्। पित्तलं रूक्षतीक्ष्णोष्णं लवणानुरसं कटु॥८२॥
कृमिशोफोदरानाहशूलपाण्डुकफानिलान्। गुल्मारुचिविषश्वित्रकुष्ठार्शांसि जयेल्लघु॥८३॥

Urine of go (cow), aja (goat), avi (sheep), mahisha (buffalo), gaja (elephant), ashva (horse), ushtra (camel) and khara (donkey) is –

Pittalam – aggravates Pitta,

Ruksha – not unctous, dry,

Tikshna – penetrating deep,

Ushna – hot in potency,

Katu with lavanaanurasa – pungent with salt as its secondary taste.

It is indicated in

Krimi – worms,

Shopha – oedema,

Udara – abdominal enlargement,

Anaha – abdominal distension,

Shoola – colic,

Pandu – anaemia,

Kaphaanilan – aggravation of Kapha and Vata,

Gulma – abdominal tumours,

Aruchi – loss of taste,

Visha – poisoning,

Shvitra – leucoderma,

Kushta – skin diseases,

Arsha – haemorrhoids and is

Laghu – easy to digest.

तोयक्षीरेक्षुतैलानां वर्गर्मद्यस्य च क्रमात्। इति द्रवैकदेशोऽयं यथास्थूलमुदाहृतः ॥८४॥

The liquids included in Toya varga (types of water), Kshiravarga (types of milk), Ikshuvarga (types of sugarcane), Tailavarga (types of oils), and Madyavarga (fermented beverages) have been broadly described in this chapter.

इतिश्रीवैद्यपतिसिंहगुप्तसूनुवाग्भटविरचितायामष्टाङ्गहृदयसंहितायां   सूत्रस्थाने द्रवद्रव्यविज्ञानीयोनामपञ्चमोऽध्यायः ॥५॥

Thus ends the chapter called Dravadravyadi vijnaniyam, the fifth in Sutrasthana of AstangaHrudayam composed by SrimadVaghata, son of Sri Vaidyapati Simhagupta.

6

अन्नस्वरूपविज्ञानीयमध्यायम् (annaswarupa vijnaniyam adhyayam)

The sixth chapter of Astanga Hridaya is called Annaswaroopa Vijnaneeya Adhyaya. It deals with details of different food materials. The chapter covers corn, grains, legumes, pulses, prepared foods, non veg foods, leafy vegetables, fruits, salts and medicinal herbs.

अथातोऽन्नस्वरूपविज्ञानीयमध्यायं व्याख्यास्यामः । इति ह स्माहुरात्रेयादयो महर्षयः ।
Maharshi Atreya and other sages pledge that henceforth they would be explaining the chapter named 'Annasvarupavijnaniyam'.

Shuka DhanyaVarga – Group of cereals:
Shalidhanyas – Types of rice:
रक्तो महान् सकलमस्तूर्णकः शकुनाहृतः।
सारामुखो दीर्घशूको रोध्रशूकः सुगन्धिकः।।१।।
पुण्ड्रः पाण्डुः पुण्डरीकः प्रमोदो गौरसारिवौ।
काञ्चनो महिषः शूको दूषकः कुसुमाण्डकः।।२।।
लाङ्गला लोहवालाख्यः कर्दमाः शीतभीरुकाः।
पतङ्गास्तपनीयाश्च ये चान्ये शालयः शुभाः।।३।।
Rakta (red), Mahan (big sized rice), Kalama, Turnaka, Shakunahruta, Saaramukha, Deerghashuka (having long sharp spike at the ends), Rodhrashuka, Sugandhika (having good smell), Pundra, Pandu, Pundarika, Pramoda, Gaura (white rice), Sariva, Kanchana (golden colored rice),

Mahisha, Shuka, Dushaka, Kusumandaka, Langala, Lohavala, Kardama, Sheetabheeruka, Patanga, Stapaneeya (bright red colored rice) – these varieties of rice are good for consumption.

Qualities, health benefits of rice:

स्वादुपाकरसः स्निग्धा वृष्या बद्धाल्पवर्चसः|
कषायानुरसाः पथ्य लघवो मूत्रल हिमाः||४||

Swadu rasa – sweet taste,

Swadupaka – sweet taste conversion after digestion,

Snigdha – unctuous,

Vrushya – is a natural aphrodisiac,

Baddhalpavarchasah – causes mild constipation, decreases the volume of faeces,

Kashaya anurasa – mild astringent taste,

Pathya – suitable for daily consumption,

Laghu – light to digest,

Mutrala – diuretic, increases urine volume,

Hima – coolant.

Raktashali – Red variety of rice:

शूकजेषु वरस्तत्र रक्तस्तृष्णात्रिदोषहा|

Red variety of rice (Raktashali) is the best among the cereals. It relieves thirst (trishna) and balances all the three Doshas (tridoshaha).

Mahan and Kalama Varieties of rice:

माहांस्तमनु कलमस्तं चाप्यनु ततः परे||५||

Mahan and Kalama are successively inferior in qualities when compared to Raktashali (red variety of rice).

The other varieties are inferior to kalama with respect to its qualities.

Yavaka, Hayana, Pamshu, Vashpa, Naishadha varieties of rice:

यवका हायनाः पांसुबाष्पनैषधकादयः|
स्वादूष्णा गुरवः स्निग्धाः पाकेऽम्लाः श्लेष्मपित्तलाः||६||
सृष्टमूत्रपुरीषाश्च पूर्वं पूर्वं च निन्दिताः|

Yavaka, Hayana, Pamshu, Vashpa, Naishadha varieties of rice are

Svadu – sweet,

Ushna – hot in potency,

Guru – hard to digest,

Snigdha – unctuous, oily,

Amlapaka – undergoes sour taste conversion after digestion,

Shleshma pittala – increases Kapha and Pitta,

Srushta mutra pureesha – increases bulk and volume of urine and faeces.

Their qualities increase in their successive order i.e., yavaka is inferior and naisadhaka is superior in terms of quality.

Vrihi dhanya:

Shashtika Shali – Paddy which matures in 60 days:

स्निग्धो ग्राही लघुः स्वादुदुस्त्रिदोषघ्नः स्थिरो हिमः॥७॥

षष्टिको व्रीहिषु श्रेष्ठो गौरश्चासितगौरतः।

Shashtikashali – the paddy which matures in 60 days is best (sreshta) among all paddies. It is

Snigdha – unctuous, oily,

Grahi – absorbent,

Laghu – light to digest,

Svadu – sweet,

Tridoshaghna – balances all the three Doshas,

Sthira – brings about stability,

Hima –coolant.

It is of two types – Gaura (white) and Asita–gaura (blackish white).

Other varieties of rice:

ततः क्रमान्महाव्रीहिकृष्णव्रीहिजतूमुखाः॥८॥

कुक्कुटाण्डकलावाख्यपारावतकशूकराः।

गन्धनाः कुरुविन्दाश्च गुणैरल्पान्तराः स्मृताः।

Next inferior to shashtika is mahavrihi, next to that is krishnavrihi and the others such as jatumukha, kukkutandaka, lavaka, paravataka, sukara, varaka, uddalaka, ujvala, cina, sarada, dardura, gandhana and kuruvinda.

स्वादुरम्लविपाकोऽन्यो व्रीहिः पित्तकरो गुरुः॥१०॥

बहुमूत्रपुरीषोष्मा, त्रिदोषस्त्वेव पाटलः।

The other varieties of rice are –

Svadu – sweet in taste,

Amla – sour at the end of digestion,

Pittakara – increases Pitta and

Guru – hard to digest.

Bahu mutra purishaushma – It increases volume of urine, faeces, increases body heat and causes imbalance of Tridosha.

Trina dhanyas – Millets – group of grains obtained from grass like plants:

कङ्गुकोद्रवनीवारश्यामाकादि हिमं लघु॥११॥

तृणधान्यं पवनकृल्लेखनं कफपित्तहृत्।

Kangu, Kodrava, Neevara, Shyamaka are different varieties of Trina dhanya. These are –

Hima – cold in potency,

Laghu – easily digestible,

Pavanakrit – increases Vata,

Ulekhanam – Lekhana (scraping) and

Kaphapittahrit – pacifies Kapha and Pitta.

Priyangu and Koradusha:

भग्नसन्धानकृत्तत्र प्रियङ्गुर्बृंहणी गुरुः॥१२॥

कोरदूषः परं ग्राही स्पर्शे शीतो विषापहः।

Priyangu helps in fracture healing (bhagnasandhanakrit), is nutritive, nourishing (bruhmana) and hard to digest (guru).

Koradusha is grahi (absorbent), sparshosheeta (cool to touch) and vishapaha (anti–poisonous).

Yava – Barley:

रूक्षः शीतो गुरुः स्वादुः सरो विड्वातकृद्यवः॥१३॥ वृष्यः स्थैर्यकरो मूत्रमेदःपित्तकफान् जयेत्।

पीनसश्वासकासोरुस्तम्भकण्ठत्वगामयान्॥१४॥ न्यूनो यवादनुयवः रूक्षोष्णो वंशजो यवः।

Yava (Barley) is –

Rooksha – dry,

Sheeta – cold,

Guru – Heavy to digest,

Svadu – sweet,

Sara – promotes bowel movements, laxative,

Vit–vatakrut – it increases the bulk of faeces and causes flatus,

Vrushya – natural aphrodisiac,

Stairyakrut – increases body stability,

Useful in –

Mutra – urinary disorders,

Meda – disorders of fat metabolism,

Pitta and Kapha imbalance disorders,

Peenasa – running nose, rhinitis,

Shwasa – Asthma, COPD, wheezing, breathing difficulty,

Kasa – cough, cold,

Urusthamba – thigh stiffness,

Kantaroga – diseases of throat,

Twakroga – skin diseases.

Anuyava (a small sized barley variety) is inferior in qualities to that of Yava.

Venuyava (seeds of bamboo) is ruksha (non– unctuous) and ushna (hot in potency).

Godhuma – Wheat:

वृष्यः शीतो गुरुः स्निग्धो जीवनो वातपित्तहा||१५|| सन्धानकारी मधुरो गोधूमः स्थैर्यकृत्सरः|

पथ्या नन्दीमुखी शीता कषायमधुरा लघुः||१६||

Wheat is –

Vrushya – natural aphrodisiac,

Sheeta – cold,

Guru – Heavy to digest,

Snigdha – unctuous, oily,

Jivaneeya – enlivening,

Vatapittaha – pacifies Vata and Pitta,

Sandhanakari – heals fractures and wounds,

Madhura – sweet,

Sthairyakrut – increases body stability,

Sara – promotes bowel movements,

Pathya – can be consumed on a daily basis.

Nandimukhi variety of wheat is good for health. It is

Sheeta – cold,

Kashaya madhura– astringent and sweet in taste,

Laghu – light to digest.

Joorna – Sorghum:

निःसारावातलारूक्षाजूर्णाध्मानकरासरा||१६+१||

Joorna is –
Nisara–lacks nutrition,
Vatala – aggravates vata,
Ruksha – causes dryness,
Adhmanakara – causes abdominal distension and
Sara – is laxative.

Shimbi dhanya varga – Group of legumes and pulses:
मुद्गाढकीमसूरादि शिम्बीधान्यं विबन्धकृत्|
कषायं स्वादु सङ्ग्राहि कटुपाकं हिमं लघु||१७||
मेदःश्लेष्मास्त्रपित्तेषु हितं लेपोपसेकयोः|

Mudga (green gram), Adhaki (pigeon pea/red gram), Masura (lentil) and other varieties belong to the group called Shimbidhanya (those having pods/legumes).

They possess the following properties –
Vibandhakrut –causes constipation,
Kashaya, Swadu – astringent and sweet in taste,
Grahi – absorbent,
Katuvipaka – pungent taste conversion after digestion,|
Hima – Sheeta – cold in potency,
Laghu – easily digestible,
Mitigate meda (fat), sleshma (kapha), asra (blood) and pitta,
Suited for use as lepa (external application) and seka (bathing the body parts) etc.

Mudga, Kalaya:
वरोऽत्र मुद्गोऽल्पचलः, कलायस्त्वतिवातलः||१८||
Varo atramudga – Among them, mudga (green gram) is best,
Alpachalaha – it causes mild increase of chala (vata).
Kalaya (garden pea/round pea) is ati vatala – increases Vata excessively.

Chanaka – Chickpea:
असृक्पित्तहरोरूक्षोवातलश्चणकःस्मृतः||१८१+१||
Chanaka is –
Asrikpittahara – relieves bleeding disorders,
Ruksha – causes dryness and

Vatala – aggravates Vata.

Raja masha – Cow pea:
राजमाषोऽनिलकरो रूक्षो बहुशकृद्गुरुः|
Rajamasha (cow pea) is
Anilakara – increases Vata,
Ruksha – causes dryness,
Bahu shakrit– produces more faeces and is
Guru – hard to digest.

Kulatha – Horse gram:
उष्णाः कुलत्थाः पाकेऽम्लाः शुक्राश्मश्वासपीनसान्||१९||
कासार्शःकफवातांश्च घ्नन्ति पितास्रदाः परम्|
Kulatha (horse gram) is
Ushna – hot in potency,
Amlapaka – sour at the end of digestion,
Shukra – cleanses semen.
It cures –
Ashma – urinary stones, / shukrashma – stones in semen
Shwasa – Asthma, COPD, wheezing, breathing difficulty,
Peenasa – running nose, rhinitis,
Kasa – cough,
Arshas – haemorrhoids,
Kapha and Vata diseases.
It increases pittasra (bleeding disorders).

Nishpava – Indian butter bean / cow–peas
निष्पावो वातपितास्रस्तन्यमूत्रकरो गुरुः||२०||
सरो विदाही दृक्शुक्रकफशोफविषापहः|
Nishpava aggravates Vata, Pitta, bleeding disorders,
It increases stanya (breast milk production) and is mutrakara (promotes urine formation).
It is
Guru – Heavy to digest,
Sara – promotes bowel movements,
Vidahi – increases burning sensation,
It is not good for drik (eyes) and shukra (semen) quality.

It decreases Kapha, shopha (inflammation) and is vishapaha (useful in poisoning).

Masha – Black gram benefits:

माषः स्निग्धो बलश्लेष्ममलपित्तकरः सरः||२१|| गुरूष्णोऽनिलहा स्वादुः शुक्रवृद्धिविरेककृत्|

Black gram is

Snigdha – unctuous,

Balya – increases strength,

Sleshmapittakara – increases Kapha and Pitta,

Sara – laxative,

Guru – not easily digestible,

Ushna – hot in potency,

Anilaha – Vatahara – mitigates Vata,

Svadu – Madhura – sweet in taste,

Shukravruddhikara, virekakrut – increases semen and promotes ejaculation strength.

फलानि माषवद्विद्यात्काकाण्डोलात्मगुप्तयोः||२२||

Fruits of Kakandola and Atmagupta (Mucuna pruriens) are similar to Masha (black gram) in qualities.

Tila – Sesame seeds:

उष्णस्त्वच्यो हिमः स्पर्शे केश्यो बल्यस्तिलो गुरुः|
अल्पमूत्रः कटुः पाके मेधाऽग्निकफपित्तकृत्||२३||

Tila (sesame seed) is

Ushna – hot in potency,

Tvachya – good for the skin,

Sheetasparsha – cold to touch,

Keshya – good for hairs,

Balya – strengthening,

Guru – hard to digest,

Alpamutra – decreases urine output,

Katupaka – pungent at the end of digestion,

Medhakrut – increases intelligence,

Agnikrut – increases digestive function,

Kaphapittakrit – increases kapha and pitta.

Uma – Linseed:
स्निग्धोमा स्वादुतिक्तोष्णा कफपित्तकरी गुरुः|
दृक्शुक्रहृत्कटुः पाके, तद्वद्बीजं कुसुम्भजम्||२४||
The seed of Uma (linseed) is
Snigdha – unctuous,
Swadutikta – sweet and bitter in taste,
Ushna – hot in potency,
Kaphapittakari – increases kapha and pitta,
Guru – hard to digest,
Drikshukrahrit – not good for vision and semen,
Katupaka – pungent taste conversion at the end of digestion.
The seeds of Kusumbha (safflower) also have similar properties.

माषोऽत्र सर्वेष्ववरो, यवकः शूकजेषु च|
Masa (black gram) in the group of simbija (legumes) and yavaka (small
barley) in the group of sukaja (cereals) are inferior.

Nava Dhanya – Fresh grains:
नवं धान्यमभिष्यन्दि, लघु संवत्सरोषितम्||२५||
शीघ्रजन्म तथा सूप्यं निस्तुषं युक्तिभर्जितम्|
Fresh grains (just harvested) are
Abhisyandi– causes excess exudation from tissue pores and block them,
Samvatsaroshitam – those old by one year are laghu (easily digestible).
Those which grow quickly (Shigrajanma), those which are removed from
their husk (nistusha), those that are properly fried (bharjita) are also easy
to digest (laghu).

Kritannnavarga– Group of cooked cereals:
यवगोधूममाषाश्चितलाश्चाभनविाहताः
मण्डपेयाविलेपीनामोदनस्य च लाघवम्||२६||
[Manda, peya, vilepi and odana are preparations of rice or other grains
cooked in water.
Manda – The thin fluid resembling water, drained out immediately after
boiling is known as manda;
Peya – slightly thicker to manda but still only liquid is peya;
Vilepi – the next stage with more of solid grains and less of fluid is called

vilepi and

Odana – the last stage which is solid without fluid portion is known as odana.]

Manda, peya, vilepi and odana are more easily digestible in their preceding order of enumeration.

Manda – is easiest to digest.

Odana – is comparatively harder to digest.

यवगोधूममाषाश्चतिलाश्चाभिनवाहिताः।
पुराणाविरसाःसूक्ष्मानतथार्थकरामताः ॥२६१+१॥

Barley, wheat, black gram and sesame seeds are best used when fresh (within one year time period). When they are old, they become Virasa – lose taste and lack nutritional value.

Manda – Rice boiled water:

यथापूर्वं शिवस्तत्र मण्डो वातानुलोमनः।
तृड्ग्लानिदोषशेषघ्नः पाचनो धातुसाम्यकृत्॥२७॥
स्रोतोमार्दवकृत्स्वेदी सन्धुक्षयति चानलम्।

Amongst these, Manda is the best.

It has the following properties –

Vatanulomana – causes easy movement of faeces and flatus,

Relieves trit (thirst) and glani (exhaustion),

Sheshadoshagna – It nullifies residual doshas,

Pachana – helps in digestion,

Dhatu samyakrit – restores the normalcy of the tissues,

Srotomardavakrit – causes softness of the channels,

Svedi – causes perspiration and

Sandukshayati ca analam – kindles the digestive fire.

Peya – Rice gruel:

क्षत्तृष्णाग्लानिदौर्बल्यकुक्षिरोगज्वरापहा॥२८॥ मलानुलोमनी पथ्या पेया दीपनपाचनी।

Peya (more liquid, less solid) relieves

Kshut – hunger,

Trishna – thirst,

Glani – exhaustion,

Dourbalya – debility,

Kukshiroga – diseases of the abdomen and

Jwara – fevers.
It brings about
Mala anulomana – easy elimination of faeces,
Pathya – is wholesome,
Deepana – kindles appetite and
Pachana – helps in digestion.

Vilepi – Thick rice gruel:

विलेपी ग्राहिणी हृद्या तृष्णाघ्नी दीपनी हिता||२९||

व्रणाक्षिरोगसंशुद्धदुर्बलस्नेहपायिनाम्|

Vilepi (less liquid more solid) is

Grahi – withholds discharge of fluids from the body,constipative,

Hridya – good for the heart,

Trishnagni– relieves thirst,

Deepani – kindles appetite,

Hita – ideal for all, especially for those suffering from

Vrana – ulcers,

Akshiroga – eye diseases,

Samshudha – those who have been administered Panchakarma purification therapies,

Durbala – who are weak and

Sneha payinam – who have been given fats for drinking as part of Snehana therapy (before Panchakarma).

Odana – cooked rice:

सुधौतः प्रसुतः स्विन्नोऽत्यक्तोष्मा चौदनो लघुः||३०||

यश्चाग्नेयौषधक्वाथसाधितो भृष्टतण्डुलः|

विपरीतो गुरुः क्षीरमांसाद्यैर्यश्च साधितः||३१||

Odana (cooked rice) prepared with grains which have been washed well (sudhauta), in which the entire water has evaporated and which is devoid of hot fumes is easy to digest (laghu);

Likewise that prepared in a decoction of agneyaoushada (medicinal substances of hot potency) or that prepared with brishtatandula (fried grains) are also easily digestible (laghu);

Preparations opposite to these and those that are prepared by addition of Kshira (milk), mamsa (meat) etc., are hard to digest (guru).

इति द्रव्यक्रियायोगमानाद्यैः सर्वमादिशेत्|

In this manner, the effect of grains, kinds of processing, admixtures, quantity and other aspects should be determined.

Mamsa rasa – Meat soup:

बृंहणः प्रीणनो वृष्यश्चक्षुष्यो व्रणहा रसः||३२||

Mamsa rasa (meat soup) is

Brihmana – nourishing,

Preenana – gives satisfaction,

Vrushya – aphrodisiac,

Chakshushya – good for the eye (vision) and

Vranaha – heals ulcers and wounds.

Mudgasupa – Soup of green gram:

मौद्गस्तु पथ्यः संशुद्धव्रणकण्ठाक्षिरोगिणाम्|३३|

Mudgasupa (soup of green gram) is –

Pathya – good for health,

It is indicated in

Samshudha – for those who have undergone Panchakarma purification therapies,

Vrana – ulcers,

Kantaroga – diseases of the throat and

Akshiroga – diseases of the eyes.

Kulattha Supa – Horse gram soup:

वातानुलोमी कौलत्थो गुल्मतूनीप्रतूनिजित्||३३||

Kulattha Supa (horse gram soup) is

Vatanulomi – initiates normal downward movement of Vata.

Useful in

Gulma – abdominal tumours and

Tuni, pratuni – types of pain of the groin region.

Eatables prepared from Tila (sesame):

तिलपिण्याकविकृतिः शुष्कशाकं विरूढकम्|

शण्डाकीवटकं दृग्ध्नं दोषलं ग्लपनं गुरु||३४||

Eatables prepared from Tila (sesame), Pinyaka (residue of sesame seed after the oil is extracted), Shushkashaka (dried leafy vegetables), Virudadhanya (germinated grains), shandakivataka (balls of fried rice dried in sun and then fried in oil) are

Drignam–damage the eyes/vision,
Doshala – aggravates doshas,
Glapanam – cause debility and
Guru – are hard to digest.

Rasala:

रसाला बृंहणी वृष्या स्निग्धा बल्या रुचिप्रदा।
Rasala (curds churned and added with pepper powder and sugar) is
Bruhmani–increases body weight,
Vrishya – aphrodisiac,
Snigdha – unctuous,
Balya – improves strength and
Ruchiprada – improves taste.

Panaka – Vegetable / fruit juice:

श्रमक्षुत्तृट्क्लमहरं पानकं प्रीणनं गुरु।।३५।।
विष्टम्भि मूत्रलं हृद्यं यथाद्रव्यगुणं च तत्
Panaka is –
Shrama hara – relieves exhaustion,
Kshut hara – relieves hunger,
Trit hara – relieves thirst,
Klama hara – relieves fatigue,
Prinanam – gives satisfaction,
Guru – hard to digest,
Vishtambi – constipative,
Mutrala – is diuretic and
Hridya – good for the heart.
Its properties depend on the material from which it is prepared

प्रभूताभ्यन्तरमलो माषसूप: परं स्मृत: ।।
विद्याद्यूषे रसे सूपेशाके चैवोत्तरोत्तरम्।।
गौरवं तनुसान्द्राम्लस्वादुष्वेषु पृथक्तथा।
Masha (black gram) excessively increases Abhyantara mala (faeces).
Yusha, rasa, supa and shaka are successively guru (heavy for digestion), i.e.
yusha is the lightest and shaka is the heaviest for digestion.
Similarly, each of these preparations when tanu (thin), sandra (thick), amla
(sour) and swadu (sweet) are successively more and more guru (heavy for

digestion).

Laja – Fried paddy:

लाजास्तृट्छर्द्यतीसारमेहमेदःकफच्छिदः ॥३६॥
कासपित्तोपशमना दीपना लघवो हिमाः।

Laja is prepared by frying paddy. It relieves

Trit – thirst,

Chardi – vomiting,

Atisara – diarrhoea,

Meha – diabetes, urinary disorders,

Meda – obesity,

Kaphaupashamana – mitigates Kapha,

Kasaupashamana – relieves cough,

Pitta upashamana – relieves Pitta,

Deepana – increases appetite,

Laghu – easy to digest and

Hima – cold in potency.

Prithuka – Parboiled and flaked paddy:

पृथुका गुरवो बल्याः कफविष्टम्भकारिणः ॥३७॥

Prithuka (prepared by boiling paddy for a short while and pounding it with pestle and mortar) is

Guru – hard to digest,

Balya – strengthening,

Kaphakara – increases Kapha,

Vishtamba – causes constipation.

Dhana – Fried barley and other grains:

धाना विष्टम्भिनी रूक्षा तर्पणी लेखनी गुरुः।

Dhana (made by frying barley which is soaked in water and saktu (flour) either raw or fried) is

Vishtambhi – constipative,

Ruksha – dry,

Tarpani – satisfying,

Lekhani – scarifying and

Guru – hard to digest.

Saktu – Corn flour/ fried barley

सक्तवो लघवः क्षुत्तृट्श्रमनेत्रामयव्रणान्||३८||

घ्नन्ति सन्तर्पणाः पानात्सद्य एव बलप्रदाः|

नोदकान्तरितान्न द्विर्न निशायां न केवलान्||३९||

न भुक्त्वा न द्विजैश्छित्वा सक्तूनद्यान्न वा बहून्|

Saktu (corn flour) is –

Laghu – easy to digest,

Relieves kshut (hunger), trit (thirst), shrama (fatigue), netramaya (eye diseases) and vrana (wounds),

Santarpana – is nutritious,

Sadyaevabalaprada – provides instant strength.

Na udakaantarita – corn flour should not be eaten without drinking water in between,

Na dvi – should not be consumed twice in a day,

Na nisha – should not be consumed at night,

Na kevala – should not be taken solely, without other kinds of foods.

Na bhuktva – should not be consumed after meals,

Na dvijaischitva – it should not be chewed and

Na bahun – it should not be consumed in excess quantities.

Pinyaka – Oil cakes:

पिण्याको ग्लपनो रूक्षो विष्टम्भी दृष्टिदूषणः||४०||

Pinyaka (residue of sesame, groundnut and other oil seeds, after extracting the oil from it) produces

Glapana – fatigue,

Ruksha – dryness,

Vishtambhi– constipation and

Drikdushana – vitiates vision.

रौक्ष्यादिवष्टम्भते कोष्ठे विष्टम्भित्वादिवदह्यते।

विदाहात्कुरुते ग्लानिं पिण्याको निशिसेवितः ||४०+१ ||

Pinyaka (oil cakes) when consumed at night produces roukshya (dryness) which leads to vishtambha (constipation). Vishtambha further leads to vidaha (burning sensation) which leads to glani (fatigue).

Vesavara – Meat cooked with spices:

वेसवारो गुरुः स्निग्धो बलोपचयवर्धनः|

मुद्गादिजास्तु गुरवो यथाद्रव्यगुणानुगाः||४१||

Vesavara (meat, cut into minute bits, added with spices like pepper, ginger etc, and roasted or fried) is

Guru – hard to digest,

Snigdha – is unctuous,

Balaupachayavardhana – increases strength and builds the body.

Vesavara prepared from mudga (green gram) and others is guru (hard to digest) and possess properties similar to the material from which it is prepared.

Steaming, baking etc.

कुकूलकर्परभ्राष्ट्रकन्द्वङ्गारविपाचितान्|
एकयोनींल्लघून्विद्यादपूपानुत्तरोत्तरम्||४२||

Eatables cooked by kukula (steaming), karpara (baked on hot mud or iron pan), brashtra (in a vessel kept over a stove), kanda (inside a hearth) and angara (baked by placing on burning coal directly) are easy to digest in the successive order of their enumeration.

This means, eatables prepared directly over coal is easier to digest than eatables cooked by steaming.

Mamsavarga – Group of meats
Mrigavarga (deer etc.):

हरिणैणकुरङ्गर्क्षगोकर्णमृगमातृकाः|
शशशम्बरचारुष्कशरभाद्या मृगाः स्मृताः||४३||

Harina (antelope, fawn), Ena (black antelope), Kuranga (type of deer), Arksa (white footed antelope), Gokarna (Deer antelope), Mrigamatrika (red coloured hare like deer), Shasha (rabbit), Shambara (deer with branched horns), Charushka (gazelle), Sarabha (eight footed animal) etc. are known as Mriga.

Viskiravarga – group of birds which scratch the earth in search of food:

लाववार्तीकवर्तीररक्तवर्त्मकककुक्कुभाः|
कपिञ्जलोपचक्राख्यचकोरकुरुबाहवः||४४||
वर्तको वर्तिका चैव तितिरिः क्रकरः शिखी|
ताम्राचूडाख्यबकरगोनर्दगिरिवर्तिकाः||४५||
तथा शारपदेन्द्राभवरटाद्याश्च विष्किराः|

Lava (bustard quail), Vartika (bush quail), Vartira (rain quail), Raktavartma (red eyed owl), Kukkubha (wild cock), Kapinjala (black partridge), Upachakra (small greek pheasant), Chakora (greek pheasant), Kurubahava, Vartaka (button quail), Vartika (bush quail), Tittiri (grey partridge), Krakara (black partridge), Sikhi (peacock), Tamracuda (domestic cock), Bakara (small crane), Gonarda (siberian crane), Girivartika (mountain quail), Sharapada (a kind of sparrow), Indrabha (hedge sparrow), Varata (goose) etc belong to the group known as Viskira (birds which scratch the ground in search of food).

Pratudavarga – Group of birds which peck the food with beak

Pratuda – birds which peck the food with beak:

जीवञ्जीवकदात्यूहभृङ्गाह्वशुकसारिकाः||४६||

लट्वाकोकिलहारीतकपोतचटकादयः|

प्रतुदाः

Jivanijivaka (Greek partridge), Datyuha (gallinule), Bhrunagahwa (shrike), Suka (parakeet), Sarika (mynah), Latva (wild sparrow), Kokila (cuckoo), Harita (grey pigeon), Kapota (wood pigeon), Chataka (house sparrow) etc. belong to the group of Pratuda (birds which peck the food with beak).

Bileshaya – Group of creatures that live in burrows

भेकगोधाहिश्वाविदाद्या बिलेशयाः||४७||

Bheka (frog), godha (iguana lizard), Ahi (snake), swavid (hedgehog) etc. are Bileshaya (group of animals living in burrows).

Prasahavarga – Creatures which catch their food by teeth, tear it and eat:

गोखराश्वतरोष्ट्राश्वद्वीपिसिंहर्क्षवानराः|

मार्जारमूषकव्याघ्रवृकबभ्रुतरक्षवः||४८||

लोपाकजम्बुकश्येनचाषवान्तादवायसाः

शशघ्नीभासकुररगृध्रोलूककुलिङ्गकाः||४९||

धूमिका मधुहा चेति प्रसहा मृगपक्षिणः|

Go (cow), Khara (ass, donkey), Aswatara (mule), Ustra (camel), Ashwa (horse), Dwipi (leopard), Simha (lion), Aruksha (deer), Vanara (monkey), Marjala (cat), Musaka (rat, mice), Vyaghra (tiger), Vrka (jackal), Babhru (large brown mongoose), Tarksu (hyena), Lopaka (fox), Jambuka (jackal), Syena (hawk), Casa (blue joy), Vantada (dog), Vayasa (crow), Sasaghni (golden eagle), Bhasa (bread vulture), Kurara (osprey), Grdhra (vulture), Uluka (owl), Kulingaka (sparrow hawk), Dhumika(owlet), Madhuha (honey buzzard), these and other animals and birds belong to the group known as Prasaha (which catch their food by the teeth, tear it and eat).

Mahamriga – Large animals:

वराहमहिषन्यङ्कुरुरुरोहितवारणाः||५०||
सृमरश्चमरः खड्गो गवयश्च महामृगाः|

Varaha (boar), Mahisha (buffalo), Nyanku (dog deer), Rohita (big deer), Ruru (swamp deer), Varana (elephant), Srmara (Indian wild boar), Chamara (yak), Khadga (rhinoceros) and Gavaya (goyal ox) are known as Mahamriga (animals having huge body).

Apcharavarga – Water birds:

हंससारसकादम्बवककारण्डवप्लवाः||५१||
बलाकोत्क्रोशचक्राह्वमद्गुक्रौञ्चादयोऽप्चराः|

Hamsa (swan), Sarasa (Indian crane), Kadamba (grey legged goose), Baka (heron), Karandava (white breasted goose), Palva (pelican), Balaka (crane), Utkrosa (mattard), Chakrahva (ruddy sheldrake), Madgu (small cormorant), Krouncha (pound heron) etc. are know as Apcara (water birds).

Matsyavarga – Group of fishes:

मत्स्या रोहितपाठीनकूर्मकुम्भीरकर्कटाः||५२||
शुक्तिशङ्खोद्रशम्बूकशफरीवर्मिचन्द्रिकाः|
चुलूकीनक्रमकरशिशुमारतिमिङ्गिलाः||५३||
राजीचिलिचिमाद्याश्च मांसमित्याहुरष्टधा|

Rohita (red fish), Pathina (boal), Kurma (tortoise), Kumbhira (gavial, alligator), Karkata (crab), Sukti (pearl mussel), Sankha (conch shell), Urdu (otter), Sambuka (comman snail), Safari (large glistening fish), Varmicandrika (a kind of cat fish), Culuki (propoise, seahog), Pakra (crocodile), Makara (crocodile), Sisumara (dolphin), Timingala (whale, shark), Raji (snake fish), Cilicima (red striped fish) and others belongs to group of matsya (fishes).

Thus eight kinds (sources) of mamsa (meat) are enumerated.

योनिष्वजावी व्यामिश्रगोचरत्वादनिश्चते||५४||

Goat (aja) and sheep (avi) are not included in any particular group because they are seen everywhere irrespective of any particular yoni (locality of origin).

आद्यान्त्या जाङ्गलानूपा मध्यौ साधारणौ स्मृतौ|
Out of the eight groups mentioned above, the first three (Mriga, Viskriya and Pratuda) are also known as Jangala;
The last three (Mahamriga, Jalacara and Matsya), are also called Anupa;
The middle two (Bilesaya and Prasaha) are known as Sadharana.
Qualities of meat belonging to Jangala group of animals:

तत्र बद्धमलाः शीता लघवो जाङ्गला हिताः||५५||
पित्तोत्तरे वातमध्ये सन्निपाते कफानुगे|
Meat of the Jangala group causes
Badha mala – constipation,
Sheeta – cold (in potency),
Laghu – easily digestible.
This meat is suitable in vitiation of tridosha (sannipata) with predominance of Pitta, moderate increase of Vata and mild increase of Kapha.

Meat of Sasha (rabbit):
दीपनः कटुकः पाके ग्राही रूक्षो हिमः शशः||५६||
The flesh of shasha (rabbit), is
Deepana – enhances hunger,
Katupaka – pungent after digestion,
Grahi – water absorbent and
Hima – cold in potency.

Meat of Vartaka (button quail):
ईषदुष्णगुरुस्निग्धा बृंहणा वर्तकादयः|
The flesh of the Vartaka (button quail) and others are
Ishatushna – slightly hot in potency,
Guru – hard to digest,
Snigdha – unctuous and
Brihmana – makes the body stout.

Meat of Tittiri (sparrow):
तित्तिरिस्तेष्वपि वरो मेधाग्निबलशुक्रकृत्||५७||
ग्राही वर्ण्योऽनिलोद्रिक्तसन्निपातहरः परम्|

Tittiri (sparrow) meat is still better.

It enhances –

Medha – intelligence,

Agni – power of digestion,

Bala – strength,

Sukra – semen,

It is –

Grahi – withholds discharges of fluids from the body,

Varnya – improves the skin complexion,

Sannipatahara – effectively mitigates sannipata (vitiation of tridoshas) with increase of vata.

As it is seen across Jangala (dry, arid land) and anupadesha (moist, marshy land), it has the properties of snigdha (unctuous), ushna (hot potency), guru (heavy for digestion) and is Brihmana (nutritive, nourishing).

Meat of Shikhi (Peacock):

नातिपथ्यः शिखी पथ्यः श्रोत्रस्वरवयोद्दशाम्||५८||

The flesh of shikhi (peacock) is –

Na atipathya – not very wholesome,

but it is good for the ears (srotra), voice (svara), to slow down aging (vaya), and eyes (drik).

Meat of Kukkuta (cock):

तद्वच्च कुक्कुटो वृष्यः ग्राम्यस्तु श्लेष्मलो गुरुः।

Flesh of cock (wild fowl), is similar to that of peacock;

it is Vrishya – aphrodisiac;

that of the domesticated (gramya) fowl increases kapha and is guru (hard to digest).

Meat of Krakara (black partridge):

मेधाऽनलकरा हृद्याः क्रकराः सोपचक्रकाः||५९||

Flesh of krakara (black partridge) is

Medhakara – increases intelligence,

Analakara – improves digestion,

Hridya – is good for the heart (or the mind);

Similar is the flesh of upachakraka.

Meat of Kanakapota:

गुरुः सलवणः काणकपोतः सर्वदोषकृत्|

Meat of kana kapota is

Guru – hard to digest,

Sa lavana – slightly salty and

Sarvadoshakrit – increases all the doshas.

Meat of Chataka:

चटकाः श्लेष्मलाः स्निग्धा वातघ्नाः शुक्रलाः परम्||६०||

Meat of cataka is

Sleshmala – increases kapha,

Snigdha – unctuous,

Vataghna – mitigates vata and

Shukrala param – best to increase semen.

Flesh of animals of the next succeeding groups (bilesaya, prasaha, mahamriga, jalachara and matsya)

गुरूष्णस्निग्धमधुरा वर्गाश्चातो यथोत्तरम्|

मूत्रशुक्रकृतो बल्या वातघ्नाः कफपित्तलाः||६१||

Flesh of animals of the next succeeding groups (bilesaya, prasaha, mahamriga, jalachara and matsya) are successively more and more

Guru – hard to digest,

Ushna – hot in potency,

Snigdha – unctuous,

Madhura – sweet,

Mutrakrita – increases urine,

Shukrakrita – increases semen,

Balya – strengthening,

Vatagna – mitigates vata and

Kaphapittala – increases kapha and pitta.

Meat of Mahamriga (large animals):

शीता महामृगास्तेषु, क्रव्यादप्रसहाः पुनः|

लवणानुरसाः पाके कटुका मांसवर्धनाः||६२||

जीर्णार्शोग्रहणीदोषशोषार्तानां परं हिताः|

Flesh of the Mahamrigas (big animals) are

Sheeta – cold in potency generally;

Among them the flesh of carnivorous (kravyada) and prasaha animals have Lavanaanurasa – salty secondary taste,

Katupaka – pungent taste conversion at the end of digestion,

Mamsavardhana – increases the muscle bulk,

It is indicated in persons suffering from long standing haemorrhoids (jeernaarshas), duodenal diseases (grahani dosha) and emaciation (shosha).

Meat of Goat (Aja):

नातिशीतगुरुस्निग्धं मांसमाजमदोषलम्||६३||

शरीरधातुसामान्यादनभिष्यन्दि बृंहणम्|

Goat's meat is –

Na atisheetam – not very cold in potency,

Guru – hard to digest,

Snigdham – unctuous,

Adoshalam – does not aggravate the doshas,

Sharira dhatu samanyad – identical to the doshas of the human body,

Anabhisyandi – does not cause increase of secretions in the tissue channels,

Brihmana – nourishing, causes weight gain.

Meat of sheep (Avi):

विपरीतमतो ज्ञेयमाविकं बृंहणं तु तत्||६४||

The properties of meat of Avi (sheep) are opposite in nature to that of goat but is brihmana (causes weight gain).

Gomamsa (flesh of cow, bull, bullock):

शुष्ककासश्रमात्यग्निविषमज्वरपीनसान्|

कार्श्यं केवलवातांश्च गोमांसं सन्नियच्छति||६५||

Gomamsa (flesh of cow, bull, bullock) cures

Shushkakasa – dry cough,

Shrama – exhaustion,

Atyagni – excess hunger,

Vishamajwara – intermittent fevers,

Pinasa – chronic nasal catarrh,

Karshya – emaciation and

Kevalavataroga – diseases caused by increase of vata independently.

Flesh of Mahisa (Buffalo):

उष्णो गरीयान्महिषः स्वप्नदाढर्यबृहत्त्वकृत्|

Flesh of Mahisa (buffalo) is

Ushna – hot,

Guru – not easily digestible,

Swapnakrit – produces sleep,

Dardyakrit – increases strength and

Bahutvakrit–increases stoutness of the body.

Flesh of Varaha (pig):

तद्वद्वराहः श्रमहा रुचिशुक्रबलप्रदः||६६||

Flesh of varaha (pig) is similar to that of buffalo. It is

Shramaha – relieves fatigue, and increases

Ruchi – taste,

Shukra – semen and

Bala – strength.

Flesh of Matsya (Fish):

मत्स्याः परं कफकराः चिलिचीमस्त्रिदोषकृत्|

Fish in general tends to greatly increase Kapha. Chilichima fish tends to increase all the three doshas.

Best birds

लावरोहितगोधैणाः स्वे स्वे वर्गे वराः परम्||६७||

Meat of lava (swallow), rohita (a fresh water fish), godha (iguana) and ena (black antelope) are best in their respective groups.

मत्स्यादिपक्षिणांचैवगुरूण्यण्डानिचादिशेत्।
तानिस्निग्धानिवृष्याणिस्वादुपाकरसानिच||६७१+१||

The eggs of fishes and birds are heavy in nature (Guru), unctuous (Snigdha), aphrodisiac (Vrushya), have sweet taste (Swadu Rasa) and undergo sweet taste conversion after digestion (SwaduPaka).

Meats which are suitable and unsuitable for consumption:

मांसं सद्योहतं शुद्धं वयःस्थं च भजेत् त्यजेत्|
मृतं कृशं भृशं मेद्यं व्याधिवारिविषैर्हतम्||६८||

The following types of meat can be used for consumption:

Sadyohatam – meat of animals which have just been killed,

Shuddha – which are uncontaminated and

Vayastham – of young animals only should be used as food;

Meat that should not be used for consumption:

Svayammritam – Meat of naturally dead animals,

Krisha – that are very emaciated,

Medyam – which are very fatty,

and of those animals which are dead due to vyadhi (diseases), vari (water) and visha (poison) should be rejected.

पुंस्त्रियोः पूर्वपश्चार्धे गुरुणी, गर्भिणी गुरुः|

लघुर्याषिच्चतुष्पात्सु, विहङ्गेषु पुनः पुमान्||६९||

शिरःस्कन्धोरुपृष्ठस्य कट्याः सक्थ्नोश्च गौरवम्|

तथाऽऽमपक्वाशययोर्यथापूर्वं विनिर्दिशेत्||७०||

शोणितप्रभृतीनां च धातूनामुत्तरोत्तरम्|

मांसाद्गरीयो वृषणमेढ्रवृक्कयकृद्गुदम्||७१||

Meat obtained from the parts above the umbilicus of male animals, from the parts below the umbilicus of female animals and that obtained from pregnant animals are all guru (hard to digest).

Among the quadrupeds, the flesh of females is laghu (easily digestible) whereas the flesh of males is laghu among birds.

Flesh obtained from the shira (head), skanda (neck), uru (thighs), prishta (back), kati (waist), sakthi (forelegs), amashaya (stomach) and pakvashaya (intestines) are hard to digest in the reverse order of enumeration i.e., flesh obtained from shira (head) is the most heaviest for digestion and that obtained from pakvashaya the least.

Among dhatus (tissues), rakta (blood), mamsa (muscle), meda (fat) etc. are successively more and more guru;

Vrishana (testicles), medra (penis), vrikka (kidneys), yakrit (liver) and guda (rectum) are harder to digest than the flesh.

ShakaVarga – Group of leafy vegetables:

शाकं पाठाशठीसूषासुनिषण्णसतीनजम्|

त्रिदोषघ्नं लघु ग्राहि सराजक्षववास्तुकम्||७२||

Patha (Cissampelos pareira), Shati (Hedychium spicatum), Srusha, Sunishanna, Satinaja in general are

Tridoshagna – mitigates all the three doshas,

Laghu – are easily digestible and

Grahi – absorbent.

सुनिषण्णोऽग्निकृद्वृष्यस्तेषु राजक्षवः परम्।
ग्रहण्यर्शोविकारघ्नः वर्चोभेदि तु वास्तुकम्॥७३॥

Among the above mentioned shaka (vegetables),
Sunishanna increases hunger (agnikrit) and is aphrodisiac (vrishya);
Rajakshava is still better and cures duodenal diseases (grahanivikara) and haemorrhoids (arshas);
Vastuka breaks up the hard faeces (varchobhedi).

Kakamachi (Solanum nigrum), Cangeri (Oxalis corniculata):

हन्ति दोषत्रयं कुष्ठं वृष्या सोष्णा रसायनी।
काकमाची सरा स्वर्या चाङ्गेर्यम्लाऽग्निदीपनी॥७४॥
ग्रहण्यर्शोऽनिलश्लेष्महितोष्णा ग्राहिणी लघुः।

Kakamachi (Solanum nigrum) is
Hantidoshatrayam – mitigates the three doshas,
Useful in
Kushta – skin diseases,
Vrishya – is aphrodisiac,
Ushna – hot in potency,
Rasayanam – rejuvenator,
Sara – causes easy movement of faeces and
Svarya – is good for the voice.
Changeri (Oxalis corniculata) is –
Amla – sour in taste,
Agni deepani – kindles digestion,
Useful in
Grahani – duodenal diseases,
Arsha – haemorrhoids and
Anilasleshma – increased vata and kapha,
Ushna – hot in potency,
Grahi – withholds elimination of fluids and
Laghu – is easily digestible.

पटोलसप्तलारिष्टशाङ्गेर्ष्टावल्गुजाऽमृताः॥७५॥
वेत्राग्रबृहतीवासाकुतिलीतिलपर्णिकाः।
मण्डूकपर्णीकिर्कोटकारवेल्लकपर्पटाः॥७६॥
नाडीकलायगोजिह्वावावार्ताकं वनतिक्तकम्।

करीरं कुलकं नन्दी कुचैला शकुलादनी||७७||
कटिल्लं केम्बुकं शीतं सकोशातककर्कशम्|
तिक्तं पाके कटु ग्राहि वातलं कफपित्तजित्||७८||

Patola, saptala, arista (neem leaves), sharngeshta (angaravalli/bharangi), Avalguja (Bakuchi), amruta (Tinospora), Vetra (shoot of vetra), Brhati (Solanum indicum), vasa (Adhatodavasica), kutilla, tilaparnika (badraka), mandukaparni (Gotu kola), Karkota, karavella (bitter gourd), parpata, nadikalaya, gojihwa (godhumi),vartaka (brhati), vanatiktaka (vatsaka/kutaja), karira, kulaka (kupila), nandi (jaya),kucaila, sakuladani (mesasrngi), katilla (raktapunarnava), kebuka (kembuka),kosataka and karkasa (kampilla) are

Sheeta – cold in potency,

Tikta rasa – bitter in taste,

Katupaka – pungent at the end of digestion,

Grahi – absorbent,

Vatalam – increase Vata and

Kaphapittajit – mitigate Kapha and Pitta.

हृद्यं पटोलं कृमिनुत्स्वादुपाकं रुचिप्रदम्|
पित्तलं दीपनं भेदि वातघ्नं बृहतीद्वयम्||७९||
कारवेल्लं सकटुकं दीपनं कफजित्परम्||८०||

Patola is

Hridya – good for the heart (or the mind),

Kriminut – destroys worms,

Svadupaka – sweet at the end of digestion and

Ruchipradam – improves taste.

The two Brihati (Brihati and Kantakari) are

Pittala – increases pitta,

Deepana – promotes hunger,

Bhedi – breaks the hard faeces and

Vatagna – alleviates Vata.

Vrusha (Vasa) cures

Vami – vomiting,

Kasa – cough,

It is the best remedy for Raktapitta – haemorrhagic diseases.

Karavella (bitter gourd) is

Katu – slightly pungent in taste,

Deepana – kindles digestion and
Kaphajit param – excellently mitigates kapha.

वार्ताकं कटु तिक्तोष्णं मधुरं कफवातजित्।
सक्षारमग्निजननं हृद्यं रुच्यमपित्तलम्॥८१॥
करीरमाध्मानकरं कषायं स्वादु तिक्तकम्।

Vartaka (brinjal) is
Katutikta – pungent, bitter in taste,
Ushna – hot in potency,
Madhura – sweet,
Kaphavatajit – mitigates kapha and vata,
Sa ksharam – is slightly alkaline,
Agni jananam – kindles digestion,
Hridyam – good for the heart,
Ruchyam – improves taste and
Apittalam – does not aggravate pitta.

Karira produces
Adhmana – distension of the abdomen,
Kashaya svadutikta – is astringent, sweet and bitter in taste.

Kosataki and Avalguja are
Bhedana – break the hard faeces and
Agni deepana – kindle digestion.

Tanduliya and Munjata:
तण्डुलीयो हिमो रूक्षः स्वादुपाकरसो लघुः।
मदपित्तविषास्रघ्नः मुञ्जातं वातपित्तजित्॥८३॥
स्निग्धं शीतं गुरु स्वादु बृंहणं शुक्रकृत्परम्।

Tanduliya is
Hima – cold in potency,
Ruksha – dry,
Swadupaka rasa – sweet in taste and also at the end of digestion and
Lagu – easily digestible.
It cures
Mada – intoxication,
Pitta – disorders due to pitta vitiation,
Visha – poison and
Asrik – disorders of blood.

Munjata properties –
Vata pittajit – mitigates vata and pitta,
Snigdha – is unctuous,
Sheeta – cold in potency,
Guru – hard to digest,
Swadu – sweet,
Brihmana – makes the body stout and
Shukrakrit – increases semen.

Palankya, Upodika (spinach) and Chanchu:
गुर्वी सरा तु पालङ्क्या मदघ्नी चाप्युपोदका||८४||
पालङ्क्यावत्स्मृतश्चञ्चुः स तु सङ्ग्रहणात्मकः|
Palankya is guru (hard to digest) and sara (laxative).
Upodika (spinach) is madagni (relieves intoxication).
Chanchu is similar to palankya and is sangrahanatmaka (withholds elimination of fluids).

Vidari:
विदारी वातपित्तघ्नी मूत्रला स्वादुशीतला||८५|| जीवनी बृंहणी कण्ठ्या गुर्वी वृष्या रसायनम्|
Vidari is
Vata pittagni – mitigates vata and pitta,
Mutrala – is diuretic,
Svadu – sweet in taste,
Sheetala – cold in potency,
Jeevani – prolongs life,
Brihmani – makes the body stout,
Kantya – good for the throat,
Guru – hard to digest,
Vrishya – aphrodisiac and
Rasayana – rejuvenator.

Jivanti:
चक्षुष्या सर्वदोषघ्नी जीवन्ती मधुरा हिमा||८६||
Jivanti is
Chakshushya – good for the eyes,
Sarvadoshagna – mitigates all the dosas,
Madhura – is sweet in taste and

Hima – cold in potency.

Phala Shaka Varga – Group of vegetables and fruits:
कूष्माण्डतुम्बकालिङ्गककर्कार्वेर्वारुतिण्डिशम्|
तथा त्रपुसचीनाकचिर्भटं कफवातकृत्||८७||
भेदि विष्टम्भ्यभिष्यन्दि स्वादुपाकरसं गुरु|
Kusmanda (ash gourd), Tumba (alabu), Kalinga, Karkaru, Evaru, Tindisa, Trapusa, Cinaka, Cirbhata are

Kaphavatakrit – causes increase of kapha and vata,

Bhedi – breaks the hard faeces,

Vishtambhi – stays long without digestion inside the stomach,

Abhishyandi – causes more secretion in the tissues,

Svadupaka rasa – sweet in taste and at the end of digestion and

Guru – not easily digestible.

Kushmanda – Ash gourd:
वल्लीफलानां प्रवरं कूष्माण्डं वातपित्तजित्||८८||
बस्तिशुद्धिकरं वृष्यम् त्रपुसं त्वतिमूत्रलम्|
Kushmanda (ash gourd) is pravara (best) among the valliphala (creepers) and

Vata pittajit – mitigates Vata and Pitta,

Vastishuddhikara – cleanses the urinary bladder and

Vrishya – aphrodisiac.

Trapusa causes more urination (atimutrala).
तुम्बं रूक्षतरं ग्राहि कालिङ्गैर्वारुचिर्भटम्||८९||
बालं पित्तहरं शीतं विद्यात्पक्वमतोऽन्यथा|
शीर्णवृन्तं तु सक्षारं पित्तलं कफवातजित्||९०||
रोचनं दीपनं हृद्यमष्ठीलाऽनाहनुल्लघु|
Tumba (alabu) is Rukshatara – very dry and Grahi – absorbent.

Kalinga, Ervaru and Cirbhita when tender (bala) are

Pittahara – mitigate pitta and

Sheeta – cold in potency.

When ripe (pakva), they possess opposite qualities.

Those which are overripe and separated from its attachment (sheernavrinta), will be

Sakshara – alkaline in taste,

Pittalam – increase pitta,

Kaphavatajit – mitigate Kapha and Vata,

Rochana – improves taste,

Deepana – improves appetite,

Hridya – good for the heart,

Ashteelanut – cures enlargement of the prostate,

Anahanut – cures distension of abdomen and is

Laghu – easily digestible.

Kanda Shaka Varga – Group of aquatic stem vegetables:

मृणालबिसशालूककुमुदोत्पलकन्दकम्||९१||

नन्दीमाषककेलूटशृङ्गाटककसेरुकम्|

क्रौञ्चादनं कलोड्यं च रूक्षं ग्राहि हिमं गुरु||९२||

Mrinala (lotus stalk), bisa (lotus root), saluki (lotus tuber), kumuda, utpalakanda, nandi, mashaka, keluta, srngataka, kaseruka, krauncadana and kalodya are

Ruksha – cause dryness,

Grahi – water absorbent,

Hima – cold in potency and

Guru – not easily digestible.

Patra Shaka Varga – Group of leafy vegetables:

कलम्बनालिकामार्षकुटिञ्जरकुतुम्बकम्|

चिल्लीलट्वाकलोणीकाकुरूटकगवेधुकम्||९३||

जीवन्तझुञ्झ्वेडगजयवशाकसुवर्चलाः|

आलुकानि च सर्वाणि तथा सूप्यानि लक्ष्मणम्||९४||

स्वादु रूक्षं सलवणं वातश्लेष्मकरं गुरु|

शीतलं सृष्टविण्मूत्रं प्रायो विष्टभ्य जीर्यति||९५||

स्विन्नं निष्पीडितरसं स्नेहाढ्यं नातिदोषलम्|

Kalamba, Nalika (kapotacarana), marsa, kutinjara, kutumbaka, cilli (vastuka), latvaka, lonika, karutaka, gavedhuka, jivanta, jhunjhu, edagaja, yavasaka (yavanisaka), suvarchala and aluka of different kinds, leaves of legumes used for soup and of lakshmana are

Svadu – sweet in taste,

Ruksha – slightly dry,

Salavana – salty,

Vata sleshmakara – increases Vata and Kapha,

Guru – not easily digestible,

Sheetala – cold in potency,
Srishtavinmutra – help elimination of urine and faeces,
Vishtambhi – stays long in the stomach for digestion,
They won't cause much digestive disturbances when cooked in steam, the juice squeezed out and mixed with enough oils.

Chilli, Tarkari and Varana:

लघुपत्रा तु या चिल्ली सा वास्तुकसमा मता||९६||
तर्कारीवरुणं स्वादु सतिक्तं कफवातजित्|

Chilli, which has laghupatra (small leaves) , is similar (in properties) tovastuka.
Tarkari and varana are swadu (sweet), satikta (slightly bitter) and kaphavatajit (mitigate Kapha and Vata).

Varshabhu and Kalashaka:

वर्षाभ्वौ कालशाकं च सक्षारं कटुतिक्तकम्||९७||
दीपनं भेदनं हन्ति गरशोफकफानिलान्|

Varsabhu and Kalasaka are
Sakshara – slightly alkaline,
Katutiktakam – pungent and bitter,
Deepana – improve digestion,
Bhedana – break the hard faeces.
They pacify
Gara – artificial poisoning,
Shopha – oedema,
Kaphaanila – kapha and vata.

Sprouts of Chirabilva and Shatavari:

दीपनाः कफवातघ्नाश्चिरिबिल्वाङ्कुराः सराः||९८||
शतावर्यङ्कुरास्तिक्ता वृष्या दोषत्रयापहाः|

The tender sprouts of Chirabilva are
Deepana – increase appetite,
Kaphavatagna – mitigate kapha and vata and
Sara – cause movement of bowels;
Sprouts of Satavari are
Tikta – bitter,
Vrishya – aphrodisiac and

Doshatrayapaha – mitigate the three doshas.

Flower of Shalmali:
सङ्ग्राहिशाल्मलीपुष्पंपित्तास्रघ्नंविशेषतः॥९८१+१॥
The flowers of Shalmali are
Sangrahi – absorbent,
Pittasragnam – relieves bleeding disorders.
Vamshakarira, Pattura, Kasamarda:
रूक्षो वंशकरीरस्तु विदाही वातपित्तलः॥९९॥
पत्तूरो दीपनस्तिक्तः प्लीहार्शःकफवातजित्‌।
कृमिकासकफोत्क्लेदान् कासमर्दो जयेत्सरः॥१००॥
Vamsakarira (tender shoots of bamboo) causes
Ruksha – dryness,
Vidahi – burning sensation and
Vata pittala – increase of vata and pitta.

Pattura is
Deepana – kindles digestion,
Tikta – is bitter.
It cures
Pleeha – enlargement of spleen,
Arsha – haemorrhoids and
Kaphavatajit – mitigates kapha and vata.

Kasamarda cures
Krimi – disease caused by worms,
Kasa – cough and
Kaphotkleda – increase of Kapha and is
Sara – moves the bowels.

Kousumbha:
रूक्षोष्णमम्लं कौसुम्भं गुरु पित्तकरं सरम्‌।
Kousumbha is
Ruksha – dry,
Ushna – hot in potency,
Amla – sour,
Guru – hard to digest,

Pittakara – increase Pitta and

Sara – moves the bowels.

Sarshapa (mustard):

गुरूष्णं सार्षपं बद्धविण्मूत्रं सर्वदोषकृत्||१०१||

Sarshapa (mustard) is

Guru – not easily digestible,

Ushna – hot in potency,

Badhavinmutra – binds the faeces and urine and

Sarvadoshakrit – causes increase of all the dosas.

Mulaka – Radish:

यद्बालमव्यक्तरसं किञ्चित्क्षारं सतिक्तकम्|

तन्मूलकं दोषहरं लघु सोष्णं नियच्छति||१०२||

गुल्मकासक्षयश्वासव्रणनेत्रगलामयान्|

स्वराग्निसादोदावर्तपीनसांश्च महत्पुनः||१०३||

रसे पाके च कटुकमुष्णवीर्यं त्रिदोषकृत्|

गुर्वभिष्यन्दि च स्निग्धसिद्धं तदपि वातजित्||१०४||

वातश्लेष्महरं शुष्कं सर्वम् आमं तु दोषलम्|

Tender radish:

Mulaka (radish), when bala (tender) is

Avyakta rasa – not having definite taste,

Kinchitksharasatikta – is slightly alkaline and bitter,

Doshahara – mitigates the dosas,

Laghu – easily digestible,

Ushna – hot in potency.

It cures ·

Gulma – abdominal tumours,

Kasa – cough,

Kshaya – emaciation,

Swasa – asthma,

Vrana – ulcers,

Netra galamaya – diseases of the eye and throat,

Swarasada – hoarseness of voice,

Agnisada – decreases digestive strength,

Udavarta – retrograde intestinal movements and

Pinasa – chronic nasal catarrh.

Radish, which is mature and big in size is
Katu rasa paka – pungent in taste and at the end of digestion,
Ushnavirya – hot in potency,
Tridoshakrit – increases all the three doshas,
Guru – hard to digest and is
Abhishynadi – increases secretions.

When cooked with fat, it mitigates Vata (vatajit).
The dried (shushka) one mitigates vata and kapha (vatasleshmahara).
It vitiates tridoshas when taken in raw form.

Pindalu:
कटूष्णो वातकफहा पिण्डालु: पित्तवर्धनः||१०५||
Pindalu is
Katu – pungent,
Ushna – hot in potency,
Vata kaphapaha – mitigates vata and kapha
Pitta vardhana – increases pitta.

Salanashaka Varga – Group of drugs used as spices:
कुठेरशिग्रुसुरससुमुखासुरिभूस्तृणम्|
फणिज्जार्जकजम्बीरप्रभृति ग्राहि शालनम्||१०६||
विदाहि कटु रूक्षोष्णं हृद्यं दीपनरोचनम्|
दृक्शुक्रकृमिहृतीक्ष्णं दोषोत्क्लेशकरं लघु||१०७||
Kuthera, sigru (drum stick), surasa, sumuka, asuri, bhutrna, phanijja, arjaka,
jambira etc. which comprise the Shalanashakavarga are
Grahi – water absorbent,
Vidahi – cause burning sensation during digestion,
Katu – pungent,
Ruksha – cause dryness,
Ushna – hot in potency,
Hridyam – good for the heart (or the mind),
Deepana – kindles hunger,
Rochana – improves taste.
It destroys
Drik – vision,

Shukra – semen and

Krimi – worms (intestinal parasites),

Tikshna – penetrates deep and

Dosha utkleshakara – cause slight increase of the dosas and laghu – are easily digestible.

Surasa – Holy basil benefits:

हिध्माकासविषश्वासपार्श्वरुक्पूतिगन्धहा।

सुरसः सुमुखो नातिविदाही गरशोफहा॥१०८॥

सुमुखो नातिविदाही गरशोफहा॥१०८॥

Surasa (Tulasi – Holy Basil) cures

Hidhma – hiccup,

Kasa – cough,

Visha – poison,

Swasa – asthma,

Parshvaruk – pain in the flanks and

Putigandha – bad breath.

Sumukha is

Na atividahi – does not cause much burning sensation,

Gara – cures artificial (homicidal) poison and

Shopha – oedema.

Ardrika (coriander) is

Tiktamadhura – bitter and sweet in taste,

Mutrala – diuretic and

Na ca pittakrit – does not increase pitta.

Lashuna – Garlic benefits:

लशुनो भृशतीक्ष्णोष्णः कटुपाकरसः सरः॥१०९॥

हृद्यः केश्यो गुरुवृष्यः स्निग्धो रोचनदीपनः।

भग्नसन्धानकृद्बल्यो रक्तपित्तप्रदूषणः॥११०॥

किलासकुष्ठगुल्मार्शोमेहक्रिमिकफानिलान्।

सहिध्मापीनसश्वासकासान् हन्ति रसायनम्॥१११॥

Lashuna (garlic) is

Brishatikshna – highly penetrating,

Ushna – hot in potency,

Katu rasa paka – pungent in taste, and at the end of digestion,

Sara –facilitates easy bowel movements,

Hridya – good for the heart (or the mind),

Keshya – good for hairs,

Guru – hard to digest,

Vrishya – aphrodisiac,

Snigdha – unctuous,

Rochana – improves taste,

Deepana – improves digestion,

Bhagnasandhanakrit – helps in union of fractures,

Balya – gives strength,

Rakta pitta pradushana – greatly vitiates the blood and pitta.

It cures

Kilasa – leucoderma,

Kushta – skin diseases,

Gulma – abdominal tumours,

Arsha – heamorrhoids,

Meha – diabetes,

Krimi – worms,

Kaphaanilan – diseases caused by Kapha and Vata,

Hidhma – hiccup,

Pinasa – chronic nasal catarrh,

Swasa– asthma, dyspnoea and

Kasa – cough.

Asrapittakrit – it increases bleeding disorders.

Palandu – Onion Benefits:

पलाण्डुस्तद्गुणन्यूनः श्लेष्मलो नातिपित्तलः।

Palandu (onion) is inferior in qualities compared to Lashuna (garlic). It is
Sleshmala – increases Kapha,
Na atipittala – does not intensely vitiate Pitta.

Grinjanaka – Carrot benefits:

कफवातार्शसां पथ्यः स्वेदेऽभ्यवहृतौ तथा॥११२॥
तीक्ष्णो ग्रञ्जनको ग्राही पित्तिनां हितकृन्न सः।

Grinjanaka (carrot) is best suitable for persons suffering from haemorrhoids of Kapha and Vata origin, for sweda (fomenting the pile masses) and for eating.
It is

Tikshna – penetrating,
Grahi – water absorbent and
Pittanam hitakrit na – not suitable to those who have Pitta predominance.

Surana – Yam benefits:
दीपनः सूरणो रुच्यः कफघ्नो विशदो लघुः||११३||
विशेषादर्शसां पथ्यः भूकन्दस्त्वतिदोषलः|
Surana (Yam) is
Deepana – kindles digestion,
Ruchya – improves taste,
Kaphagna – mitigates Kapha,
Vishada – lucid,
Laghu – easily digestible.
Visheshatarshasampathya – it is especially good for haemorrhoids.

Bhukanda causes an increase of all the dosas to a great extent.
पत्रे पुष्पे फले नाले कन्दे च गुरुता क्रमात्||११४||
वरा शाकेषु जीवन्ती सार्षपं त्ववरं परम्|
Leaves (patra), flowers (pushpa), fruits (phala), tubular leaves (nala) and
tubers (kanda) are heavy to digest (guru) in their successive order, i.e.
leaves are lightest for digestion and tubers are the heaviest.
Jivanti is the best and Sarshapa (mustard) is the worst among the leafy
vegetables.

PhalaVarga – Group of fruits:
Draksha – Grapes benefits:
द्राक्षा फलोत्तमा वृष्या चक्षुष्या सृष्टमूत्रविट्||११५||
स्वादुपाकरसा स्निग्धा सकषाया हिमा गुरुः|
निहन्त्यनिलपित्तास्रतिक्तास्यत्वमदात्ययान्||११६||
तृष्णाकासश्रमश्वासस्वरभेदक्षतक्षयान्|
Draksa (grapes) is
Phalottama – best among fruits,
Vrishya – is aphrodisiac,
Chakshushya – good for the eyes,
Srishta mutra vit – helps elimination of urine and faeces,
Swadupaka rasa – sweet in taste and at the end of digestion,
Snigdha – unctuous,

Sakashaya – slightly astringent,
Hima – cold potency,
Guru – hard to digest.
It cures
Diseases of vata, pitta and rakta,
Tiktasyata – bitter taste in the mouth,
Madatyaya – intoxication,
Trishna – thirst,
Kasa – cough,
Srama – fatigue,
Swasa – dyspnoea, respiratory conditions,
Swarabheda – hoarseness of voice,
Kshata – injury to the lungs and
Kshaya – emaciation.

Dadima – Pomegranate Benefits:

उद्रिक्तपित्ताञ्जयति त्रीन्दोषान्स्वादु दाडिमम्||११७||
पित्ताविरोधि नात्युष्णमम्लं वातकफापहम्|
सर्वं हृद्यं लघु स्निग्धं ग्राहि रोचनदीपनम्||११८||

Dadima (pomegranate) mitigates the greatly increased Pitta in particular (udriktapittanjayati) and the other dosas also but to a lesser extent.
It is swadu (sweet);
The amla (sour) variety of dadima (pomegranate) is
Pittavirodhi – does not increase Pitta,
Na atyushnam – not very hot in potency and
Vata kaphapaham – mitigates Vata and Kapha.
All varieties of Dadima (pomegranate) are
Hridya – good for the heart,
Laghu – easily digestible,
Snigdha – unctuous,
Grahi – withholds elimination of fluids,
Rochana – stimulates appetite and
Deepana – stimulates digestion.

मोचखर्जूरपनसनारिकेलपरूषकम्|
आम्रातताल्काश्मर्यराजादनमधूकजम्||११९||
सैवीरबदराइकोल्लफल्गुश्लेष्मातकोद्भवम्|

वातामाभिषुकाक्षोडमुकूलकनिकोचकम्||१२०||
उरुमाणं प्रियालं च बृंहणं गुरु शीतलम्|
दाहक्षतक्षयहरं रक्तपित्तप्रसादनम्||१२१||
स्वादुपाकरसं स्निग्धं विष्टम्भि कफशुक्रकृत्|

Mocha (plantain), kharjura (dates) panasa (jack fruits) narikela (coconut), parusaka, amrataka, tala, kasmarya, rajadana, madhuka, sauvira, badara, ankola, phalgu, slesmataka, vatama, abhisuka, aksoda, mukulaka, nikocaka, urumanam and priyala are

Brihmana – make the body stout,

Guru – not easily digestible,

Sheetala – cold in potency.

It relieves

Daha – burning sensation,

Kshata – injury to the lungs,

Kshaya – emaciation.

Rakta pitta prasadanam – purifies Rakta (blood) and Pitta.

Svadupaka rasa – sweet in taste and also at the end of digestion,

Snigdha – unctuous,

Vishtambhi – stay long in the stomach without digestion,

Kaphashukrakrit – increases kapha and semen.

Fruits of Parushaka, Tala and Kashmarya:

वातघ्नं पित्तजननमामं विद्यात्परूषकम्||
तदेवपक्वं मधुरं रक्तपित्तनिवर्हणम्|
फलं तु पित्तलं तालं सरं काश्मर्यजं हिमम्||१२२||
शकृन्मूत्रविबन्धघ्नं केश्यं मेध्यं रसायनम्|

Parushaka–

Tender fruits of Parushaka pacify Vata and increase Pitta.

Ripe fruits of Parushaka are Madhura (sweet) and cure raktapitta (bleeding disorders).

Fruit of Tala (toddy) is

Pittala – increases Pitta,

Sara – moves the bowels.

Fruit of **Kasmarya** is
Hima – cold in potency,
Shakrinmutravibhandagnam – relieves the obstruction of faeces and urine,
Keshya – good for the hairs,
Medhya – increases intelligence and
Rasayanam – is a rejuvenator.

Fruits of Vatama (almond), Priyala (Chironji) and Kola (jujube fruit):
वातामाद्युष्णवीर्यं तु कफपित्तकरं सरम्||१२३||
परं वातहरं स्निग्धमनुष्णं तु प्रियालजम्|
प्रियालमज्जा मधुरो वृष्यः पित्तानिलापहः||१२४||
कोलमज्जा गुणैस्तद्वत्तृट्छर्दिःकासजिच्च सः|

Vatama (almond) etc. are
Ushnavirya – hot in potency,
Kaphapittakara – increase Kapha and Pitta,
Sara – laxative.

Priyala (Buchanania lanzan) is
Vataharam param – mitigates vata effectively,
Snigdha – is unctuous,
Anushnam – not very hot in potency.
Its majja (flesh) is
Madhura – sweet,
Vrishya – aphrodisiac,
Pittanilapaha – mitigates pitta and vata.

Kola majja (fleshy part of the kola) is similar to that of Priyala in properties, and relieves
Trit – thirst,
Chardi – vomiting and
Kasa – cough.

Bilva – Bael fruit Benefits:
पक्वं सुदुर्जरं बिल्वं दोषलं पूतिमारुतम्||१२५||
दीपनं कफवातघ्नं बालं, ग्राह्युभयं च तत्|

Bilvaphala (bael fruit) when pakva (ripe) is
Durjaram – hard to digest,
Doshalam – aggravates the doshas and
Putimarutam – produces flatus with bad odour.
Unripe (bala) bilva fruit is
Deepana – kindles digestion,
Kaphavatagna – mitigates Vata and Kapha.
Both ripe and unripe varieties are grahi (water absorbent).

Kapitha fruit:
कपित्थमामं कण्ठघ्नं दोषलं, दोषघाति तु||१२६||
पक्वं हिध्मावमथुजित्, सर्वं ग्राहि विषापहम्|

Ama kapittha (unripe Kapittha) is
Kantagnam – bad for the throat,
Doshalam – increases the three doshas.
Ripe (pakva) fruit is
Doshaghati – mitigates the dosas.
It relieves
Hidhma – hiccup,
Vamathu – vomiting.
Both ripe and unripe varieties are
Grahi – water absorbent and
Vishapaha – antipoisonous.

Jambava – Jamun fruit benefits:
जाम्बवं गुरु विष्टम्भि शीतलं भृशवातलम्||१२७||
सङ्ग्राहि मूत्रशकृतोरकण्ठ्यं कफपित्तजित्|
Jambava (Jamun fruit) is
Guru – not easily digestible,
Vishtambhi – stays long inside the stomach,
Sheetalam – cold in potency,
Brishavatalam – greatly aggravates Vata,
Sangrahi mutra shakrito – absorbs moisture from urine and faeces,
Akantyam – bad for throat and
Kaphapittanut – mitigates kapha and pitta.

Bala Amra – Tender unripe mango:

वातपित्तासृक्कृद्बालं, बद्धास्थि कफपित्तकृत्॥१२८॥

गुर्वाम्रं वातजित्पक्वं स्वाद्वम्लं कफशुक्रकृत्।

Bala amra (tender unripe mango) is

Vatakrit – increases Vata,

Pittasrakrit – causes bleeding disorders.

When its seed is fully formed and mature (badhaasthi), it is KaphaPittakrit (increases Kapha and Pitta).

When it is ripe (pakva) it is

Guru – not easily digestible,

Vatajit – mitigates vata,

Svaduamlam – sweet and sour in taste,

Kaphashukrakrit – increases Kapha and semen.

Fruits of Vrukshamla, Shamya and Pilu:

वृक्षाम्लं ग्राहि रूक्षोष्णं वातश्लेष्महरं लघु॥१२९॥

शम्या गुरूष्णं केशघ्नं रूक्षम् पीलु तु पित्तलम्।

कफवातहरं भेदि प्लीहार्शःकृमिगुल्मनुत्॥१३०॥

सतिक्तं स्वादु यत्पीलु वात्युष्णं तत्त्रिदोषजित्।

Vrksamla (Garcinia fruits) is

Grahi – absorbent,

Ruksha – dry,

Ushna – hot in potency,

Vata sleshmahara – mitigates Vata and Kapha and

Laghu – easily digestible.

Samya (fruit of Sami) is

Guru – not easily digestible,

Ushna – hot in potency,

Keshagnam – destroys the hairs and

Ruksham – causes dryness.

Pilu

Pittalam – increases Pitta,

Kaphavataharam – mitigates Kapha and Vata,

Bhedi – is purgative.

It cures

Pleeha – diseases of the spleen,

Arsha – haemorrhoids,

Krimi – worms,

Gulma – abdominal tumours.

That variety of pilu which has tiktasvadu (bitter– sweet) taste is not very hot in potency (natyushnam) and mitigates all three dosas (tridoshajit).

Shushka Vrikshamla – Dried Kokum butter fruit:

तृष्णाघ्नं उष्णमम्लायाः फलं पित्तकरं सरम्॥१२९१+१॥

The dried fruit of vrikshamla is

Trishnagnam – alleviates excessive thirst,

Ushnam – hot in potency,

Amla – sour in taste,

Pittakaram – increases Pitta and

Sara – helps in easy bowel movements.

Matulunga fruit (Citron fruit)

त्वक्तिक्तकटुका स्निग्धा मातुलुङ्गस्य वातजित्॥१३१॥

बृंहणं मधुरं मांसं वातपित्तहरं गुरु।

लघु तत्केसरं कासश्वासहिध्मामदात्ययान्॥१३२॥

आस्यशोषानिलश्लेष्मविबन्धच्छर्द्यरोचकान्

गुल्मोदरार्शःशूलानि मन्दाग्नित्वं च नाशयेत्॥१३३॥

The skin (tvak) of matulunga (citron) fruit is

Tiktakatuka – bitter and pungent in taste,

Snigdha – unctuous and

Vatajit – mitigates Vata.

Its fleshy (mamsa) part is

Brihmana – makes the body stout,

Madhura – is sweet in taste,

Vata pittahara – mitigates Vata and Pitta and

Guru – is not easily digestible.

Its kesara (tendril) is

Laghu – easily digestible.

It cures

Kasa – cough,

Swasa – asthma,

Hidhma – hiccup,

Madatyaya – alchoholic intoxication,

Asyashosha – dryness of the mouth,
Anilasleshma – disorders of Vata and Kapha,
Vibandha – constipation,
Chardi – vomiting,
Arochaka – loss of taste,
Gulma – abdominal tumours,
Udara – ascites,
Arsha – haemorrhoids,
Shoola – colic and
Mandagni – weakened digestive capacity.

Naranga (orange)

मधुरं किञ्चिदम्लं च हृद्यं भक्तप्ररोचकम्।
गुरुवातप्रशमनं विद्यान्नारङ्गजं फलम्॥१३३+१॥

Orange (Naranga) fruit is
Madhura – sweet,
Kinchitamlam – slightly sour,
Hridyam – good for the heart,
Bhaktaprarochakam–improves taste of dishes, when used as an ingredient.
Improves tasting capacity of tongue.
Guru – not easily digestible and
Vata prashamanam – alleviates Vata.

Bhallataka – Marking nut:

भल्लातकस्य त्वङ्मांसं बृंहणं स्वादु शीतलम्।
तदस्थ्यग्निसमं मेध्यं कफवातहरं परम्॥१३४॥

The outer rind (tvak) and fleshy part (mamsa) of bhallataka fruit is
Brihmana – makes the body stout,
Svadu – sweet in taste,
Sheetala – cold in potency.
Its seed (asthi) is just like fire (agni) in properties,
Medhya – increases intelligence and
Kaphavataharam param – excellently mitigates kapha and vata.

Fruits of Palevata and Aruka (peach):

स्वाद्वम्लं शीतमुष्णं च द्विधा पालेवतं गुरु।
रुच्यमत्यग्निशमनम् रुच्यं मधुरमारुकम्॥१३५॥

पक्वमाशु जरां याति नात्युष्णगुरुदोषलम्|
Palevata fruit is of two varieties –
One is Svadu (sweet in taste) and Sheeta (cold in potency), and the other is
Amla (sour in taste) and Ushna (hot in potency).
Both the varieties are
Guru – hard to digest,
Ruchyam – improve taste and
Atyagnishamanam – cure diseases due to excess digestive activity.
Aruka fruit that is pakva (ripe) is
Ruchya – improves taste,
Madhura – sweet,
Ashujaram – undergoes digestion quickly,
Natyushnam – not very hot in potency,
Guru – hard to digest and
Doshalam – increases the dosas.

Fruits of Draksha, Parushaka and Karamardaka:

द्राक्षापरूषकं चार्द्रमम्लं पित्तकफप्रदम्||१३६||
गुरूष्णवीर्यं वातघ्नं सरं सकरमर्दकम्|
तथाऽम्लं कोलकर्कन्धुलकुचाम्रातकारुकम्||१३७||
ऐरावतं दन्तशठं सतूदं मृगलिण्डिकम्|

Undried (ardra) Draksa (grapes), Parusaka and Karamardaka are
Amla – sour,
Pitta kaphapradam – increase pitta and kapha,
Guru – hard to digest,
Ushnavirya – hot in potency,
Vatagna – mitigate vata and
Sara – laxative.
Kola, karkandhu, lakuca, amrataka, aruka, airavata, dantasatha, satuda and
mrigalindika are also amla (sour in taste) and have properties similar to the
above described fruits.

Shushka Phala Varga – Group of Dry Fruits:

नातिपित्तकरं पक्वं शुष्कं च करमर्दकम्||१३८||
दीपनं भेदनं शुष्कमम्लीकाकोलयोः फलम्|
तृष्णाश्रमक्लमच्छेदि लघ्विष्टं कफवातयोः||१३९||

Karamardaka(Bengal currant) fruit ripened (pakva) and dried (shushka) does not intensely vitiate Pitta.

Fruits of Amlika (tamarind) and Kola (jujube) are

Deepana – improves digestion,

Bhedana – cause purgation.

It cures

Trishna – thirst,

Shrama – exhaustion,

Klama – fatigue,

Laghu – are easily digestible and

Kaphavatayo – mitigates kapha and vata.

Ripened and dried fruit of Kola (jujube)

स्वाद्वम्लं लघुकोलं तु शुष्कं जीर्णं च दीपनम्॥१३९१+१॥

The ripened and dried fruit of Kola (jujube) is

Swadu amla – sweet and sour,

Laghu – easily digestible and

Deepana – improves appetite.

फलानामवरं तत्र लकुचं सर्वदोषकृत्।

Lakuca phala (Money jack fruit) is qualitatively inferior among all the fruits and increases tridosas.

Dried Naranga (Orange):

वातघ्नं दुर्जरं प्रोक्तं नारङ्गं कफकृद्गुरु।

तृष्णाशूलकफोत्क्लेदच्छर्दि श्वासनिवारणम्॥१४०१+१॥

The dried fruit of Naranga is

Vatagna – alleviates Vata,

Durjaram–difficult to digest,

Kaphakrit – increases Kapha,

Guru – not easily digestible.

It cures

Trishna – excessive thirst,

Shoola – colic,

Kaphotkleda–vitiates Kapha,

Chardi – vomiting,

Swasa – dyspnoea, asthma.

Narikela – Coconut:

नारिकेलं गुरुस्निग्धं पित्तघ्नं स्वादुशीतलम्।
बलमांसकरं हृद्यं बृंहणं वस्तिशोधनम्॥१४०१+२॥

Narikela is

Guru – not easily digestible,

Snigdha – unctuous,

Pittagnam – alleviates Pitta,

Svadu – sweet in taste,

Sheetalam – cold in potency,

Balamamsakara – improves strength and muscle bulk,

Hridyam – good for the heart,

Brihmanam – Nourishing,

Basti shodhanam – cleanses the urinary bladder.

Varjya – Qualities of food articles that are worth rejecting:

हिमानलोष्णदुर्वातव्याललालादिदूषितम्॥१४०॥
जन्तुजुष्टं जले मग्नमभूमिजमनार्तवम्।
अन्यधान्ययुतं हीनवीर्यं जीर्णतयाऽति च॥१४१॥
धान्यं त्यजेत्तथा शाकं रूक्षसिद्धमकोमलम्।
असञ्जातरसं तद्वच्छुष्कं चान्यत्र मूलकात्॥१४२॥
प्रायेण फलमप्येवं तथाऽऽमं बिल्ववर्जितम्।

Grains which have been spoiled by hima (mist), anila (heavy breeze), ushna (heat of sunlight), durvata (polluted air), and lala (saliva) of snake and other reptiles;

which are infested with jantu (insects and pests);

which have remained under water for long time (jalemagnam);

not grown in the field meant for it (abhumijam);

which are unseasonal (anarthavam);

mixed with other grains (anyadhanyayutam);

which have lost their properties (hinaviryam);

having become very old (jeernatayaati)

should be rejected.

Vegetables (shaka) prepared without addition of fat (snehadravya);

which are very hard even after cooking (akomalam);

tender vegetables which have not developed their normal taste (asanjata rasa);

which have become dry (shushkam) should not be used except mulaka (radish).

Unripe (ama) fruits are not suitable for use except bilva (bael fruit).

Aushada Varga – Group of medicinal herbs:

Lavana Varga – Group of salts:

विष्यन्दि लवणं सर्वं सूक्ष्मं सृष्टमलं मृदु||१४३||

वातघ्नं पाकि तीक्ष्णोष्णं रोचनं कफपित्तकृत्|

All types of salts are

Vishyandi – produce more secretions in the tissues,

Sukshma – enter into minute pores,

Srishta mala – help in soft/easy movement of faeces,

Vatagnam – mitigate vata,

Paki – help in digestion,

Tikshna – penetrating,

Rochanam – improves appetite and

Kaphapittakrit – aggravate kapha and pitta.

Saindhava lavana – Rock salt:

सैन्धवं तत्र सस्वादु वृष्यं हृद्यं त्रिदोषनुत्||१४४||

लघ्वनुष्णं दृशः पथ्यमविदाह्यग्निदीपनम्|

Saindhava salt (rock salt) is

Sasvadu – lightly sweet,

Vrishyam – aphrodisiac,

Hridyam – good for the heart (or mind),

Tridoshanut – mitigates all the three doshas,

Laghu – easily digestible,

Anushnam – not hot in potency,

Drisha – good for vision,

Pathya – good for health,

Avidahi – does not cause burning sensation during digestion and

Agni deepana – kindles digestion.

Sauvarchala lavana – Sochal salt / black salt

लघु सौवर्चलं हृद्यं सुगन्ध्युद्गारशोधनम्||१४५||

कटुपाकं विबन्धघ्नं दीपनीयं रुचिप्रदम्|

Sauvarcala (black salt) is

Laghu – easily digestible,

Hridyam – good for the heart (or mind),
Sugandhi – possesses good smell,
Udgarashodhanam – purifies belching,
Katupakam – pungent at the end of digestion,
Vibhandagnam – relieves constipation,
Deepaniyam – kindles digestion and
Ruchipradam – improves taste.

Vida lavana:

ऊर्ध्वाधःकफवातानुलोमनं दीपनं बिडम्||१४६||
विबन्धानाहविष्टम्भशूलगौरवनाशनम्|

Vida lavana brings about
Urdhvakaphaanulomana – evacuation of Kapha in upward direction,
Adhavatanulomana – evacuation of Vata in downward direction,
Deepana – kindles digestion.
It cures
Vibandha – constipation,
Anaha – abdominal distension,
Vishtambha – constipation,
Shoola – colic and
Gaurava – heaviness.

Samudra, Audbhidha, Krishna, Romaka and Pamsulavana:

विपाके स्वादु सामुद्रं गुरु श्लेष्मविवर्धनम्||१४७||
सतिक्तकटुकक्षारं तीक्ष्णमुत्क्लेदि चौदि्भदम्|
कृष्णे सौवर्चलगुणा लवणे गन्धवर्जिताः||१४८||
रोमकं लघु, पांसूत्थं सक्षारं श्लेष्मलं गुरु|

Samudra lavana (common salt) is
Svaduvipaka – sweet at the end of digestion,
Guru – not easily digestible and
Sleshmavivardhanam – aggravates kapha.

Audbhida lavana is

Satikta – slightly bitter,
Katukakshara – pungent and alkaline in taste,
Tikshna – penetrates deep and
Utkledi – increases the secretions.

Krishna lavana (black variety of salt) has properties similar to souvarcala but is devoid of gandha (fragrance).
Romaka is laghu – easily digestible
Pamsu lavana is
Saksharam – slightly alkaline,
Sleshmalam – aggravates kapha and
Guru – not easily digestible.

लवणानां प्रयोगे तु सैन्धवादि प्रयोजयेत्||१४९||
The usage of salts should be in the respective order of saindhava, sauvarchala, vida, samudra, audbidha, krishna, romaka and pamsulavana.

Yavakshara – Alkali prepared from barley:
गुल्महृद्ग्रहणीपाण्डुप्लीहानाहगलामयान्|
श्वासार्शःकफकासांश्च शमयेद्यवशूकजः||१५०||
Yavakshara (alkali prepared from barley) mitigates
Gulma – abdominal tumours,
Hridamaya – diseases of the heart,
Grahani – duodenal diseases,
Pandu – anaemia,
Pleeha – splenic disorders,
Anaha – distension of the abdomen,
Gala roga – diseases of the throat,
Swasa – asthma, dyspnoea,
Arsha – haemorrhoids and
Kaphakasa – cough arising from Kapha.

Kshara – Alkali:
क्षारः सर्वश्च परमं तीक्ष्णोष्णः कृमिजिल्लघुः|
पित्तासृग्दूषणः पाकी छेद्यहृद्यो विदारणः||१५१||
अपथ्यः कटुलावण्याच्छुक्रौजःकेशचक्षुषाम्|
All ksharas (alkalis) are
Teekshna – penetrating,
Ushna – very hot in potency,
Krumijit – destroy worms,
Laghu – easily digestible,
Pitta Asrukdushana – vitiate pitta and blood,

Paki – helps in digestion, causes healing of wounds,

Chedya – help break up hard masses,

Ahrudya – not good for the heart,

Vidarana – punctures the tissues.

As it possesses Katu (pungent) and lavana (salty) tastes, it is detrimental to shukra (semen), ojas (essence of the tissues), kesha (hairs) and chakshu (eyes).

Hingu – Asafoetida:

हिङ्गु वातकफानाहशूलघ्नं पित्तकोपनम्||१५२||

कटुपाकरसं रुच्यं दीपनं पाचनं लघु|

Hingu (asafoetida) is

Vatakaphagnam – mitigates Vata, Kapha,

Anahagnam – cures distension of the abdomen,

Shoolagnam – relieves colic,

Pittakopanam – aggravates pitta,

Katupakarasam – pungent in taste and at the end of digestion,

Ruchyam – enhances taste,

Deepanam –enhances appetite,

Pachanam – enhances digestion and

Laghu – is easily digestible.

Hareetaki – Terminalia chebula:

कषाया मधुरा पाके रूक्षा विलवणा लघु||१५३||

दीपनी पाचनी मेध्या वयसः स्थापनी परम्|

उष्णवीर्या सराऽऽयुष्या बुद्धीन्द्रियबलप्रदा||१५४||

कुष्ठवैवर्ण्यवैस्वर्यपुराणविषमज्वरान्|

शिरोऽक्षिपाण्डुहृद्रोगकामलाग्रहणीगदान्||१५५||

सशोषशोफातीसारमेदमोहवमिक्रिमीन्|

श्वासकासप्रसेकार्शःप्लीहानाहगरोदरम्||१५६||

विबन्धं स्रोतसां गुल्ममूरुस्तम्भमरोचकम्|

हरीतकी जयेद्व्याधींस्तांस्तांश्च कफवातजान्||१५७||

Haritaki is

Kashaya rasa – astringent taste,

Madhura vipaka – sweet at the end of digestion,

Ruksha – causes dryness,

Vilavana – devoid of lavana (possesses the remaining five tastes),

Laghu – easily digestable,
Deepani – kindles hunger,
Pachani – helps in digestion,
Medhya – improves intelligence,
Vayasahasthapani – best to retain youth,
Ushnavirya – hot in potency,
Sara – laxative,
Ayushya – bestows long life,
Buddhi indriyabalaprada – strengthens the mind and the sense organs.
It cures
Kushta – skin diseases,
Vaivarnya – discolouration,
Vaisvarya – disorders of voice,
Purana vishamajvara – chronic intermittent fevers,
Shiro roga – diseases of the head,
Akshiroga – diseases of the eyes,
Pandu – anaemia,
Hridroga – heart diseases,
Kamala – jaundice,
Grahanigada – disease of the duodenum,
Shosha – emaciation,
Shopha – oedema,
Atisara – diarrhoea,
Meha – urinary disorders, diabetes,
Moha – fainting,
Vami – vomiting,
Krimi – worms (intestinal parasites),
Swasa – dyspnoea,
Kasa – cough,
Praseka – excess salivation,
Arsha – haemorrhoids,
Pleeha – disease of the spleen,
Anaha – distension of the abdomen,
Gara – artificial poisoning,
Udara – enlargement of the abdomen,
Vibhandam srothasam – obstruction of channels,
Gulma – abdominal tumours,
Urusthamba – stiffness of the thighs,

Arochaka – lack of taste (anorexia) and
many other diseases arising from (aggravation of) kapha and vata.

Amalaka (Emblica officinalis) and Aksha (Terminalia bellirica):
तद्वदामलकं शीतमम्लं पित्तकफापहम्|
कटु पाके हिमं केश्यमक्षमीषच्च तद्गुणम्||१५८||
Amalakais similar to Haritaki in properties, but is sheeta (cold in potency)
and mitigates pitta and kapha.
Aksha (vibhitaka) is
Katupaka – pungent at the end of digestion,
Hima – cold in potency,
Keshya – good for hairs and
possesses properties similar (to haritaki and amalaka) but in slightly lesser
degrees.

Triphala benefits:
इयं रसायनवरा त्रिफलाऽक्ष्यामयापहा|
रोपणी त्वग्गदक्लेदमेदोमेहकफास्रजित्||१५९||
Thus, Triphala (haritaki, amalaki and vibhitaki), is
Rasayanavara – the best rejuvenator of the body,
Akshiamayapaha – cures diseases of the eyes,
Ropani – heals wounds.
It cures
Tvakgada – skin diseases,
Kleda – excess moisture of the tissues,
Meda – obesity,
Meha – diabetes,
Aggravation of kapha and Asra (blood).

Trijata and Chaturjata:
सकेसरं चतुर्जातं त्वक्पत्रैलं त्रिजातकम्|
पित्तप्रकोपि तीक्ष्णोष्णं रूक्षं रोचनदीपनम्||१६०||
Twak (Cinnamon), Patra (Cinnamon leaf) and Ela (Cardamom) together
are known as Trijataka and
these along with Kesara forms Chaturjata.
These are
Pittaprakopi – aggravate pitta,
Tikshna – are penetrating,

Ushna – hot in potency,

Ruksha – cause dryness,

Deepana – improve appetite and

Rochana – improves taste.

Maricha – Black Pepper:

रसे पाके च कटुकं कफघ्नं मरिचं लघु।

Black pepper is

Katu rasa paka – pungent taste and at the end of digestion,

Kaphagna – mitigates kapha and

Laghu – is easily digestible.

Pippali – Long Pepper:

श्लेष्मला स्वादुशीताऽऽर्द्रा गुर्वी स्निग्धा च पिप्पली॥१६१॥

सा शुष्का विपरीताऽतः स्निग्धा वृष्या रसे कटुः।

स्वादुपाकाऽनिलश्लेष्मश्वासकासापहा सरा॥१६२॥

न तामत्युपयुञ्जीत रसायनविधिं विना।

Pippali (long pepper), in its ardra (undried) state is

Sleshmala – aggravates kapha,

Swadu – is sweet in taste,

Sheeta – cold in potency,

Guru – not easily digestible and

Snigdha – is unctuous.

Pippali (long pepper) in its shushka (dry) form, possesses opposite qualities. It is

Snigdha – unctuous,

Vrishya – aphrodisiac,

Katu rasa – pungent in taste,

Swadupaka – sweet at the end of digestion,

Anilasleshmapaha – mitigates Vata and Kapha.

It cures

Swasa – asthma,

Kasa – cough and is

Sara – laxative.

Long pepper should not be used in excess, for long periods, without following the regimen of rejuvenation therapy (rasayanavidhi).

Nagara – Ginger:

नागरं दीपनं वृष्यं ग्राहि हृद्यं विबन्धनुत्||१६३||

रुच्यं लघु स्वादुपाकं स्निग्धोष्णं कफवातजित्|

तद्वदार्द्रकमेतच्च त्रयं त्रिकटुकं जयेत्||१६४||

स्थौल्याग्निसदनश्वासकासश्लीपदपीनसान्|

Nagara (dry ginger) is

Deepana – increases hunger,

Vrishya – is aphrodisiac,

Grahi – water absorbent,

Hridya – good for the heart (or the mind),

Vibandhanut – relieves constipation,

Ruchyam – improves taste,

Laghu – easily digestible,

Swadupaka – sweet at the end of digestion,

Snigdha – unctuous,

Ushna – hot in potency and

Kaphavatajit – mitigates kapha and vata.

Similar in properties is Ardraka (fresh, undried ginger).

Trikatu–

Maricha (pepper), Pippali (long pepper) and Nagara (ginger) together are known as Trikatu.

It relieves

Sthoulya – obesity,

Agnisada – weakened digestive strength,

Swasa – asthma,

Kasa – cough,

Slipada – filariasis and

Pinasa – chronic nasal catarrh.

Chavika and Pippalimoola:

चविकापिप्पलीमुलं मरिचाल्पान्तरं गुणैः||१६५||

Chavika (Piper chaba) and Pippalimula (long pepper root) possess properties similar to Marica (black pepper) but are slightly inferior to it.

Chitraka – Leadwort:

चित्रकोऽग्निसमः पाके शोफार्शःकृमिकुष्ठहा।

Chitraka (leadwort) is

Agni samapaka – is similar to fire in digesting things.

It cures

Shopha – oedema,

Arsha – haemorrhoids,

Krimi – worms and

Kushta – skin diseases.

Panchakola:

पञ्चकोलकमेतच्च मरिचेन विना स्मृतम्॥१६६॥

गुल्मप्लीहोदरानाहशूलघ्नं दीपनं परम्।

All the above, excluding marica, i.e. pippali, pippalimula, cavya, citraka and nagara are known as panchakolaka.

It cures

Gulma – abdominal tumours,

Pleeha – disease of the spleen,

Udara – enlargement of the abdomen,

Anaha – distensionof abdomen,

Shoola – abdominal colic and is

Deepanam param – best to improve hunger and digestion.

Mahat Panchamoola:

बिल्वकाश्मर्यतर्कारीपाटलाटिण्टुकैर्महत्॥१६७॥

जयेत्कषायतिक्तोष्णं पञ्चमूलं कफनिलौ।

Bilwa, kasmarya, tarkari, patala and tintuka are together known as Mahatpanchamula. It is

Kashaya tikta – astringent and bitter in taste,

Ushna – hot in potency and

Kaphaanilajayet – mitigate kapha and anila (vata).

Hrasva Panchamoola:

ह्रस्वं बृहत्यंशुमतीद्वयगोक्षुरकैः स्मृतम्॥१६८॥

स्वादुपाकरसं नातिशीतोष्णं सर्वदोषजित्॥

Brihatidwaya (brihati and kantakari), amsumatidwaya (saliparni and prsniparni) and gokshuraka are together known as Hrasvapanchamula (Laghupanchamoola). It is

Svadupaka rasa – sweet in taste and at the end of digestion,
Na atisheetaushnam – neither very hot nor very cold in potency and
Sarvadoshajit – mitigates all the three dosas.

Madhyama Panchamoola:

बलापुनर्नवैरण्डशूर्पपर्णीद्वयेन तु||१६९||
मध्यमं कफवातघ्नं वातिपित्तकरं सरम्|

Bala, punarnava, eranda, surpaparnidvaya (masaparni and mudgaparni) together constitute Madhyamapanchamula. It is
Kaphavatagnam – mitigates kapha and vata,
Na atipittakaram – does not greatly aggravate pitta and
Sara – is laxative.

Jivana Panchamoola:

अभीरुवीराजीवन्तीजीवकर्षभकैः स्मृतम्||१७०||
जीवनाख्यं तु चक्षुष्यं वृष्यं पित्तानिलापहम्|

Abhiru (Asparagus racemosus), Vira, Jivanti, Jivaka and Rsabhaka together form the Jivanapancamula. It is
Chakshushyam – good for the eyes,
Vrishyam – aphrodisiac and
Pitta anilapaham – mitigates pitta and anila (vata).

Trina Panchamoola:

तृणाख्यं पित्तजिद्दर्भकासेक्षुशरशालिभिः||१७१||

Trnakhya (trnapancamula) consists of Darbha, Kasha, Iksu, Sara and Sali, and it mitigates Pitta (pittajit).

शूकशिम्बीजपक्वान्नमांसशाकफलौषधैः|　　　　वर्गितैरन्नलेशोऽयमुक्तो
नित्योपयोगिकः||१७२||

Thus, were described, in brief, the substances used daily as food, in groups such as suka, simbi, pakvanna, mamsa, saka, phala and ausadha.

इति　　　　श्रीवैद्यपतिसिंहगुप्तसूनुश्रीमद्वाग्भटविरचितायमष्टाङ्गहृदयसंहितायां
सूत्रस्थानेऽन्नस्वरूपविज्ञानियो नाम षष्ठोऽध्यायः||६||

Thus ends the chapter called Annasvarupavijnaniyam, the sixth in Sutrasthana of AstangaHrudaya composed by SrimadVaghata, son of Sri VaidyapatiSimhagupta.

7

अन्नरक्षाध्यायम्
(annaraksha adhyayam)

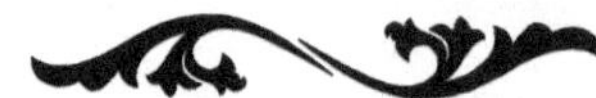

The 7th chapter of the Sutrasthana of Ashtanga Hridayam is named 'Anna Raksha Vidhi Adhyaya'. Anna means food, Raksha means protection. This chapter explains royal physician and his role in protecting the king from poisoned foods, features of poisoned foods and drinks, incompatible food combinations, effects and treatments, introduction to the three pillars of life i.e. food, sleep and celibacy and healthy sleeping rules.

अथातो अन्नरक्षाध्यायं व्याख्यास्यामः इति ह स्माहुरात्रेयादयो महर्षयः ।
Atreya and other sages pledge that they will henceforth be explaining the chapter named annarakshavidhi adhyaya (protection of foods).

Pranacharya (royal physician) and his residence:
राजा राजगृहासन्ने प्राणाचार्यं निवेशयेत् ।
सर्वदा स भवत्येवं सर्वत्र प्रतिजागृविः ॥ १ ॥
The king should arrange for the residence of the royal physician near the palace (Rajagriha asana) so that the physician can be vigilant about all things at all times.

अन्नपानं विषाद्रक्षेद्विशेषेण महीपतेः ।
योगक्षेमौ तदायत्तौ धर्माद्या यन्निबन्धनाः ॥ २ ॥

The foods (anna) and drinks (pana) of the king should be protected from poison (visha), because the King's health and welfare depends on his food and drink and the health and welfare of the country is dependent on the King.

Vishayukta odana - Features of poisoned foods and drinks:

ओदनो विषवान्सान्द्रो यात्यविस्राव्यतामिव ।
चिरेण पच्यते पक्वो भवेत्पर्युषितोपमः ॥ ३ ॥
मयूरकण्ठतुल्योष्मा मोहमूर्छाप्रसेककृत् ।
हीयते गन्धवर्णाद्यैः क्लिद्यते चन्द्रिकाचितः ॥ ४ ॥

Boiled or cooked rice (odana) mixed with poison becomes

Sandra – thick and

Avisravyatam – a form wherein the contents do not overflow out of the vessel,

Chirena pachyate – takes a lot of time to get cooked,

After being cooked it becomes

Paryushitopama – similar to stale food,

Mayura kanta tulya ushma - boiled rice if poisoned will emit blue coloured steam resembling the colour of a peacock's neck.

It causes

Moha – delusion,

Murcha – fainting,

Praseka – excessive salivation.

Hiyate varna gandhadhyaih – quickly loses its colour, odour etc

Klidyate – becomes watery, sticky and

Chandrikachita - full of shining particles (appears and shines just like scattered drops of oil over a layer of water).

Vishayukta Vyanjanani - Features of poisoned side dishes:

व्यञ्जनान्याशु शुष्यन्ति ध्यामक्वाथानि तत्र च ।
हीनातिरिक्ता विकृता छाया दृश्येत नैव वा ॥ ५ ॥

The side-dishes that are poisoned

Ashu shushyati - get dried up quickly,

Dhyamakwathani – become dirty,

Hina atirikta vikrita chaya drishyeta naiva va - deficient (reduced), excess (enlarged) or malformed (abnormal) reflective images of one's own self are seen or not seen at all.

फेनोर्ध्वराजिसीमन्ततन्तुबुद्बुदसम्भवः ।
विच्छिन्नविरसाः रागाः खाण्डवाः शाकमामिषम् ॥ ६ ॥

Phena (froth) and urdhva raji (lines) appear on the surface (of the side dishes dirtied by contact of poison).

Simanta (cracks - dish breaks into fragments), tantu (slimy thread like structures) and budbuda (bubbles) are likely to appear.

Vichinna (separation of liquid and solid portions) and

Virasa (appearance of bad taste) is seen in dishes like

Raga - sweetened syrups,

Khandava - sweet puddings,

Shakam – vegetables and

Amisham – meat.

Appearance of lines of different colors on different poisoned side dishes and materials:

नीला राजी रसे ताम्रा क्षीरे दधनि दृश्यते ।
श्यावापीतासिता तक्रे घृते पानीयसन्निभा ॥ ७ ॥

When poisoned,

Nila raji rase – blue lines appear on meat soup,

Tamra ksheere – coppery red lines appear on milk,

Dadhani drishyate shyava – black lines appear on curds,

Peeta sita takre – yellowish white lines appear on buttermilk,

Grite paneeya sannibha – lines appearing like water are seen on ghee.

मस्तुनि स्यात्कपोताभा राजी कृष्णा तुषोदके ।
काली मद्याम्भसोः क्षौद्रे हरितैलेऽरुणोपमा ॥ ८ ॥

Mastuni syat kapothabha – lines resembling colour of pigeon appear on supernatant liquid layer of the curds (whey),

Raji krishna tushodake – bluish black lines appear on sour drink prepared from the husk of barley,

Kali madyambhaso - black lines appear on wines and water,

Kshaudre harit – green coloured lines appear on honey,

Taile arunopama – crimson lines appear on oil.

Effect of poison on other edibles and materials:

पाकः फलानामामानां पक्वानां परिकोथनम् ।

द्रव्याणामार्द्रशुष्काणां स्यातां म्लानिविवर्णते ॥ ९ ॥

Pakam phalanam amanam - unripe fruits ripen fast,

Pakvanam parikothanam – the ripe fruits become overripe and get decomposed,

The substances which are ardra (wet) and shushka (dry) become mlani (dull) and vivarna (discoloured) respectively.

मृदूनां कठिनानां च भवेत् स्पर्शविपर्ययः ।
माल्यस्य स्फुटिताग्रत्वं म्लानिर्गन्धान्तरोद्भवः ॥ १० ॥

Mridu (soft) and katina (hard) substances obtain opposite feel (sparsha viparyaya) i.e. soft substances become hard and hard substances become soft.

The flowers of the garland (mala) get split at the end (sphutitha agra), appear dull and faded (mlani) and obtain an unnatural smell (gandhantarodbhava).

ध्याममण्डलता वस्त्रे, शदनं तन्तुपक्ष्मणाम् ।
धातुमौक्तिककाष्ठाश्मरत्नादिषु मलाक्तता ॥ ११ ॥
स्नेहस्पर्शप्रभाहानिः सप्रभत्वं तु मृन्मये ।

When in contact with poison,

Dhyama mandalata vastre – dirty patches appear on clothes,

Shadanam tantu pakshmanam – the threads and hems of clothes fallout,

Vessels prepared from dhatu (metals), mouktika (pearls), kashta (wood), ashma (stone), ratnadi (precious stones etc) become dirty and

Sneha sparsha prabha hani - lose their unctuousness and lustre.

Saprabhatvam tu mrinmaye – mud vessels gain good look and lustre in spite of being lustreless.

Vishada lakshana - Features of the person who poisons things:
विषदः श्यावशुष्कास्यो विलक्षो वीक्ष्यते दिशः ॥ १२ ॥
स्वेदवेपथुमांस्त्रस्तो भीतः स्खलति जृम्भते ।

The person who is about to poison someone will have

Shyava shushka asya – discoloured and dry face,

Vilaksho veekshate dishaha – eccentrically looks in all directions,

Sveda vepathuman – sweating and tremors,

Trasta – tired,

Bheeta – frightened,

Skhalati – slips while talking and walking and
Jrumbhate – yawns frequently.

Vishayukta ahara pariksha - Testing of poisoned foods:
प्राप्यान्नं सविषं त्वग्निरेकावर्तः स्फुटत्यति ॥ १३ ॥
शिखिकण्ठाभधूमार्चिरनर्चिर्वोग्रगन्धवान् ।
On contact with food mixed with poison (savisha) the fire (agni)
Ekavrita - emits flame as a single pile, either towards the right or towards
the left,
Sphutati ati – emits crackling sounds,
Shikhi kantabha dhoomarchi – the colour of the smoke and flame resembles
the colour of peacock's neck (glistening blue colour) and
Anarchi va – sometimes the fire may not give up flames at all and it will
Ugra gandhavan – eliminate a strong and foul smell.

म्रियन्ते मक्षिकाः प्राश्य काकः क्षामस्वरो भवेत् ॥ १४ ॥
उत्क्रोशन्ति च दृष्ट्वैतत् शुकदात्यूहशारिकाः ।
After consuming poisoned food,
Mriyate makshika - the bees die,
Kakaha kshamasvaro bhavet – the crow's voice becomes feeble and
depleted,
The birds which will cry out loudly (utkroshanti) on seeing the poisoned
food are
Shuka - parrots,
Datyuha - gallinule bird and
Sarika – mynah.

हंसः प्रस्खलति ग्लानिर्जीवञ्जीवस्य जायते ॥ १५ ॥
चकोरस्याक्षिवैरग्यं क्रौञ्चस्य स्यान्मदोदयः
On poisoning,
Hamsa praskalati – the swan fumbles while walking,
Glani jivam jivasya jayate – the jivajivaka bird either gets exhausted or dies,
Chakorasya akshi vairagyam - chakora bird's (a type of partridge) eyes turn
red,
Kraunchasya syat madodayaha - the pond heron gets intoxicated.

कपोतपरभृद्दक्षचक्रवाका जहत्यसून् ॥ १६ ॥

उद्वेगं याति मार्जारः शकृन्मुञ्चति वानरः ।

The pigeon (kapota), cuckoo (parabriddaksha) and chakravaka bird quickly lose their life (jahati asoon) on seeing or eating poisoned food,
The cat (marjara) gets excited / confused (udvegam) and
The monkey (vanara) defecates (shakrit munchati).

हृष्येन्मयूरस्तद्दृष्ट्या मन्दतेजो भवेद्विषम् ॥ १७ ॥

On seeing poisoned food, the peacock (mayura) becomes excited and overjoyed. As a result, the poison becomes mild, losing its intensity.

Method of rejecting the poisoned food:

इत्यन्नं विषवज्ज्ञात्वा त्यजेदेव प्रयत्नतः ।
यथा तेन विपद्येरन्नपि न क्षुद्रजन्तवः ॥ १८ ॥

Iti annam vishavat jnatva – After knowing and confirming the poisoned food and after having considered that food equivalent to poison,
Tyajet evam prayatnataha - one should reject the food judiciously
Yatha tena vipadyerannapi na kshudra jantavaha - while taking care that the rejected and discarded poisoned food should neither be available to nor harm even the smallest (kshudra) of living organisms (jantu).

Visha Annaja Vikara - Diseases caused by poisoned food:

स्पृष्टे तु कण्डूदाहोषाज्वरार्तिस्फोटसुप्तयः ।
नखरोमच्युतिः शोफः सेकाद्या विषनाशनाः ॥ १९ ॥
शस्तास्तत्र प्रलेपाश्च सेव्यचन्दनपद्मकैः ।
ससोमवल्कतालीशपत्रकुष्ठामृतानतैः ॥ २० ॥

The touch of poisoned foods produces
Kandu - itching,
Dahosha - burning sensation all over the body and at the site of touch,
Jwara - fever,
Arti - pain,
Sphota - eruptions,
Supta - loss of tactile sensation,
Nakha roma chyuti - falling of nails and hairs and
Shopha - swelling.
The treatment shall be Seka (washing or pouring over the entire body or site of contact of poisoned food) using water processed with anti-poisonous drugs,

Pralepa (application of paste) of
Sevya (Ushira),
Candana (sandalwood),
Padmaka – Wild Himalayan Cherry – Prunus puddum / cerasoides,
Somavalka,
Talisa Patra – Cinnamomum tamala,
Kushta - Saussurea lappa,
Amrita - Tinospora cordifolia and
Nata – Valeriana wallichi.

Local effect of poison in oral cavity:
लाला जिह्वौष्ठयोर्जाड्यमूषा चिमिचिमायनम् ।
दन्तहर्षो रसाज्ञत्वं हनुस्तम्भश्च वक्त्रगे ॥ २१ ॥
सेव्याद्यैस्तत्र गण्डूषाः सर्वं च विषजिद्धितम् ।
Poisoned food inside the mouth causes
Lala - excess of salivation,
Jihwa oshtayo jadyam - inactivity of the tongue and lips,
Usha - burning sensation,
Chimichimayanam – tingling sensation in the mouth,
Dantaharsha - tingling sensation of the teeth,
Rasajnatvam - inability to perceive taste and
Hanusthambha - stiffness of the lower jaw.
The treatment shall be gandusha (retention of medication in oral cavity) with water processed with Sevya – Vetiveria zizanioides and other drugs mentioned earlier and all other therapies for the mouth which are anti-poisonous

Amashaya-Pakvashayagata Visha - Effect of poisonous food in the stomach and intestines, symptoms:
आमाशयगते स्वेदमूर्छाध्मानमदभ्रमाः ॥ २२ ॥
रोमहर्षो वमिर्दाहश्चक्षुर्हृदयरोधनम् ।
बिन्दुभिश्चाचयोऽङ्गानां पक्वाशयगते पुनः ॥ २३ ॥
अनेकवर्णं वमति मूत्रयत्यतिसार्यते ।
तन्द्रा कृशत्वं पाण्डुत्वमुदरं बलसङ्क्षयः ॥ २४ ॥

Amashayagata Visha – Effects of poison in the stomach:
Sweda - sweating,

Murcha - fainting,
Adhmana - flatulence,
Mada - toxicity,
Bhrama - giddiness,
Romaharsha - horripilation,
Vami - vomiting,
Daha - burning sensation,
Chakshu hrudaya rodhanam - loss of movement of the eyes and heart and
Bindubhi achaya anganam - appearance of black dots all over the body.

Pakvashayagata Visha – Effects of poison in the intestine:
Aneka varnam vamati - vomiting of many colours,
Mutrayati - excess of urination,
Atisara - diarrhoea,
Tandra - drowsiness,
Krishatvam - emaciation,
Pandutvam - pallor,
Udara - enlargement of the abdomen and
Balasamkshaya - loss of strength.

Treatment of conditions caused by poisonous food in the stomach and intestines:
तयोर्वान्तविरिक्तस्य हरिद्रे कटभीं गुडम् ।
सिन्धुवारकनिष्पावबाष्पिकाशतपर्विकाः ॥ २५ ॥
तण्डुलीयकमूलानि कुक्कुटाण्डमवल्गुजम् ।
नावनाञ्जनपानेषु योजयेद्विषशान्तये ॥ २६ ॥
In both these conditions (poisoned food in stomach and intestine) after
administering emesis (vamana) and purgation (virechana) therapies,
Turmeric (haridra), Katabi (Berberis aristata, Celastrus paniculata) and
jaggery (guda),
Sinduvarita (Vitex negundo), nishpava (cowpea / flat bean), bashpika
(Gardenia gummifera), shataparvika (Acorus calamus),
Roots of tanduliyaka (Amaranthus viridis), kukkuta andam (egg of hen),
avalguja (Psoralea corylifolia) – all these drugs should be used in the form
of
Navana – nasal medication,
Anjana – collyrium,

Pana – as drinks (decoction prepared from these herbs).
These methods help relieve the effect of poison.

Hrid Vishodhana, Gara Visha Chikitsa - Treatment to detoxify the heart and to treat chronic poisoning:

विषभुक्ताय दद्याच्च शुद्धयोर्ध्वमधस्तथा ।
सूक्ष्मं ताम्ररजः काले सक्षौद्रं हृद्विशोधनम् ॥ २७ ॥
शुद्धे हृदि ततः शाणं हेमचूर्णस्य दापयेत् ।
न सज्जते हेमपाङ्गे पद्मपत्रेऽम्बुवद्विषम् ॥ २८ ॥
जायते विपुलं चायुर्गरेऽप्येष विधिः स्मृतः ।

A person who has been poisoned should be administered the following
Shudhya urdhvam adha – emesis and purgation to remove the remnant
poison in the gut, after proper cleansing,
Ash of copper (tamra raja) should be administered mixed in honey
(kshaudra) to cleanse and detoxify the heart (hrit).
Following proper cleansing of the heart (by administration of copper ash),
the ash of gold (hema churna) is administered for a long period in the dose
of 3 grams (one shaana).
In Hemapanga (a person who has been administered gold for a long period),
the poison will not do any harm.
In fact the poison (visha) will not remain in the body just like a water
(ambu) drop doesn't stay on a lotus leaf (padma patra) for a long time.
Such a person gains longevity of life (vipulam ca ayu).
Gara visha or chronic poisoning also may be treated on the same lines.

Viruddha Ahara - Incompatible foods:

विरुद्धमपि चाहारं विद्यादिविषगरोपममम् ॥ २९ ॥

On many occasions, consuming two food items together or a particular type
of food processing may render the food toxic. It is known as incompatible
food (virudha ahara). Even incompatible foods should be considered similar
to poison / artificial poisoning.

Examples of Viruddha Ahara or incompatible foods:

आनूपमामिषं माषक्षीरक्षौद्रविरूढकैः ।
विरुध्यते सह बिसैर्मूलकेन गुडेन वा ॥ ३० ॥
विशेषात् पयसा मत्स्या मत्स्येष्वपि चिलीचिमः ।

Anupam amisham (meat of animals living in marshy regions) is incompatible when consumed with masha (black gram), kshaudra (honey), ksheera (milk) and virudaka (germinated grains).

Bisa (lotus stem), mulaka (radish) or guda (jaggery) is incompatible with matsya (fish).

Taking matsya (fish) with paya (milk) is incompatible.

Even among the fishes, the Chilichima variety of fish is incompatible with milk.

विरुद्धमम्लं पयसा सह सर्वं फलं तथा ॥ ३१ ॥

तद्वत् कुलत्थवरककङ्गुवल्लककुष्टकाः ।

भक्षयित्वा हरितकं मूलकादि पयस्त्यजेत् ॥ ३२ ॥

All amla (sour) substances are virudha (incompatible) with paya (milk).

All sour fruits are also incompatible with milk.

Kulatha (horse gram), varaka (shama millet), kangu (Callicarpa macrophylla), valla (flat Indian bean), makushtaka (peanut type) also are incompatible with milk.

After consuming haritaka (green leafy vegetables) and moolaka (radish), paya (milk) should be avoided.

वाराहं श्वाविधा नाद्याद्दध्ना पृषतकुक्कुटौ ।

आममांसानि पित्तेन माषसूपेन मूलकम् ॥ ३३ ॥

अविं कुसुम्भशाकेन बिसैः सह विरूढकम् ।

माषसूपगुडक्षीरमध्वाज्यैर्लकुचं फलम् ॥ ३४ ॥

फलं कदल्यस्तक्रेण दध्ना तालफलेन वा ।

कणोषणाभ्यां मधुना काकमाची गुडेन वा ॥ ३५ ॥

सिद्धां वा मत्स्यपचने पचने नागरस्य वा ।

सिद्धामन्यत्र वा पात्रे कामातामुषितां निशाम् ॥ ३६ ॥

The below mentioned types of combination of foods and methods of processing are said to be incompatible –

Varaha (pork) along with shvavidha (porcupine) meat;

Kukkuta (chicken) and prishata (spotted deer) along with dadhi (curds);

Ama mamsa (uncooked meat) along with pitta (bile);

Mulaka (radish) along with masha supa (black gram);

Avi (sheep) meat along with kusumbha shaaka (leaves of kusumbha herb);

Virudaka (germinated grains) along with Bisa (lotus stem);

Lakucha Phala (money jack fruit) along with masha supa (black gram soup), guda (jaggery), ksheera (milk), madhu (honey) or ajya (ghee);

Kadali phala (banana) along with takra (buttermilk);

Dadhi (curds) along with Tala phala (Palm date);

Pippali (long pepper), Maricha (black pepper) and honey;

Kakamachi - black nightshade fruit (Solanum nigrum) with guda (jaggery);

Kakamachi fruit processed in the same vessel, in which matsya (fish) was processed;

Kakamachi fruit processed in the same vessel in which nagara (ginger) was processed;

Kakamachi fruit processed in any other vessel but kept overnight should not be used since it is incompatible.

Wrong processing methods:

मत्स्यनिस्तालितस्नेह साधिताः पिप्पलीस्त्यजेत् ।

कांस्ये दशाहमुषितं सर्पिरुष्णं त्वरुष्करे ॥ ३७ ॥

भासे विरुध्यते शूल्यः कम्पिल्लस्तक्रसाधितः ।

ऐकध्यं पायससुराकृशराः परिवर्जयेत् ॥ ३८ ॥

The following food combinations and processing methods are also incompatible –

Pippali (long pepper) processed in the oil used for frying matsya (fish);

Sarpi (ghee) kept in a kamsya (bronze) vessel for more than 10 days;

Consumption of hot substances or hot procedures like sun bath, exposure to heat etc is not recommended while consuming Bhallataka (Semecarpus anacardium, Marking Nut);

Meat of bhasa bird (white headed vulture) should not be roasted;

Kampilla (Mallotus philippensis) prepared in takra (buttermilk);

Taking payasa (traditional Indian sweet pudding prepared in milk base), sura (fermented herbal drink, resembling beer) and krishara (dish prepared using rice and green gram) together is incompatible.

Wrong mixtures:

मधुसर्पिर्वसातैलपानीयानि द्विशात्रिशः ।

एकत्र वा समांशानि विरुध्यन्ते परस्परम् ॥ ३९ ॥

भिन्नांशे अपि मध्वाज्ये दिव्यवार्यनुपानतः ।

मधुपुष्करबीजं च मधुमैरेयशार्करम् ॥ ४० ॥

मन्थानुपानः क्षौरेयो हारिद्रः कटुतैलवान् ।

When madhu (honey), sarpi (ghee), vasa (meat fat), taila (sesame oil) and paniya (beverages) are mixed in quantities of twos, threes or all together, in sama amsha (equal quantities) will become virudha (mutually incompatible).

Madhu (honey) along with ajya (ghee), even in bhinna amsha (unequal proportions), should not be consumed along with divya vari (rain water).

Honey along with seeds of Pushkara,

Honey, along with Maireya (wine of dates) and sugar (sharkara),

Milk drinks along with Mantha (solution of corn flour),

Yellow coloured mushroom (haaridra) with mustard oil is incompatible.

उपोदकातिसाराय तिलकल्केन साधिता ॥ ४१ ॥

Upodaka (Indian spinach) processed along with tila kalka (paste of sesame seeds), when consumed, causes atisara (diarrhoea) and hence is incompatible.

वलाका वारुणीयुक्ता कुल्माषैश्च विरुध्यते ।
भृष्टा वराहवसया सैव सद्यो निहन्त्यसून् ॥ ४२ ॥

Meat of valaka bird consumed with date wine (Varuni), green gram and other pulses cooked together (Kulmasha) is incompatible.

Meat of valaka bird fried in pork fat (varaha vasa) instantly takes away the life when consumed, hence is incompatible.

तद्वत् तित्तिरिपत्राढ्यगोधालावकपिञ्जलाः ।
एरण्डेनाग्निना सिद्धास्तत्तैलेन विमूर्छिताः ॥ ४३ ॥

Meat of tittiri (partridge), patradhya (peacock), godha (iguana lizard), lava (common quail) and kapinjala (francolin partridge) cooked by burning the wood of eranda (castor plant) or processed (fried) in eranda taila (castor oil) is lethal.

हारीतमांसं हारिद्रशूलकप्रोतपाचितम् ।
हरिद्रवह्निना सद्यो व्यापादयति जीवितम् ॥ ४४ ॥
भस्मपांसुपरिध्वस्तं तदेव च समाक्षिकम् ।।

The meat of harita bird pierced with wood of haridra (turmeric) and cooked over haridra vahni (the flame of turmeric) is lethal.

The meat of the same bird cooked by smearing it with bhasma (ash) and pamsu (sand) when consumed mixed with makshika (honey) becomes lethal.

Definition of Viruddha (incompatible):

यत्किञ्चिद्दोषमुत्क्लेश्य न हरेत्तत् समासतः ॥ ४५ ॥

Yat kinchit - anything (food or activity)

Dosham utkleshya - that causes increase of doshas but

Na haret - does not expel them (doshas) out of the body

Tat samasataha - is concisely called

Viruddham - Viruddha or incompatible

Treatment of Viruddha Ahara Janya Vikara (conditions caused due to consumption of incompatible food):

विरुद्धं शुद्धिहरत्रेष्टा शमो वा तद्विरोधिभिः ।

द्रव्यैस्तैरेव वा पूर्वं शरीरस्याभिसंस्कृतिः ॥ ४६ ॥

The treatment for conditions arising due to consumption of incompatible foods include

Shodhana – purification procedure – Panchakarma,

Shamana – palliative treatment,

Virodha chikitsa – symptom based treatment.

Health should be restored quickly by using foods that have opposite qualities to that of incompatible foods.

People in whom incompatible foods will not cause ill-effects:

व्यायामस्निग्धदीप्ताग्निवयःस्थबलशालिनाम् ।

विरोध्यपि न पीडायै सात्म्यमम्लं च भोजनम् ॥ ४७ ॥

Ill effects of incompatible foods will not be seen in the following

Vyayama - who exercise regularly,

Snigdha - who are habituated to oily fatty food,

Deeptagni - who have good digestion power,

Vayastha - in the young and

Bala – those who are strong.

In those, who are habituated (satmya) to incompatible food and in those who have been taking small quantities of incompatible food for a long period of time, the ill effects will not be seen.

Satmikarana Krama (Method of accustomization)

पादेनापथ्यमभ्यस्तं पादपादेन वा त्यजेत् ।

निषेवेत हितं तद्वदेकदिव्रत्यन्तरीकृतम् ॥ ४८ ॥

Padena apathyam abhyastham - unhealthy and unwholesome things (foods, drinks, activities) which have become accustomed due to constant practice and long use, should be discontinued in quarterly proportions,

Pada padena va tyajet – they should be rejected or discontinued gradually, quarter by quarter (one fourth portion at a time should be discontinued) and not at once.

Nisheveta hita tadvat – similarly, healthy and wholesome things should be gradually practiced, quarter by quarter with

Ekadvitrayantarikritam – intervals of 1, 2 or 3 days

Effect of breaking the method of accustomization:

अपथ्यमपि हि त्यक्तं शीलितं पथ्यमेव वा ।

सात्म्यासात्म्यविकाराय जायते सहसान्यथा ॥ ४९ ॥

When apathya (unhealthy practises) is discontinued or when one starts indulging in pathya (healthy practises), many diseases manifest due to satmya (suitability) and asatmya (non-suitability) respectively especially when one discontinues apathya and starts following pathya suddenly, not following the rules and regulations (wherein it is advised to withdraw unhealthy things and practice healthy things gradually, quarter by quarter).

Effect of krama satmikarana (gradual accustomization):

क्रमेणापचिता दोषाः क्रमेणोपचिता गुणाः ।

नाप्नुवन्ति पुनर्भावमप्रकम्प्या भवन्ति च ॥ ५० ॥

The morbidity and ill effects of incompatible foods accumulated in the body over a period of time, when eliminated gradually and the accumulation of good qualities due to gradual indulgence of compatible foods and practices will help in gradual destruction of bad qualities and prevents the recurrence of ill effects and in gradual increase of good qualities, leading to robust health.

अत्यन्तसन्निधानानां दोषाणां दूषणात्मनाम् ।

अहितैर्दूषणं भूयो न विद्वान्कर्तुमर्हति ॥ ५१ ॥

The doshas which are in the proximity of the dushyas (body and tissues) which already have a tendency to contaminate the body elements should not be further contaminated by the intake of unhealthy things by a wise person who knows everything.

Trayopastambha - Three pillars of life:

आहारशयनाब्रह्मचर्यैर्युक्त्या प्रयोजितैः ।
शरीरं धार्यते नित्यमागारमिव धारणैः ॥ ५२ ॥
आहारो वर्णितस्तत्र तत्र तत्र च वक्ष्यते ।

Traya means three, upastambha means pillars. Trayopastambha includes ahara, shayana and abrahmacharya, which are considered as the three pillars which support the body.

Ahara - food,

Shayana - sleep and

Abrahmacharya - non-celibacy

When skilfully applied or practised will support the body constantly, just like a house is supported by its pillars.

The concept of ahara has been contextually explained at various places in the treatise, and also in the relevant contexts of the chapters to come.

Nidra – Sleep:

निद्रायत्तं सुखं दुःखं पुष्टिः कार्श्यं बलाबलम् ॥ ५३ ॥
वृषता क्लीबता ज्ञानमज्ञानं जीवितं न च ।

Dependent on sleep are the below mentioned entities

Sukham – happiness,

Dukham - unhappiness,

Pushti – nourishment,

Karshyam - emaciation,

Bala – strength,

Abala - debility,

Vrishata - sexual power,

Klibata - impotence,

Jnanam – knowledge,

Ajnanam - ignorance,

Jivitam - life and

Na jivitam - its absence (death).

अकालेऽतिप्रसङ्गाच्च न च निद्रा निषेविता ॥ ५४ ॥
सुखायुषी पराकुर्यात्कालरात्रिरिवापरा ।

Sleeping at improper time (akala), excessive sleep (atiprasangat) or lack of sleep (na ca nidra) when practiced regularly, will destroy happiness (sukha) and longevity (ayusha) just like the kala ratri or the night of destruction (kalaratri) will cause the destruction of the world.

Ratri Jagarana and Diva Swapna Guna (qualities of awakening at night and day sleep):

रात्रौ जागरणं रूक्षं स्निग्धं प्रस्वपनं दिवा ॥ ५५ ॥

अरूक्षमनभिष्यन्दि त्वासीनप्रचलायितम् ।

Ratri jagarana – Keeping awake at nights is ruksha - causes dryness inside the body,

Divasvapna – sleeping during daytime is snigdha - unctuous and

Taking a nap while sitting comfortably (during the day) is aruksha (does not cause dryness) and anabishyandi (not unctuous).

Rtu and divaswapna (day sleep during different seasons):

ग्रीष्मे वायुचयादानरौक्ष्यरात्र्यल्पभावतः ॥ ५६ ॥

दिवास्वप्नो हितोऽन्यस्मिन् कफपित्तकरो हि सः ।

In grishma (summer), there will be chaya (accumulation) of vayu (vata), the season too will be hot (Northern solstice) and ruksha (dryness will be more),

The nights (length) are also short; therefore divaswapna (day sleep) is hita (beneficial) during summer, whereas sleeping during day time in other seasons (excluding greeshma or summer) is kapha pittakara (will increase kapha and pitta).

Divaswapna yogya – Indications for day sleep:

मुक्त्वा तु भाष्ययानाध्वमद्यस्त्रीभारकर्मभिः ॥ ५७ ॥

क्रोधशोकभयैः क्लान्तान् श्वासहिध्मातिसारिणः ।

वृद्धबालाबलक्षीणक्षततृट्शूलपीडितान् ॥ ५८ ॥

अजीर्ण्यभिहतोन्मत्तान् दिवास्वप्नोचितानपि ।

धातुसाम्यं तथा ह्येषां श्लेष्मा चाङ्गानि पुष्यति ॥ ५९ ॥

Day sleeping is beneficial in the below mentioned conditions –

Those who are exhausted due to excessive

Bhashya - speaking,

Yana - travelling,

Adhva - walking,

Madya - excessive consumption of wine,

Stri - excessive sexual indulgence,

Bhara - carrying heavy loads,

Karma - heavy physical activities,

Krodha - anger,

Shoka – grief,

Bhaya - fear,

those suffering from

Swasa – asthma (breathing disorders)

Hidhma – hiccup,

Atisara - diarrhoea,

Vriddha - aged people,

Bala - children,

Abala - those debilitated,

Ksheena – the emaciated,

Kshata - those suffering from injury,

Trit - thirst,

Shoola - abdominal pain,

Ajeerni – those suffering from indigestion,

Abhihata - those assaulted,

Unmatta - those intoxicated and

Divaswapnochitan - those who are habituated to sleeping during the day.

Reason: The day sleep brings about dhatusamya (normalcy of tissues) in the above said conditions.

The sleshma (kapha) which is increased and nourished by day sleep in turn nourishes the body (anganam pushyati).

Contraindications for day sleep:

बहुमेदः कफाः स्वप्युः स्नेहनित्याश्च नाहनि ।
विषार्तः कण्ठरोगी च नैव जातु निशास्वपि ॥ ६० ॥

The following persons are contraindicated for day sleep

Bahu meda - excessive accumulation of fat in their body (obese),

Bahu kapha - those in whom kapha is aggravated and

Sneha nitya - those who are accustomed to taking oily foods daily.

Those suffering from

Visha - poisoning and

Kanta roga - throat diseases should not even sleep at night.

Akala shayana janya vikara – Effect of untimely sleep and management:

अकालशयनान्मोहज्वरस्तैमित्यपीनसाः ।
शिरोरुक्शोफहृल्लासस्रोतोरोधाग्निमन्दताः ॥ ६१ ॥

तत्रोपवासवमनस्वेदनावनमौषधम् ।

Effects of sleeping at improper time (akala shayana) include

Moha - delusion,

Jwara - fever,

Staimitya - lassitude,

Pinasa - nasal catarrh,

Shiroruk - headache,

Shopha - oedema,

Hrillasa - nausea,

Srotorodha - obstruction to the channels of the body and pores of the tissues and

Agnimandata - weakness of digestive fire.

Treatment to combat ill effects of untimely sleep includes

Upavasa - fasting,

Vamana - emesis,

Sweda - sudation and

Navana - nasal medications.

Treatment for ati nidra (excessive sleep):

योजयेदतिनिद्रायां तीक्ष्णं प्रच्छर्दनाञ्जनम् ॥ ६२ ॥

नावनं लङ्घनं चिन्तां व्यवायं शोकभीक्रुधः ।

एभिरेव च निद्राया नाशः श्लेष्मातिसङ्क्षयात् ॥ ६३ ॥

In case of ati nidra (excessive sleep), one should administer

Tikshna prachardana - strong emetics,

Anjanam - collyrium,

Navanam - nasal drops,

Langhanam - fasting,

Chinta - worry,

Vyavayam - sexual intercourse,

Shoka - grief,

Bhi - fear and

Krudha - anger.

By these measures kapha gets decreased (sleshma abisamkshayat) which in turn reduces sleep.

Effect of Nidra Nasha (loss of sleep):

निद्रानाशादङ्गमर्द गौरवजृम्भिकाः ।

जाड्यग्लानिभ्रमापक्तितन्द्रा रोगाश्च वातजाः ॥ ६४ ॥

Loss of sleep leads to

Angamarda - squeezing pain in the body parts,

Gaurava - heaviness of the head,

Alasya – drowsiness,

Jrimbhika - too much of yawning,

Jadyam - lassitude,

Glani - exhaustion (even without strain),

Bhrama - giddiness,

Apakti - indigestion,

Tandra - stupor and

Vataja roga - diseases of Vata origin.

Pathology of unconsciousness, fainting:

कफोऽल्पो वायुनोद्धूतो धमनीः सन्निरुध्य तु ।

कुर्यात् सञ्ज्ञापहां तन्द्रां दारुणां मोहकारिणीम् ॥ ६४+१ ॥

Aggravated Kapha along with Vata Dosha, obstructs (Sanniruddhya) the nervous system / blood vessels supplying to brain (Dhamani) and causes

Sanjnapaha – unconsciousness

Daruna Tandra – extreme fatigue, lassitude, sleepiness

Moha – coma.

Yathakalam nidra – Advocation of timely sleep:

यथाकालमतो निद्रां रात्रौ सेवेत सात्म्यतः ।

असात्म्यजागरादर्धं प्रातः स्वप्यादभुक्तवान् ॥ ६५ ॥

The person should sleep at proper time, especially at night time (ratrau), daily, as much as desirable and become habituated (satmya) to it.

If he has kept awake at night (jagarat) due to non-habituation (not accustomed to staying awake at night), he should sleep for half that period (half period of the time for which he was awake or half period of time which he usually sleeps at night as habituated), on the next morning, without taking food (abhuktavan).

Manda nidra chikitsa – treatment of loss of sleep:

शीलयेन्मन्दनिद्रस्तु क्षीरमद्यरसान्दधि ।

अभ्यङ्गोद्वर्तनस्नानमूर्धकर्णाक्षितर्पणम् ॥ ६६ ॥

कान्ताबाहुलताश्लेषो निर्वृतिः कृतकृत्यता ।

मनोऽनुकूला विषयाः कामं निद्रासुखप्रदाः ॥ ६७ ॥

ब्रह्मचर्यरतेर्ग्राम्यसुखनिःस्पृहचेतसः ।
निद्रा सन्तोषतृप्तस्य स्वं कालं नातिवर्तते ॥ ६८ ॥

Those suffering from very little sleep (or no sleep at all), should indulge in the use of

Ksheera - milk,

Madya - wine,

Rasa - meat soup and

Dadhi - curds,

Abhyanga - oil massage,

Udvartana – powder massage,

Snana - bath,

Murdha karna akshi tarpanam - anointing the head, ears and eyes with nourishing oils,

Kanta bahulata slesho - comforting embrace by the arms of the wife,

Nivritti kritakrityata - harbouring the feeling of satisfaction of having done good deeds and

Mano anukula vishaya - resorting to things which are comforting to the mind as much as desired;

These bring about the pleasure of good sleep.

For those who follow the regimen of celibacy (brahmacharya), who are disinterested in sexual pleasures and who are contented with happiness (santosha), sleep will not be very late than its regular time.

Abrahmacharya (Non-celibacy) - Rules and regulations for sex:

ग्राम्यधर्मं त्यजेन्नारीमनुत्तानां रजस्वलाम् ।
अप्रियामप्रियाचारां दुष्टसङ्कीर्णमेहनाम् ॥ ६९ ॥
अतिस्थूलकृशां सूतां गर्भिणीमन्ययोषिताम् ।
वर्णिनीमन्ययोनिं च गुरुदेवनृपालयम् ॥ ७० ॥
चैत्यश्मशानाहननचत्वराम्बुचतुष्पथम् ।
पर्वाण्यनङ्गं दिवसं शिरोहृदयताडनम् ॥ ७१ ॥
अत्याशितोऽधृतिः क्षुद्वान्दुःस्थिताङ्गः पिपासितः ।
बालो वृद्धोऽन्यवेगार्तस्त्यजेद्रोगी च मैथुनम् ॥ ७२ ॥

One should avoid having sex with a woman

Anuttanam - who is not lying down in supine position (with her face facing upwards),

Rajasvalam – who is menstruating,

Apriyam apriyachara - who is disliked and whose acts are displeasing,

Dushta sankirna mehanam – whose private parts (sex organs) are dirty and who is troublesome,

Ati sthula krisha – who is very obese or very emaciated,

Sutam garbhinim – who has recently delivered a child or who is pregnant,

Anya yoshitam – a woman other than his wife,

Varninim – who is a nun (dedicated female student who lives in hermitage or monastery).

One should avoid sex -

Anya yoni ca – with other animals like goat, buffalo etc,

Guru deva nripalayam – in the abode of the teacher (school), gods (temple) and kings (palace),

Chaitya shmashaana ayatana chatvambu chatushpadam – in monasteries, burial grounds, places of torture and of sacrifice and at the place of meeting of four roads,

Parvanyanangam divasam - during days of special significance (new moon, full moon, eclipse, festivals, mourning days and others), in organs which are non-sexual (mouth, anus etc.) and also on days forbidden for sex,

Shiro hridaya tadanam – one should not hit the head or chest (heart) while having sex, i.e. one should avoid violence during sex,

Atyashito adhriti kshudvan – after heavy meals, without keen interest in sex, or when hungry,

Dusthitha anga - when his body is in uncomfortable positions,

Pipasita - when thirsty,

Balo vriddho – with children and with old women,

Anya vegarta – when troubled by other urges such as urine, faeces etc

Tyajet rogi ca maithunam – when he himself is a patient.

Rutu and Gramyadharma (sexual intercourse in different seasons):
सेवेत कामतः कामं तृप्तो वाजीकृतां हिमे ।
त्र्यहाद्वसन्तशरदौ पक्षाद्वर्षानिदाघयोः ॥ ७३ ॥

In Hemanta and Shishira seasons (winter and late winter), one can indulge in copulation daily, as much as he likes, after making use of aphrodisiacs (vajikritam).

In Vasanta (spring) and Sarat (autumn) seasons, one can have sex once in three days.

Asamyak maithuna janya vikara – Ill-effects of improper indulgence in sexual intercourse:

भ्रमक्लमोरुदौर्बल्यबलधात्विन्द्रियक्षय: ।

अपर्वमरणं च स्यादन्यथा गच्छतः स्त्रियम् ॥ ७४ ॥

The symptoms of improper indulgence in sexual intercourse with a woman are

Bhrama - giddiness,

Klama - exhaustion,

Uru dourbalya - weakness of thighs,

Bala kshaya - loss of strength,

Dhatu kshaya - depletion of tissues,

Indriya kshaya - loss of acuity of senses and

Aparvamaranam - premature death.

Samyata maithuna - Qualities obtained by disciplined indulgence in sexual intercourse:

स्मृतिमेधायुरारोग्यपुष्टीन्द्रिययशोबलैः ।

अधिका मन्दजरसो भवन्ति स्त्रीषु संयताः ॥ ७५ ॥

When one indulges in sexual intercourse with women in a disciplined way, he is bestowed with rich qualities like

Smriti - good memory,

Medha - intelligence,

Ayu - longevity,

Arogya - health,

Pushti indriya - nourishment, acuity of sense organs / restoration and fortification (richness in terms of quality and quantity) of semen,

Yasha - reputation,

Bala - strength and

Manda jara - slow ageing (established youth).

Gramyadharma uttara karma - Post sex rejuvenation measures:

स्नानानुलेपनहिमानिलखण्डखाद्य शीताम्बुदुग्धरसयूषसुराप्रसन्नाः ।

सेवेत चानु शयनं विरतौ रतस्य तस्यैवमाशु वपुषः पुनरेति धाम ॥ ७६ ॥

After the sexual act, one feels depleted of vigour. To overcome that, he should indulge in one or more of

Snana - bath,

Anulepana - applying scented pastes,

Hima anila - exposure to cool breeze,

Kandadyaha - eating dishes prepared from sugar candy,

Sheeta ambu - drinking cold water,

Dugdha - milk,

Rasa - meat juice,

Yusha - soup,

Sura - fermented liquor prepared from grains and

Prasanna - clear supernatant fluid of Sura.

After having consumed the above said, one should go to sleep. With this, the lost vigour of the body will be restored and replenished. The vigour will quickly return back to its abode (body), once again.

Benefits attained by the King who is in the protection of a wise physician:

श्रुतचरितसमृद्धे कर्मदक्षे दयालौ भिषजि निरनुबन्धं देहरक्षां निवेश्य ।

भवति विपुलतेजःस्वास्थ्यकीर्तिप्रभावः स्वकुशलफलभोगी भूमिपालश्चिरायुः ॥ ७७ ॥

With his physician who is well conversant with the scriptures and its practices, efficient in work, kind in nature having implicitly reposed the protection of his body, without any hesitation or doubt, will attain

Vipula teja - great valour,

Swasthya - health,

Keerthi - fame,

Prabhava - influence,

Svakushala phalabhogi - capacity to enjoy the fruits of all his actions and deeds (earned due to his capacity and skills) and

Chirayu - longevity of life.

इति श्री वैद्यपतिसिंहगुप्तसूनु वाग्भटविरचितायां अष्टाङ्गहृदय संहितायां सूत्रस्थाने अन्नसंरक्षणीयो नाम सप्तमोऽध्यायः ॥

Thus ends the 7th chapter of Ashtangahridaya Samhita, Sutrasthana, named Annaraksha Vidhi, written by Shrimad Vagbhata, son of Shri Vaidyapati Simhagupta.

8

मात्राशितीयमध्यायम्
(matrashitiyam adhyayam)

The 8th chapter of Sutrasthanam of Ashtanga Hridayam is named Matrashiteeya Adhyaya. In this chapter the following topics are covered –
The right quantity of food to be taken,
Right time of food intake,
Types of indigestion and their treatment,
Qualities and types of after drinks,
Right method of food intake etc.

अथातो मात्राशितीयमध्यायं व्याख्यास्यामः | इति ह स्माहुरात्रेयादयो महर्षयः |
Atreya and other sages pledge that they would henceforth be explaining the chapter named Matrashiteeya adhyaya.

Matrayukta ahara sevana – Need for taking food in proper quantity:
मात्राशी सर्वकालं स्यान्मात्रा ह्यग्नेः प्रवर्तिका|
मात्रां द्रव्याण्यपेक्षन्ते गुरूण्यपि लघून्यपि||१||
One should always consume food in proper quantities. When taken in the right quantities, the food activates and kindles the agni (digestion power). The foods that we consume may be guru (heavy to digest) or laghu (light to digest). Both guru and laghu forms of food depend on its quantity, i.e. they should be consumed in proper quantities so that they undergo proper

digestion.

Method of taking guru (hard to digest) and laghu (light to digest) foods:

गुरूणामर्धसौहित्यं लघूनां नातितृप्तता|

मात्राप्रमाणं निर्दिष्टं सुखं यावद्विजीर्यति||२||

The foods which are guru (heavy to digest) should be consumed up to half of one's capacity i.e. only till half of satiation level is achieved (Ardhasouhityam)

The foods which are laghu (light to digest) should be consumed till one is not totally satiated i.e. intake of food should be stopped before it reaches one's full capacity (Na atitriptata).

MatraPramana (proper quantity of food) can be defined as that quantity of food which undergoes digestion easily (without producing any ill effects).

Effects of Heena MatraAhara (Food taken in less quantity):

भोजनं हीनमात्रं तु न बलोपचयौजसे|

सर्वेषां वातरोगाणां हेतुतां च प्रपद्यते||३||

Hinamatraahara (the food consumed in less quantity) does not increase

Bala – strength,

Upachaya – nourishment or

Ojas – radiance, luster.

Gradually it becomes a hetu (causative factor) for all diseases of Vata origin.

Effects of Ati Matra Ahara (food taken in excessive quantity):

अतिमात्रं त्वशनं त्रीनपि दोषान् प्रकोपयेत्|

पीड्यमाना हि वाताद्या युगपत्तेन कोपिताः||४||

आमेनान्नेन दिष्टेन तदेवाविश्य कुर्वते|

विष्टम्भयन्तोऽलसकं च्यावयन्तो विसूचिकाम्||५||

अधरोत्तरमार्गाभ्यां सहसैवाजितात्मनः|

When food is consumed in excess (atimatra), it quickly vitiates all the three doshas.

The ingested food doesn't get digested properly.

At the same time, vata and other doshas get vitiated.

When obstructed by undigested food, vata and other doshas get vitiated at the same time.

As a result of indigestion and due to elapse of time of digestion, ama (caused due to undigested food) is formed.

The vitiated doshas are once again contaminated by ama and get lodged along with the ama or undigested food.

The vitiated doshas cause Alasaka due to the blockage of the channels of the body caused by the contaminated food.

The same doshas cause Visuchika by expelling the indigested food simultaneously and repeatedly from lower (anal) and upper (oral) passages. Both these conditions occur mainly in ajitatmana (people who are not self controlled).

Alasaka:

प्रयाति नोर्ध्वं नाधस्तादाहारो न च पच्यते||६||
आमाशयेऽलसीभूतस्तेन सोऽलसकः स्मृतः|

The condition in which the food neither comes out from the upper route (naurdhvam) in the form of vomiting nor from the downward route (naadha) in the form of defecation nor undergoes digestion (na ca pachyate), but stays stagnated in the stomach (amashaya) is called Alasaka.

Visuchika:

विविधैर्वेदनोद्भेदैर्वाय्वादिभृशकोपतः||७||
सूचीभिरिव गात्राणि विध्यतीति विसूचिका|

A condition in which various types of pain (vividhavedana) get manifested due to sudden aggravation (bhrishakopa) of Vayu and other doshas is called Visuchika. In this, the pain appears as though the whole body (gatra) is being pricked by many suchis (needles) and hence the name.

Visuchika symptoms based on Dosha predominance:

तत्र शूलभ्रमानाहकम्पस्तम्भादयोऽनिलात्||८||
पित्ताज्ज्वरातिसारान्तर्दाहतृट्प्रलयादयः|
कफाच्छर्द्यङ्गगुरुतावाक्सङ्गष्ठीवनादयः||९||

In Visuchika, different set of symptoms are manifested when each dosha predominates in the disease –

When Vata is predominantly aggravated in visuchika, it causes

Shoola – abdominal pain,

Bhrama–delusion, giddiness,

Anaha – bloating of abdomen,

Kampa – tremors,

Sthambhadi – stiffness etc. symptoms.

When Pitta is predominantly aggravated in visuchika, it causes
Jwara – fever,
Atisara – diarrhoea,
Antardaha – internal burning sensation,
Trit – excessive thirst,
Pralayadi – unconsciousness etc symptoms.
When Kapha is predominantly aggravated in visuchika, it causes
Chardi – vomiting,
Angaguruta – heaviness of the body,
Vaksanga – difficulty to speak,
Shteevanadi – excessive salivation etc symptoms.

Manifestation of symptoms of Alasaka:

विशेषाद्दुर्बलस्याल्पवह्नेर्वेगविधारिणः।
पीडितं मारुतेनान्नं श्लेष्मणा रुद्धमन्तरा॥१०॥
अलसं क्षोभितं दोषैः शल्यत्वेनैव संस्थितम्।
शूलादीन् कुरुते तीव्रांश्छर्द्यतीसारवर्जितान्॥११॥

In Visuchika manifesting specially in
Durbala – people who are weak,
Alpavahne – having low digestion capacity and
Vega vidharina – those are habituated to suppressing the natural urges of the body,
the free movements of Vata in the body are blocked by anna (food). This stagnated food further gets obstructed in the stomach by the vitiated Sleshma (Kapha), and becomes alasa (lazy) and kshobhita (inactivated) in the stomach. This food gets further agitated by Vata, Pitta and Kapha and stays in the stomach itself in the form of a shalya (foreign body) leading to shoola (severe abdominal colic) and many such serious symptoms, but without chardi (vomiting) and atisara (diarrhoea).

Dandalasaka:

सोऽलस अत्यर्थदुष्टास्तु दोषा दुष्टाम्बद्धखाः।
यान्तस्तिर्यक्तनुं सर्वा दण्डवत्स्तम्भयन्ति चेत्॥१२॥
दण्डकालसकं नाम तं त्यजेदाशुकारिणम्।

The above explained is known as Alasaka.
Severely vitiated doshas, being blocked in the channels of the body which are filled and contaminated by ama, move obliquely (tiryak) in abnormal

pathways in the body, afflicts the entire body making it stiff like a log of wood (dandavatsthambayanti) and hence is called Dandakalasaka.

This condition should be denied treatment since it tends to quickly cause death.

Ama visha (indigested food poison):

विरुद्धाध्यशनाजीर्णशीलिनो विषलक्षणम्||१३||

आमदोषं महाघोरं वर्जयेद्विषसंज्ञकम्|

विषरूपाशुकारित्वादिविरुद्धोपक्रमत्वतः||१४||

People who regularly indulges in

Virudhashana – incompatible foods,

Adhyashana – excessive intake of foods and

Ajeernasheelino – eating food in spite of prevailing indigestion,

develop amadosa which is similar to visha (poison) in nature.

This condition is called amavisha (undigested food poison).

In this, treatment should be refused since the condition is mahaghora (dreadful, troublesome, causes severe pain and agony), visharupa (has similarity with poison), ashukari (tends to cause death quickly) and requires virudhaupakrama (treatments of opposite nature for poison and ama)

Alasaka Chikitsa – Treatment for Alasaka:

अथाममलसीभूतं साध्यं त्वरितमुल्लिखेत्|

पीत्वा सोग्रापटुफलं वार्युष्णं योजयेत्ततः||१५||

स्वेदनं फलवर्तिं च मलवातानुलोमनीम्|

नाम्यमानानि चाङ्गानि भृशं स्विन्नानि वेष्टयेत्||१६||

In sadhya (curable) forms of alasaka, firstly ullekhana (emesis) should be administered. For this, the person has to drink ushnavari (hot water) mixed with powder of Acorus calamus, black salt and Randia dumetorum (Emetic Nut).

Following this, the patient should be administered svedana (sudation therapy) and phalavarti (suppositories prepared from medicines) which help in anulomana (downward movement) of mala (faeces) and vata (flatus).

The parts of the body which have become rigid (namyamananiangani) due to the effect of ama, should be subjected to swedana (fomentation) and veshtana (wrapping with clothes / bandaging)

Ingredients of Phalavarti (suppositories):
मदनं पिप्पलीकुष्ठं वचागौराश्चसर्षपाः।
गुडक्षारसमायुक्ता फलवर्तिः प्रशस्यते॥१६१+१॥
The following are the ingredients of Phalavarti –
Madana – Randia dumetorum – emetic nut,
Pippali – Piper longum – long pepper,
Kushta – Saussurea lappa,
Vacha – Acorus calamus,
Gaurasarshapa – Sinapis alba – White mustard,
Guda – jaggery and
Kshara–Yavakshara – Alkali prepared from Barley.

Visuchikachikitsa – Treatment for vishucika:
विसूच्यामतिवृद्धायां पाष्ण्योर्दाहः प्रशस्यते।
तदहश्चोपवास्यैनं विरिक्तवदुपाचरेत्॥१७॥
In the advanced (ativriddha) stage of vishucika, branding by fire (cauterization) over the heel is recommended.
On the same day, the patient has to fast (upavasa) and should be taken care of as the one who has undergone purgation therapy (viriktavat) i.e. all the post virechana procedures and treatments including samsarjana karma (dietetic regimen in the form of gruels etc) should be administered.

Contra–indication of medicines in those suffering from Ajirna (indigestion):
तीव्रार्तिरपि नाजीर्णी पिबेच्छूलघ्नमौषधम्।
आमसन्नोऽनलो नालं पक्तुं दोषौषधाशनम्॥१८॥
निहन्यादपि चैतेषां विभ्रमः सहसाऽऽतुरम्।
In spite of presence of tivra arti (severe pain), the patient suffering from ajirna (indigestion) should not consume shoolagna aushada (pain killing medicines) because the anala (digestive fire) debilitated by ama (improperly processed metabolites) will be unable to digest the doshas, aushadha (medicines) and ashana (food).
These three i.e. doshas, medicines and food which cannot be digested or converted by the debilitated fire will cause severe troubles and kill the patient in quick time.

Indication of medicine when the food is digested:

जीर्णाशने तु भैषज्यं युञ्ज्यात् स्तब्धगुरूदरे||१९||
दोषशेषस्य पाकार्थमग्नेः सन्धुक्षणाय च|

When the food is being digested properly (jirnaashanam) and in the presence of stiffness and heaviness of abdomen (stabdha guru udara), medicines shall be administered to digest the residual doshas (shesha doshas) and to stimulate the digestive fire (agni sandhukshana).

Apatarpana (lightening) treatments for diseases caused by ama:

शान्तिरामविकाराणां भवति त्वपतर्पणात्||२०||
त्रिविधं त्रिविधे दोषे तत्समीक्ष्य प्रयोजयेत्|

The diseases caused by ama or undigested food is relieved by administration of Apatarpana (lightening therapies i.e. langhana).

The three types of Apatarpana i.e. langhana, langhana–pachana and shodhana should be applied in three types of dosha vitiation i.e.

Langhana – in mild dosha vitiation,

Langhana pachana – in moderate dosha vitiation and

Shodhana – in severe dosha vitiation.

These three types of apatarpana shall be judiciously administered in three types of doshas after properly analyzing the desha (place), kala (time), agni (digestion power) etc. factors.

Administration of three types of langhana in three types of doshas:

तत्राल्पे लङ्घनं पथ्यं, मध्ये लङ्घनपाचनम्||२१||
प्रभूते शोधनं, तदिध मूलादुन्मूलयेन्मलान्|

When doshas (ama) are alpa (less in quantity), only langhana (fasting) will be suitable.

If doshas (ama) are present in madhya (moderate) proportions then langhana–pachana (fasting combined with medicines which increase digestion capacity) are suitable.

When doshas (ama) are present in prabhuta (large) proportions, shodhana (purification like Panchakarma therapies) should be administered.

The above said three types of apatarpana when judiciously administered in the three types of amadoshas respectively, will expel out the doshas and ama from their roots (moola).

Treatment principle for diseases:

एवमन्यानपि व्याधीन् स्वनिदानविपर्ययात्||२२||
चिकित्सेदनुबन्धे तु सति हेतुविपर्ययम्|
त्यक्त्वा यथायथं वैद्यो युञ्ज्याद्व्याधिविपर्ययम्||२३||

Similarly, the principle of relieving the causative factors should be adopted in other diseases too.

However, if the diseases persist for a longer time or recur, then the cause specific treatment should be given up and treatments which are opposite to the disease should be adopted by the physicians immediately. This is called *Vyadhi Viparyaya Chikitsa* (treatment which is against the disease).

Alternatively, *Tadarthakari Chikitsa* (treatments though not actually opposite to either the cause or diseases still produce the desired result), should be adopted.

Pakva Dosha Chikitsa (treatment of doshas devoid of ama):

तदर्थकारि वा, पक्वे दोषे त्विद्धे च पावके|
हितमभ्यञ्जनस्नेहपानबस्त्यादि युक्तितः||२४||

When the doshas become pakva (ripened) after the digestion of ama and when the digestive activity is restored completely to normalcy, then beneficial measures like

Abhyanjana – oil massage,

Snehapana – oleation,

Basti – medicated enema therapy etc

should be judiciously administered.

Ajirna Bheda (different types of digestion)

Ama ajirna:

अजीर्णं च कफादामं तत्र शोफोऽक्षिगण्डयोः|
सद्योभुक्त इवोद्गारः प्रसेकोत्क्लेशगौरवम्||२५||

Indigestion caused by vitiated kapha is known as Amajirna. It is characterized by

Shophoakshigandayo – swelling of the eye sockets and cheeks,

Sadyobhuktaivaudgara – pure belching similar to those which come up immediately after meals,

Praseka – excessive salivation,

Utklesha – nausea and

Gaurava – heaviness of the body.

Vishtabdhaajirna:

विष्टब्धमनिलाच्छूलविबन्धाध्मानसादकृत्|

Vishtabdhajirna is the indigestion caused by vitiated vata. It is characterized by

Shoola – pain in the abdomen,

Vibandha – constipation,

Adhmana – flatulence and

Sada – debility.

Vidagdha ajirna

विष्टब्धमनिलाच्छूलविबन्धाध्मानसादकृत्|

Vidagdhajirna is the indigestion caused by vitiated pitta. It is characterized by

Trit – thirst,

Moha – fainting,

Bhrama – giddiness,

Amlodgara – sour belching and

Daha – burning sensation.

AjirnaChikitsa – Treatment for indigestion:

लङ्घनं कार्यमामे तु, विष्टब्धे स्वेदनं भृशम्|

विदग्धे वमनं, यद्वा यथावस्थं हितं भवेत्||२७||

For Ama ajirna – Langhana – fasting should be done;

For VishtabdhaAjirna – Swedana (sudation therapy) should be done;

For Vidagdha ajirna – Vamana (emesis therapy) or any therapy appropriate to the stage of disease can be done.

Vilambika:

गरीयसो भवेल्लीनादामादेव विलम्बिका|

कफवातानुबद्धाऽऽमलिङ्गा तत्समसाधना||२८||

Vilambika is another type of indigestion caused due to profound accumulation and adherence of Ama in the channels of the body. It is caused by association of Kapha and Vata and presents with all the symptoms of Ama. The treatment of vilambika is also similar to that of Ama.

RasasheshaAjirna:

अश्रद्धा हृद्व्यथा शुद्धेऽप्युद्गारे रसशेषतः|

शयीत किञ्चिदेवात्र सर्वश्चानाशितो दिवा||२९||
स्वप्यादजीर्णी, सञ्जातबुभुक्षोऽद्यान्निमतं लघु|

RasasheshaAjirna is a type of indigestion characterized by

Ashraddha – lack of enthusiasm and

Hridvyadha – discomfort in the region of the heart, in spite of the presence of shuddhaudgara (pure belching).

The person having rasasheshaajirna should sleep for some time during the day.

In all other types of indigestion also, one should sleep during the day without taking any food. Later, when hunger is manifested, he should eat small quantities of easily digestible food.

Ajirna Samanya Lakshana – General symptoms of indigestion:

विबन्धोऽतिप्रवृत्तिर्वा ग्लानिर्मारुतमूढता||३०||
अजीर्णलिङ्गं सामान्यं विष्टम्भो गौरवं भ्रमः|

The common symptoms of indigestion are

Vibandha – constipation or

Atipravritti – diarrhoea,

Glani – exhaustion,

Marutamudata – inactivity of Vata (upward movement of Vata),

Vishtambha – distension of abdomen,

Gaurava – heaviness of the body and

Bhrama – giddiness.

Ajirna anya karanani – Other causes of indigestion:

न चातिमात्रमेवान्नमामदोषाय केवलम्||३१||
द्विष्टविष्टम्भिदग्धामगुरुरूक्षहिमाशुचि|
विदाहि शुष्कमत्यम्बुप्लुतं चान्नं न जीर्यति||३२||
उपतप्तेन भुक्तं च शोकक्रोधक्षुदादिभिः|

Consumption of Atimatra (large quantities) of food causes production of Ama dosha.

Apart from that, below mentioned are the other causes that lead to indigestion –

Dvishta – foods which are disliked,

Vishtambhi – foods which cause distension of abdomen (and flatulence),

Dagdhama – foods which are over-cooked or uncooked,

Guru – foods which are not easily digestible,

Ruksha, hima, ashuchi – foods which are dry, very cold and contaminated,

Vidahi – foods which are corrosive (cause burning sensation),

Shushka – which are dried up or

Atyambuplutam – foods which are excessively soaked in water.

The food consumed by persons afflicted by shoka (grief), krodha (anger), kshudha (excessive hunger) etc also result in ajirna (indigestion).

DushtaAshana – Bad food habits:

मिश्रं पथ्यमपथ्यं च भुक्तं समशनं मतम्||३३||

विद्यादध्यशनं भूयो भुक्तस्योपरि भोजनम्|

अकाले बहु चाल्पं वा भुक्तं तु विषमाशनम्||३४||

त्रीण्यप्येतानि मृत्युं वा घोरान् व्याधीन्सृजन्ति वा|

Below mentioned are the three types of bad food habits –

Samashana – is consuming suitable and unsuitable foods mixed together

Adhyashana – is consuming large quantities of food even before the previously consumed food is digested

Vishamashana – is consuming less quantity or large quantity of food at improper time

All these three food habits either cause death (mrityu) or dreadful diseases (ghoravyadhi).

Ahara Vidhi – Diet regimen, method of taking food properly:

काले सात्म्यं शुचि हितं स्निग्धोष्णं लघु तन्मनाः||३५||

षड्रसं मधुरप्रायं नातिद्रुतविलम्बितम्|

स्नातः क्षुद्वान् विविक्तस्थो धौतपादकराननः||३६||

तर्पयित्वा पितॄन् देवानतिथीन् बालकान् गुरून्|

प्रत्यवेक्ष्य तिरश्चोऽपि प्रतिपन्नपरिग्रहान्||३७||

समीक्ष्य सम्यगात्मानमनिन्दन्नब्रुवन् द्रवम्|

इष्टमिष्टैः सहाश्नीयाच्छुचिभक्तजनाहृतम्||३८||

Below explained is the method of an ideal and good diet regimen.

One should consume food –

Kale – at proper time,

Satmyam – which is accustomed to one's health,

Shuchi – which is clean,

Hitam – which is pleasing,

Snigdha – which is unctuous,

Ushna – hot,

Laghu – easily digestible,

Tanmana – with due attention,

Sadrasammadhuraprayam – which contains all the six tastes with predominance of sweet taste,

Na atidrutam – neither very quickly,

Na ativilambitam – nor very slowly,

Snata – after taking bath,

Kshudvan– after appearance ofproper hunger,

Vivikthastho – sitting in solitude,

Dhauta pada karaanana – after having washed the feet, hands and face,

Tarpayitva pitrn devan athithi balakan gurun – after satisfying the manes, gods, guests, children and teachers,

Pratyavekshya tiracho api pratipanna parigrahan – after satisfying even the dependants in the house (such as servants, horses, parrots and other pets),

Samikshya samyak atmanam – after considering one's own constitution, likes and dislikes,

Anindana – without scolding or abusing the food,

Abruvan – without talking too much,

Dravam – liquid food,

Ishtam–that, which is liked,

Ishtaihisaha – in the company of liked people,

Ashniyatsuchibhaktajanahritam–that served by those who are clean and also faithful to him.

Tyajya Bhojana – Foods which need to be rejected:

भोजनं तृणकेशादिजुष्टमुष्णीकृतं पुनः।

शाकावरान्नभूयिष्ठमत्युष्णलवणं त्यजेत्॥३९॥

Food which is contaminated with trina (grass), kesha (hairs) etc, ushnikritampuna (re–heated), which consists of more of shaka (vegetables) and avaranna (undesirable grains), which is atyushna (very hot) and atilavana (very salty) should be rejected.

Foods that should not be consumed habitually:

किलाटदधिकूचीकाक्षारशुक्ताममूलकम्।

कृशशुष्कवराहाविगोमत्स्यमहिषामिषम्॥४०॥

माषनिष्पावशालूकबिसपिष्टविरूढकम्।

शुष्कशाकानि यवकान् फाणितं च न शीलयेत्॥४१॥

The following food items are not to be consumed habitually –

Kilata– dairy products which are sweet in taste,

Dadhikurchika – solid part of curds,

Kshara – alkalis,

Shukta – fermented gruels,

Ama mulaka – uncooked radish,

Krushaamisha – meat of animals which are emaciated,

Shushkaamisha – dry meat,

Varahaavi go matsyamahishaamisham – Meat of boar, sheep, cow, fish and buffalo,

Masha – black gram,

Nishpava – cowpea (flat bean),

Shaluka – rhizome of lotus,

Bisa – lotus stalk,

Pishta – flour,

Viruda – germinated grains,

Shushkashaka – dried vegetables,

Yavaka – small barley,

Phanitam – half cooked molasses.

Satmya–Pathya – Foods that can be consumed habitually, on daily basis:
शीलयेच्छालिगोधूमयवषष्टिकजाङ्गलम्।
सुनिषण्णकजीवन्तीबालमूलकवास्तुकम्॥४२॥
पथ्यामलकमृद्वीकापटोलीमुद्गशर्कराः।
घृतदिव्योदकक्षीरक्षौद्रदाडिमसैन्धवम्॥४३॥
The below mentioned foods can be consumed on a daily basis –
Shali – rice,

Godhuma – wheat,

Yava – barley,

Shashtika – rice maturing in sixty days,

Jangalam – meat of animals living in desert lands,

Sunishannaka –Blepharis edulis,

Jivanti – Leptadenia reticulata,

Balamulaka – young radish,

Vastukam – cucumber,

Pathya – Terminalia chebula,

Amalaka – Indian gooseberry,

Mridvika – dry grapes (raisins),

Patoli – pointed gourd,

Mudga – green gram,

Sharkara – sugar,

Grita – ghee,

Divyodaka – rain water or pure water,

Kshira – milk,

Kshaudra – honey,

Dadima – pomegranate and

Saindhavam – rock salt.

Use of Triphala:

त्रिफलां मधुसर्पिभ्यार्ां निशि नेत्रबलाय च|

स्वास्थ्यानुवृत्तिकृद्यच्च रोगोच्छेदकरं च यत्||४४||

Triphala should be consumed with madhu (honey) and sarpi (ghee), daily at nishi (night time), for strengthening the eyesight (netrabalaya).

Any other thing (food or medicine) which is good for promoting health and dispelling diseases should be habituated.

Foods which should be consumed at the beginning, middle and end of a meal:

बिसेक्षुमोचचोचाम्रमोदकोत्कारिकादिकम्|

अद्याद्द्रव्यं गुरु स्निग्धं स्वादु मन्दं स्थिरं पुरः||४५||

विपरीतमतश्चान्ते मध्येऽम्ललवणोत्कटम्|

Foods that should be consumed at the commencement of the meal should have the following qualities –

Guru – which are hard to digest,

Snigdha – unctuous (fatty),

Svadu – sweet,

Manda – slow and

Sthira – hard.

Example for such foods are –

Bisa – lotus,

Ikshu – sugarcane,

Mocha – plantain,

Chocha – coconut,

Amra – mango,

Modaka – sweet meat balls,

Utkarika – sweet dishes etc.

Foods of opposite qualities should be consumed at the end of the meal.
Foods which are predominantly amla (sour) and lavana (salty) should be taken in the middle of the meal.

Allotment of the stomach space for different foods:

अन्नेन कुक्षेद्र्वावंशौ पानेनैकं प्रपूरयेत्||४६||

आश्रयं पवनादीनां चतुर्थमवशेषयेत्|

The stomach should be divided into four parts.

Two parts of the stomach (half of its capacity) should be filled with solid foods.

One part of the stomach should be filled with liquids and

the remaining one part of the stomach should be kept vacant for accommodation and free circulation of air etc.

Anupana – After drinks:

अनुपानं हिमं बारि यवगोधूमयोर्हितम्||४७||

दध्नि मद्ये विषे क्षौद्रे, कोष्णं पिष्टमयेषु तु|

शाकमुद्गादिविकृतौ मस्तुतक्राम्लकाञ्जिकम्||४८||

सुरा कृशानां पुष्ट्यर्थ, स्थूलानां तु मधूदकम्|

शोषे मांसरसो, मद्यं मांसे स्वल्पे च पावके||४९||

Cold water is the ideal after–drink (Anupana) – after intake of foods prepared from

Yava – barley,

Godhuma – wheat,

Dadhi – curds,

Madya – wine,

Visha – poison and

Kshaudra – honey.

    Warm water is the ideal after–drink for

Foods which are pishtamaya (starchy),

Mastu – Supernatant liquid of curds (whey),

Takra – diluted buttermilk,

Amla kanjika – fermented gruel,

Dishes prepared from shaka (vegetables), mudga (green gram) and other legumes.

Sura (beer) is the ideal after drink for krisha (lean) person.

Madhudaka (honey mixed water) is the ideal after drink for sthula (obese)

person.

Mamsa rasa (meat soup) is the ideal after drink for shosha (the emaciated), Madya (wine) is ideal after a meal of meat and for those who have poor digestive capacity.

Milk as Anupana:

व्याध्यौषधाध्वभाष्यस्त्रीलङ्घनातपकर्मभिः|

क्षीणे वृद्धे च बाले च पयः पथ्यं यथाऽमृतम्||५०||

Milk is best suited just like amrita (nectar) for those who are debilitated by Vyadhi – diseases,

Aushada – medicines and therapies,

Adhva – walking long distances,

Bhashya – speaking,

Stri – sexual intercourse,

Langhana – fasting,

Atapa karmabhih – exposure to sun and other tiresome activities,

Ksheena – emaciated,

Bala – children and

Vriddha – the aged.

Ideal Anupana (After–drink):

विपरीतं यदन्नस्य गुणैः स्यादविरोधि च|

अनुपानं समासेन, सर्वदा तत्प्रशस्यते||५१||

An ideal anupana or after–drink is that which has

Viparitamyadannam – properties opposite of those of the foods,

Syadavirodhi – but not incompatible with them.

Such an after–drink is always valuable.

Benefits of Anupana (after–drink):

अनुपानं करोत्यूर्जां तृप्तिं व्याप्तिं दृढाङ्गताम्|

अन्नसङ्घातशौथिल्यविक्लित्तिजरणानि च||५२||

Anupana or after–drink brings about

Urja – invigoration (strength),

Tripti – contentment,

Vyapti – enables proper movement of foods inside the body and

Dridangatam – stability of body parts,

Annasangatashaithilya – helps in loosening of hard masses of food,

Viklitthi – their moistening and

Jarana – digestion.

Contra–indications of Anupana:

नोर्ध्वजत्रुगदश्वासकासोरःक्षतपीनसे।

गीतभाष्यप्रसङ्गे च स्वरभेदे च तदि्धतम्॥५३॥

Anupana should not be administered in

Urdhvajatrugada – diseases of the organs above the shoulders,

Swasa – dyspnoea, asthma,

Kasa – cough,

Urakshata – chest injury,

Pinasa – rhinitis,

For those engaged in gita (singing) and bhashya (speaking for long time) and

Swarabheda – hoarseness of voice.

Contraindications after taking liquids and food:

प्रक्लिन्नदेहमेहाक्षिगलरोगव्रणातुराः।

पानं त्यजेयुः सर्वश्च भाष्याध्वशयनं त्यजेत्॥५४॥

पीत्वा, भुक्त्वाऽऽतपं वह्निं यानं प्लवनवाहनम्।

Drinking of liquids should be avoided by

Praklinnadeha – people who are over–hydrated,

Those suffering from

Meha – urinary disorders, diabetes,

Akshiroga – diseases of eyes,

Gala roga – diseases of throat and

Vranatura – those suffering from wounds (ulcers).

The following activities are to be avoided immediately after intake of liquids –

Bhashya – speaking,

Adhva – walking long distances and

Shayana – sleeping.

The following activities are to be avoided immediately after intake of food –

Atapa – exposure to sun,

Vahni – exposure to fire,

Yana – travel in vehicles,

Plavana – swimming and

Vahanam – riding on animals.

Ahara Kala – Proper time for food consumption:

प्रसृष्टे विण्मूत्रे हृदि सुविमले दोषे स्वपथगे
विशुद्धे चोद्गारे क्षुदुपगमने वातेऽनुसरति।
तथाऽग्नावुद्रिक्ते विशदकरणे देहे च सुलघौ
प्रयुञ्जीताहारं विधिनियमितं, कालः स हि मतः॥५५॥

Food should strictly be consumed only when the below mentioned conditions prevail.

Prasrishtavinmutre – after proper elimination of faeces and urine,

Hrudisuvimale – when the mind is pleasant,

Dosha sthapathage – when the doshas are moving gently in their natural pathways (functioning normally),

Vishudhe ca udgare – when the belching is clean and pure (without foul smell or taste),

Kshudupagamane – when hunger is properly manifested,

Vateanusarathi – when the flatus is moving downward easily,

Tathaagnavudrikte – when the digestive activity is good and at its peak,

Vishadakarane – when the sense organs are functioning clearly,

Dehe ca sulaghau – when the body is light.

Food should be given in the presence of the above said conditions while following the rules, regulations and procedures of food. This is the ideal time for consumption of food.

इतिश्रीवैद्यपतिसिंहगुप्तसूनुवाग्भटविरचितायां अष्टाङ्गहृदयसंहितायां सूत्रस्थाने मात्राशितीयो नाम अष्टमोऽध्यायः ।

Thus ends the 8th chapter of Ashtangahridaya Samhita, Sutrasthana, named Matrashiteeya Adhyaya, written by Shrimad Vagbhata, son of Shri Vaidhyapati Simhagupta.

9

द्रव्यादिविज्ञानीयमध्यायम् (dravyadi vijnaniyam adhyayam)

The 9th chapter of Sutrasthana is Dravyadi Vijnaniyam Adhyayam. It deals with the properties of a dravya such as qualities, tastes, Vipaka, Veerya and Prabhava.

अथातो द्रव्यादिविज्ञानीयमध्यायं व्याख्यास्यामः इति ह स्माहुरात्रेयादयो महर्षयः ।

Atreya and other sages pledge that they would henceforth be explaining the chapter named Dravyadivijnaaneeyamadhyayam (chapter dealing with substances, their qualities and action).

Dravya Pradhanyata – Importance of substance:

द्रव्यमेव रसादीनां श्रेष्ठं, ते हि तदाश्रयाः।

पञ्चभूतात्मकं तत्तु क्ष्मामधिष्ठाय जायते||१||

Dravya – (substance / mass of the substance) is the most important factor among Rasa (tastes) and other qualities; because all these qualities (rasa, guna, virya, vipaka and prabhava) reside in the dravya (substance) only.

Dravya (substance) is composed of Panchamahabhuta (five basic elements of nature).

Among the 5 basic elements, Dravya comes into existence because the earth element forms its adishtana (base).

Prithvi or Earth as the base of Dravya:

अम्बुयोन्यग्निपवननभसां समवायतः।

तन्निर्वृत्तिर्विशेषश्च व्यपदेशस्तु भूयसा॥२॥

The substance takes its origin from ambu (water element). The substance is inevitably related with agni (fire element), pavana (air element) and nabhasa (ether / space element) through samavaya (intimate and inseparable combination).

The identification of a specific dravya is decided by the predominance of a particular element present in it.

Rasa – Primary taste:

तस्मान्नैकरसं द्रव्यं भूतसङ्घातसम्भवात्।

नैकदोषास्ततो रोगास्तत्र व्यक्तो रसः स्मृतः॥३॥

There is no substance having only eka rasa (one taste) because all the substances are made up of a combination of all five elements.

Similarly there is no roga (disease) arising out of eka dosha (a single dosha).

The taste that is vyakta (clearly perceived) during intake of dravya is called Rasa.

Anurasa – Secondary taste:

अव्यक्तोऽनुरसः किञ्चिदन्ते व्यक्तोऽपि चेष्यते।

The taste which is avyakta (not clearly manifested) or that which is kinchitvyakta (slightly perceived) at the end of a primary taste is called Anurasa or secondary taste.

Dravya, Guna and Rasa relation (relationship between substance, qualities and taste):

गुर्वादयो गुणा द्रव्ये पृथिव्यादौ रसाश्रये॥४॥

रसेषु व्यपदिश्यन्ते साहचर्योपचारतः।

Guru (heaviness) etc. qualities present in the Prithvi (earth) etc. substances are residing in the Rasa (taste of the substance); Qualities of a substance are ascribed to its Rasa (taste) because of their intimate co–existence.

Qualities of solid substances – (ParthivaDravyaLakshana):

तत्र द्रव्यं गुरुस्थूलस्थिरगन्धगुणोल्बणम्॥५॥

पार्थिवं गौरवस्थैर्यसङ्घातोपचयावहम्।

Prithvi (earth element) possess the following qualities –

Guru – heaviness,
Sthula – corpulent,
Sthira – stability,
Gandhagunolbanam– smell.

The substances having predominance of earth element possess
Gaurava – heaviness,
Sthairya – stability and
Sangata – compactness and
Upachaya – good nourishment.

Qualities of liquid substances (AapyaDravyaLakshana):

द्रवशीतगुरुस्निग्धमन्दसान्द्ररसोल्बणम्||६||
आप्यं स्नेहनविष्यन्दक्लेदप्रह्लादबन्धकृत्|

Substances predominant in water element possess
Drava – liquidity,
Sheeta – cold,
Guru – heavy to digest,
Snigdha – unctuous,
Manda – dull,
Sandra – thickness (dense) and
Rasolbanam – taste qualities in abundance.

Therefore substances having liquid as predominant element bestow
Snehana – unctuousness,
Vishyanda – secretion,
Kleda – wetness,
Prahlada – satiation (contentment) and
Bhandakrit – holding together (binding, cohesion).

Qualities of fiery substances (Agneya Dravya Lakshana):

रूक्षतीक्ष्णोष्णविशदसूक्ष्मरूपगुणोल्बणम्||७||
आग्नेयं दाहभावर्णप्रकाशपचनात्मकम्|

The substances predominant in fire element possess
Ruksha – dry,

Tikshna – sharp (penetrating),
Ushna – hot,
Vishada – non–slimy,
Sukshma – minute and
Rupagunolbanam – form (appearance) qualities in abundance.

Therefore, the substances that have fire as predominant element bestows
Daha – burning sensation,
Bha– radiance and
Varna – colour
Prakasha – brightness and
Pachana – digestion.

Qualities of airy substances (VayavyaDravyaLakshana):

वायव्यं रूक्षविशदलघुस्पर्शगुणोल्बणम्॥८॥
रौक्ष्यलाघववैशद्यविचारग्लानिकारकम्‌‌|

The substances predominant in air element possess
Ruksha – dry,
Vishada – non–slimy (clear),
Laghu – lightness and
Sparshagunolbanam – touch (tactile sensation) qualities in abundance.

Therefore, the substances predominant in air element will produce
Raukshya – dryness,
Laghava – lightness,
Vaishadya – transparency (clarity),
Vichara – movements (activities) and
Glani – exhaustion.

Qualities of ether dominant substances – NabhasaDravyaLaksana:

नाभसं सूक्ष्मविशदलघुशब्दगुणोल्बणम्‌॥९॥
सौषिर्यलाघवकरम्‌

The substances which are predominant in ether or space element possess
Sukshma – minuteness,
Vishada – transparency (clarity),
Laghu – lightness and
Shabdagunolbanam – sound (hearing) qualities in abundance.

Therefore, the substances predominant in ether element produce

Saushirya – cavitation (hollowness) and

Laghava – lightness (weightlessness).

Everything in this universe is a medicine:

जगत्येवमनौषधम्|

न किञ्चिद्विद्यते द्रव्यं वशान्नानार्थयोगयोः||१०||

Since dravya can be used in various forms and combinations, there is no dravya in the universe which cannot be used as a medicine.

Movement of dravya based on predominance of elements:

द्रव्यमूर्ध्वगमं तत्र प्रायोऽग्निपवनोत्कटम्|

अधोगामि च भूयिष्ठं भूमितोयगुणाधिकम्||११||

Generally, the substances (dravyas) predominant in agni (fire) and pavana (air) elements tend to move upwards – urdhvagamam.

The substances (dravyas) predominant in bhumi (earth) and toya (water) elements tend to move downwards – adhogami.

इति द्रव्यम् रसान् भेदैरुत्तरत्रोपदेक्ष्यते|

Hence, the Dravya has been explained. The types of Rasa (tastes) will be expounded in the following chapters.

Veerya – Potency of medicines:

वीर्यं पुनर्वदन्त्येके गुरु स्निग्धं हिमं मृदु||१२||

लघु रूक्षोष्णतीक्ष्णं च तदेवं मतमष्टधा|

Virya or potency of the drug is again said to be of eight types according to others author's opinion, therefore, the 8 types of virya enlisted below are accepted –

Guru – heaviness,

Snigdha – unctuousness (oily),

Hima – cold,

Mridu – soft,

Laghu – lightness,

Ruksha – dryness,

Ushna – hot,

Tikshna–intense, piercing, strong.

चरकस्त्वाह वीर्यं तत् क्रियते येन या क्रिया||१३||

नावीर्यं कुरुते किञ्चित्सर्वा वीर्यकृता हि सा|

According to master Charaka,veerya is that through which the action of a drug is made possible. The drug devoid of veerya does not perform any action, because all actions are possible only by the presence of veerya.

Importance of ashtavidhavirya (8 types of drug potency):

गुर्वादिष्वेव वीर्याख्या तेनान्वर्थैति वर्ण्यते||१४||

समग्रगुणसारेषु शक्त्युत्कर्षविवर्तिषु|

व्यवहाराय मुख्यत्वाद्बहवग्रग्रहणादपि||१५||

Those who include heaviness etc. eight qualities as Veerya, do so by direct implication.

Among all the 20 gunas or qualities (and also rasa, vipaka etc. entities), these 8 qualities

– remain stable in the substance

– are stronger than the rest of the qualities and are capable of inducing action by themselves,

– are important in the day–to–day routine of life,

– are obvious choices among many substances and qualities (qualities other than the 8 mentioned in veerya, tastes etc.) and also considered as the first option in all procedures.

Hence, these 8 qualities have been given importance (and considered as veerya).

Reason for Rasa etc. not being called as Veerya:

अतश्च विपरीतत्वात्सम्भवत्यपि नैव सा|

विवक्ष्यते रसाद्येषु, वीर्यं गुर्वादयो ह्यतः||१६||

So, in spite of the veerya being present in the rasa etc. entities, it will not be called as virya because of its inconsistent and invisible form and also due to the taste etc. being opposite to the reasons mentioned above. Therefore, guru etc. 8 qualities alone are considered veeryas.

Two types of Veerya:

उष्णं शीतं द्विवधैवान्ये वीर्यमाचक्षते अपि च|

नानात्मकमपि द्रव्यमग्निषोमौ महाबलौ||१७||

व्यक्ताव्यक्तं जगदिव नातिक्रामति जातुचित्|

Some other authors consider only 2 types of Veerya –

Ushna Veerya (hot potency) and

Sheeta Veerya (cold potency).

Because, though substances are of many kinds and qualities, only Agni (fire) and Soma (water) are the powerful ones.

Action of Hot Potency (Ushna Veerya):
तत्रोष्णं भ्रमतृड्ग्लानिस्वेददाहाशुपाकिता:॥१८॥
शमं च वातकफयो:

Hot potency causes
Bhrama – delusion, dizziness,
Trut – excessive thirst,
Glani – exhaustion,
Sveda – perspiration,
Daha – burning sensation,
Ashupakita – quick cooking (transformation) and
Shamam tu vatakaphayo – mitigation of Vata and Kapha.

Action of Sheeta veerya (cold potency):
करोति, शिशिरं पुन:।
ह्लादनं जीवनं स्तम्भं प्रसादं रक्तपित्तयो:॥१९॥

Sheeta Virya causes
Hladana – satiation, happiness,
Jivana – enlivening,
Sthambha – withholding, restraining and
Rakta Pitta prasada – purification of blood (rakta) and calming of Pitta.

Vipaka – Taste after digestion (post digestion effect):
जाठरेणाग्निना योगाद्यदुदेति रसान्तरम्।
रसानां परिणामान्ते स विपाक इति स्मृत:॥२०॥

When the food substances come in contact with the jataraagni (digestive fire), they will undergo a change in rasa (taste), at the end part of digestion. This change in taste that a substance undergoes is called Vipaka.

Types of Vipaka:
स्वादु: पटुश्च मधुरमम्लोऽम्लं पच्यते रस:।
तिक्तोषणकषायाणां विपाक: प्रायश: कटु:॥२१॥

Vipaka is of 3 types –
Madhura vipaka – Sweet
Amla vipaka – Sour
Katu Vipaka – Pungent

Madhura Vipaka – the svadu (sweet) and patu (salt) tastes undergo madhura vipaka after digestion.

Amla vipaka – amla (sour) taste undergoes amla vipaka after digestion.

Katuvipaka – tikta (bitter), ushana (pungent) and kashaya (astringent) tastes undergo katuvipaka after digestion.

Similarities between rasa (taste) and vipaka, mode of action of dravya on the basis of rasa, veerya etc.

रसैरसौ तुल्यफलस्तत्र द्रव्यं शुभाशुभम्।

किञ्चिद्रसेन कुरुते कर्म पाकेन चापरम्।।२२।।

गुणान्तरेण वीर्येण प्रभावेणैव किञ्चिन।

Substances act by the action of any of the following

Rasa (taste),

Vipaka (taste conversion after digestion),

Guna (the qualities that they possess),

Veerya (potency) or by

Prabhava (special effects).

Law of dominance amongst rasa, guna etc. entities contained in the substance:

यद्यद्द्रव्ये रसादीनां बलवत्त्वेन वर्तते।।२३।।

अभिभूयेतरांस्तत्तत्कारणत्वं प्रपद्यते।

विरुद्धगुणसंयोगे भूयसाऽल्पं हि जीयते।।२४।।

The one that is powerful among them (Rasa, Guna, Vipaka, Virya and Prabhava) suppresses all the other qualities to exhibit special influence and action.

In case of a combination of two opposite qualities (virudha guna), the strong one vanquishes the weak.

रसं विपाकस्तौ वीर्यं प्रभावस्तान्यपोहति।

बलसाम्ये रसादीनामिति नैसर्गिकं बलम्।।२५।।

When two opposing qualities are present in equal strength, in such a situation,

Vipaka (taste conversion after digestion) wins over Rasa (taste);

Veerya (potency) wins over Rasa (taste) and

Vipaka and Prabhava (special effect) wins over all of them (Rasa, Vipaka and Veerya).

This is the pattern of natural strength.

Definition of Prabhava:

रसादिसाम्ये यत् कर्म विशिष्टं तत् प्रभावजम्|

Special action exhibited by a substance over–ruling Rasa (taste), Guna (qualities), Vipaka (taste conversion after digestion) and Veerya (potency) is called Prabhava.

Examples for Prabhava:

दन्ती रसाद्यैस्तुल्याऽपि चित्रकस्य विरेचनी||२६||

मधुकस्य च मृद्वीका, घृतं क्षीरस्य दीपनम्|

Danti and Chitraka – Though Danti (Baliospermum montanum) is identical to Chitraka (Plumbago zeylanica) with respect to Rasa (taste) etc., Danti is a virechani (purgative) while Chitraka is not. Hence, purgation is the Prabhava of Danti.

Similarly, are Madhuka (Licorice – Glycyrrhiza glabra) and Mrdvika (grapes).

Madhuka and Mrdvika – both have similar qualities. But Mrdvika has mild purgative action, but Madhuka does not.

Milk and ghee – both possess similar qualities. But ghee is deepana (increases digestion strength) but milk does not. Hence increasing digestion strength is the prabhava (special effect) of ghee.

Vichitra Pratyayarabdha Dravya (extraordinary substances):

इति सामान्यतः कर्म द्रव्यादीनां, पुनश्च तत्||२७||

विचित्रप्रत्ययारब्धद्रव्यभेदेन भिद्यते|

The functions of Rasa (taste), Guna (property), Virya (potency), Vipaka (taste conversion after digestion) and Prabhava (special effect) have been explained.

A special category, known as VichitraPratyarabda exists, which is due to peculiar combinations of peculiar factors.

Examples of Vichitra Pratyayarabdha Dravya:

स्वादुर्गुरुश्च गोधूमो वातजिद्वातकृद्यवः||२८||

उष्णा मत्स्याः पयः शीतं कटुः सिंहो न शूकरः||

Both godhuma (wheat) and yava (barley) possess svadu (sweet) and guru (heaviness) qualities.But wheat mitigates Vata and barley aggravates it.

Matsya (fish) and paya (milk) are madhura (sweet) and guru (heavy) but still milk is sheeta (cool) and fish is ushna (hot).

Meat of simha (lion) and shukara (pig) both are madhura (sweet) and guru (heavy) but still lion meat has KatuVipaka (pungent taste conversion after digestion) and pig meat has MadhuraVipaka (sweet taste conversion after digestion).

तस्माद्रसोपदेशेननसर्वं द्रव्यमादिशेत्॥२९॥

Hence the properties of a Dravya cannot be determined based on Rasa alone.

इति श्रीवैद्यपतिसिंहगुप्तसूनुवाग्भटविरचितायां अष्टाङ्गहृदयसंहितायां सूत्रस्थाने द्रव्यादिविज्ञानीयो नाम नवमोऽध्याय: ।

Thus ends the 9th chapter of Ashtangahridaya Samhita, Sutrasthana, named Dravyadi Vijnaaneeya Adhyaya, written by Shrimad Vagbhata, son of Shri Vaidhyapati Simhagupta.

10

रसभेदीयमध्यायम्
(rasabhediyam adhyayam)

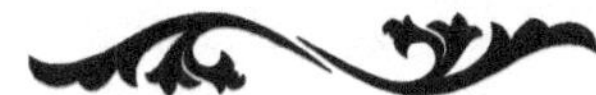

The 10th chapter of Sutrasthanam of Ashtanga Hridayam is named as Rasabhediya Adhyayam. Rasa means taste and Bheda means types. This chapter discusses in detail regarding the types of tastes and their properties.

अथातो रसभेदीयमध्यायं व्याख्यास्यामः इति ह स्माहुरात्रेयादयो महर्षयः ।
As advised by Maharshi Atreya, henceforth is described the chapter named Rasabhediyam.

Origin of tastes from the Mahabhutas (elements of nature):
क्ष्माम्भोग्निक्ष्माम्बुतेजः खवाय्वग्न्यनिलगोनिलैः।
द्वयोल्बणैः क्रमाद्भूतैर्मधुरादिरसोद्भवः॥१॥
Kshma ambho – madhura rasa / sweet taste has its origin from the predominance of earth and water,
Agni kshma – amla rasa / sour taste is formed by the combination of fire and earth elements,
Ambu teja – lavana rasa / salt taste is formed by the combination of water and fire elements,
Kha vayu – tikta rasa / bitter taste is formed by the combination of ether (space) and air elements,
Agni anila – katu rasa / pungent taste is formed by the combination of fire

and air elements,

Go anilaih – kashaya rasa / astringent taste is formed by the combination of earth and air elements.

Madhura / Swadu Rasa (sweet taste):

तेषां विद्याद्रसं स्वादु यो वक्त्रमनुलिम्पति।
आस्वाद्यमानो देहस्य ह्लादनोऽक्षप्रसादनः॥२॥
प्रियः पिपीलिकादीनाम्

Swadu / Madhura (sweet) is understood by the following properties –
Vaktram anulimpati – sticks to the oral cavity,
Asvadyamano dehasya – provides a feeling of contentment,
Hladana – gives pleasure to the body and
Akshaprasadana – gives comfort to the sense organs.
Priya pippilikadinam – It is liked even by ants.

Amla Rasa (sour taste):

अम्लः क्षालयते मुखम्।
हर्षणो रोमदन्तानामक्षिभ्रुवनिकोचनः॥३॥

Amla rasa (sour taste) is characterised by the following –
Kshalayate mukham – causes watering of the mouth,
Harshano romanam – causes horripilation,
Harshano dantanam – tingling of the teeth and
Akshi bhruva nikochanam – leads to contraction of the eyes and eyebrows.

Lavana Rasa (salt taste):

लवणः स्यन्दयत्यास्यं कपोलगलदाहकृत्

Lavana rasa (salt taste) is characterised by the following –
Syandayati asyam – causes more moisture in the mouth (increases salivation) and
Kapola gala dahakrit – burning sensation in the cheeks and throat.

Tikta Rasa (Bitter taste):

तिक्तो विशदयत्यास्यं रसनं प्रतिहन्ति च॥४॥

Tikta rasa (bitter taste) is characterised by the following
Vishadayati asyam – cleanses the mouth and
Rasanam pratihanti – destroys the organs of taste (makes perception of other tastes impossible).

Katu Rasa (pungent taste):

उद्वेजयति जिह्वाग्रं कुर्वश्चिमिचिमां कटुः।
स्रावयत्यक्षिनासास्य कपोलौ दहतीव च॥५॥

Katu rasa (pungent taste) is characterised by the following –
Udvejayati jihvagram – stimulates the tip of the tongue,
Kurvaschimichimam – causes irritation,
Sravayati akshi nasa asyam – brings out secretions from the eyes, nose and mouth and
Kapolau dahativa ca – causes burning sensation of the cheeks.

Kashaya Rasa (Astringent taste):

कषायो जडयेज्जिह्वां कण्ठस्रोतोविबन्धकृत्।

Kashaya rasa (astringent taste) is characterised by the following –
Jadayet jihvam – inactivates the tongue (diminishes capacity of taste perception) and
Kanta sroto vibhandakrit – causes obstruction of the passage in the throat.

रसानामिति रूपाणिकर्माणि

Thus explained are the symptoms of different tastes.
The functions of different tastes will be explained in the upcoming verses.

Functions of Madhura Rasa (Sweet Taste)

मधुरो रसः॥६॥
आजन्मसात्म्यात्कुरुते धातूनां प्रबलं बलम्।
बालवृद्धक्षतक्षीणवर्णकेशेन्द्रियौजसाम्॥७॥
प्रशस्तो बृंहणः कण्ठ्यः स्तन्यसन्धानकृद्गुरुः।
आयुष्यो जीवनः स्निग्धः पित्तानिलविषापहः॥८॥
कुरुतेऽप्युपयोगेन स मेदःश्लेष्मजान् गदान्।
स्थौल्याग्निसादसन्न्यासमेहगण्डार्बुदादिकान्॥९॥

Madhura rasa (sweet taste) being ajanma satmya (accustomed since birth), bestows
Dhatunam prabalam balam – greater strength to the body tissues,
It is good for
Bala – children,
Vriddha – the aged people,
Kshata – those wounded,

Kshina – the emaciated,

Varna – improves the colour,

Kesha – hairs,

Indriya – strength of sense organs and

Ojas – essence of the tissues.

It is also

Brimhana – bulk promoting,

Kantya – good for the throat,

Stanya – increases breast milk,

Sandhanakrit – unites the fractured bones,

Guru – hard to digest,

Ayushyo – promotes longevity of life,

Jivana – enlivening and

Snigdha – unctuous.

It mitigates pitta, anila (vata) and visha (poison).

By ati upayoga (excessive use), it causes

Meda sleshmajan gadan – diseases arising from vitiated meda (fat) and sleshma (kapha),

Sthoulya – obesity,

Agnisada – deficit digestion (indigestion),

Sanyasa – loss of consciousness,

Meha – diabetes, urinary disorders,

Ganda – enlargement of neck glands,

Arbudadi – malignant tumors and many such disorders.

Functions of Amla Rasa (Sour Taste):

अम्लोऽग्निदीप्तिकृत्स्निग्धो हृद्यः पाचनरोचनः।
उष्णवीर्यो हिमस्पर्शः प्रीणनः क्लेदनो लघुः॥१०॥
करोति कफपितास्रं मूढवातानुलोमनः।
सोऽत्यभ्यस्तस्तनोः कुर्याच्छैथिल्यं तिमिरं भ्रमम्॥११॥
कण्डुपाण्डुत्ववीसर्पशोफविस्फोटतृइज्वरान्।

Amla rasa (sour taste) is

Agni deeptikrit – stimulates the Agni (digestive activity),

Snigdha – unctuous,

Hridya – good for the heart,

Pachana – digestive,

Rochana – appetizer,

Ushna viryo – hot in potency,

Hima sparsha – cool to touch,

Prinana – satiates,

Kledana – causes moistening,

Laghu – it is easy for digestion,

Karoti kapha pitta asram – causes aggravation of Kapha, Pitta and Asra (blood) and

Muda vata anulomanam – makes the inactive Vata move downwards.

Sour taste if used in excess, causes

Shaithilyam – looseness of the body,

Timiram – blindness,

Bhramam – giddiness,

Kandu – itching,

Pandutva – pallor,

Visarpa – Herpes, spreading skin disease,

Shopha – swellings,

Visphota – blisters, eruptions,

Trit – thirst and

Jwara – fever

Functions of Lavana Rasa (Salt Taste):

लवणः स्तम्भसङ्घातबन्धविध्मापनोऽग्निकृत्||१२||

स्नेहनः स्वेदनस्तीक्ष्णो रोचनश्छेदभेदकृत्|

सोऽतियुक्तोऽस्रपवनं खलतिं पलितं वलिम्||१३||

तृट्कुष्ठविषवीसर्पान् जनयेत्क्षपयेद्बलम्|

Lavana rasa (salty taste) destroys

Stambha – rigidity,

Sangata – hardness,

Bandha – blocks in the channels and pores of the body.

It has the following properties –

Agnikrit – increases digestive activity,

Snehana – lubricates,

Svedana – causes sweating,

Tikshna – penetrates deep into the tissues,

Rochana – improves taste,

Cheda bhedakrit – cuts and breaks open (the growths and abscesses etc)

If used in excess, it causes

Asra pavanam – vitiation of Asra (blood) and pavanam (vata),

Kalatim – causes baldness,

Palitam – greying of hair,

Valim – wrinkles of the skin,

Trit – thirst,

Kushta – skin diseases,

Visha – effect of poison,

Visarpa – spreading skin disease and

Kshapayet balam – decreases strength of the body.

Functions of Tikta Rasa (Bitter Taste):

तिक्तः स्वयमरोचिष्णुररुचिं कृमितृड्विषम्||१४||

कुष्ठमूर्च्छाज्वरोत्क्लेशदाहपित्तकफान् जयेत्|

क्लेदमेदोवसामज्जशकृन्मूत्रोपशोषणः||१५||

लघुर्मेध्यो हिमो रूक्षः स्तन्यकण्ठविशोधनः|

धातुक्षयानिलव्याधीनतियोगात्करोति सः||१६||

Tikta rasa (bitter taste) is svayam arochishnu (by itself is not tasty), but it cures

Aruchi – anorexia,

Krimi – worms,

Trit – thirst,

Visha – poison,

Kushta – skin diseases,

Murcha – loss of consciousness,

Jwara – fever,

Utklesha – nausea,

Daha – burning sensation,

Pitta kaphan jayet – mitigates Pitta and Kapha,

Kleda upashoshana – dries up moisture,

Meda upashoshana – dries up fat,

Vasa upashoshana – dries up muscle–fat,

Majja upashoshana – dries up marrow,

Shakrit mutra upashoshana – dries up faeces and urine;

Tikta Rasa is

Laghu – easily digestible,

Medhya – increases intelligence,

Hima – cold in potency,

Ruksha – causes dryness,

Stanya vishodhana – cleanses breast milk and

Kanta vishodhana – clears the throat.

When used in excess, it causes

Dhatu kshaya – depletion of Dhatus (tissues) and

Anila vyadhi – diseases of Vata origin.

Functions of Katu Rasa (Pungent Taste):

कटुर्गलामयोदर्दकुष्ठालसकशोफजित्।

व्रणावसादनः स्नेहमेदःक्लेदोपशोषणः॥१७॥

दीपनः पाचनो रुच्यः शोधनोऽन्नस्य शोषणः।

छिनत्ति बन्धान् स्रोतांसि विवृणोति कफापहः॥१८॥

कुरुते सोऽतियोगेन तृष्णां शुक्रबलक्षयम्।

मूर्च्छामाकुञ्चनं कम्पं कटिपृष्ठादिषु व्यथाम्॥१९॥

Katu rasa (pungent taste) cures

Galamaya – diseases of throat,

Udarda – allergic rashes,

Kushta – skin diseases,

Alasaka – a type of indigestion,

Shopha – swelling (oedema),

Vranavasadana – reduces the swelling around the ulcers,

Sneha upashoshana – dries up the unctuousness,

Meda upashoshana – dries up the fat,

Kleda upashoshana – dries up the moisture,

Dipana – increases hunger,

Pachana – digestive,

Ruchya – improves taste,

Shodhana – cleansing, eliminates the Doshas,

Annasya shoshana – dries up moisture of the food,

Chinnati bhandan – breaks up hard masses,

Srotamsi vivrinoti – dilates the channels and

Kaphapaha – mitigates Kapha.

If used in excess, it causes

Trishna – thirst,

Shukra kshaya – depletion of reproductive element (sperm),

Bala kshaya – depletion of strength,

Murcha – fainting (loss of consciousness),

Akunchanam – contractures,

Kampa – tremors and

Kati prishtadishu vyatham – pain in the waist, back etc.

Functions of Kashaya Rasa (Astringent Taste):

कषायः पित्तकफहा गुरुरस्रविशोधनः।

पीडनो रोपणः शीतः क्लेदमेदोविशोषणः॥२०॥

आमसंस्तम्भनो ग्राहि रूक्षोऽति त्वक्प्रसादनः।

करोति शीलितः सोऽति विष्टम्भाध्मानहृद्रुजः॥२१॥

तृट्कार्श्यपौरुषभ्रंशस्रोतोरोधमलग्रहान्।

Kashaya rasa (astringent taste) is

Pitta kaphapaha – balances Pitta and Kapha,

Guru – it is not easily digestible,

Asra vishodhana – cleanses the blood,

Pidano ropana – causes squeezing and healing of ulcers (wounds),

Sheeta – cold in potency,

Kledamedo vishoshana – dries up the moisture and fat,

Ama – hinders the digestion of undigested food.

Grahi – is water absorbent, constipative,

Ruksha – causes dryness and

Ati twakprasadana – cleanses the skin too much.

If used in excess, it causes

Vishtambha – stasis of food without digestion,

Adhmana – flatulence, abdominal distension,

Hridruja – pain in the heart region,

Trit – thirst,

Karshya – emaciation,

Paurusha brmsha – loss of virility,

Srotorodha – obstruction of the channels and

Mala graha – constipation.

Madhura Gana – Group of sweet substances:

घृतहेमगुडाक्षोडमोचचोचपरूषकम्॥२२॥

अभीरुवीरापनसराजादनबलात्रयम्।

मेदे चतस्रः पर्णिन्यो जीवन्ती जीवकर्षभौ॥२३॥

मधूकं मधुकं बिम्बी विदारी श्रावणीयुगम्।

क्षीरशुक्ला तुगाक्षीरी क्षीरिण्यौ काश्मरी सहे॥२४॥

क्षीरेक्षुगोक्षुरक्षौद्रद्राक्षादिर्मधुरो गणः|

Ghrita – ghee,

Hema – gold,

Guda – molasses,

Akshoda – Juglans regia,

Mocha – banana (plantain),

Chocha – Bark of cinnamon,

Parushaka – Falsa fruit – Grewia asiatica,

Abhiru – Asparagus racemosus,

Vira – Roscaea procera,

Panasa – jackfruit,

Rajadana – Mimusops hexandra,

The three Bala (Bala, Atibala and Nagabala) – Sida cordifolia and its varieties,

The two Meda – Meda – Polygonatum verticillatum All, and Mahameda – Polygonatum verticillatum Allioni,

The four Parni – Shalaparni (Desmodium gangeticum), Prishniparni (Uraria picta), Mudgaparni (Phaseolus trilobus), Mashaparni (Teramnus labialis),

Jivanti – Leptadenia reticulata,

Jivaka – Malaxis acuminata D.Don / Microstylis wallichii Lindl.,

Rishabhaka – Microstylis musifera,

Madhuka – Licorice – Glycyrrhiza glabra,

Madhuka – Madhuka longifolia,

Bimbi – Coccinia grandis / indica,

Vidari – Pueraria tuberosa,

The two Sravani – Shravani (Sphaeranthus indicus), Mahashravani (Sphaeranthus africans),

Ksheerasukla – Ipomea digitata,

Tugaksiri – Bambusa arundinaceae,

The two Ksheerini – Kshirakakoli (Lilium polyphyllum), Dugdhika (Euphorbia thymifolia),

Kashmari – Gmelina arborea,

The two Saha – Kshudrasaha, Mahasaha,

Ksheera – milk,

Ikshu – sugarcane,

Gokshura – Tribulus terrestris,

Kshaudra – honey,

Draksa – grapes – Vitis vinifera etc. form the group of sweet substances.

Amla Gana – group of sour substances:

अम्लो धात्रीफलाम्लीकामातुलुङ्गाम्लवेतसम्॥२५॥

दाडिमं रजतं तक्रं चुक्रं पालेवतं दधि।

आम्रमाम्रातकं भव्यं कपित्थं करमर्दकम्॥२६॥

Examples of amla gana (group of sour substances) are –

Dhatriphala – fruit of amla – Indian gooseberry,

Amlika – tamarind,

Matulunga – Citrus medica,

Amlvetasa – Garcinia pedunculata,

Dadima – pomegranate,

Rajatam – silver,

Takram – buttermilk,

Chukram - overfermented / spoilt fermented product

Palevatam,

Dadhi – curds,

Amra – mango,

Amrataka – wild mango – Hog plum – Spondias pinnata,

Bhavyam – Dillenia indica,

Kapitham – wood apple and

Karamardakam – Carissa carandas.

Lavana Gana – group of salty substances:

वरं सौवर्चलं कृष्णं बिडं सामुद्रमौद्भिदम्।

रोमकं पांसुजं शीसं क्षारश्च लवणो गणः॥२७॥

The group of salty substances comprise of different types of salts, including –

Varam – Saindhava Lavana – rock salt,

Sauvarchalam – Sochal salt, black salt – unaqua sodium chloride,

Krishnam – Black variety of salt,

Vidam – Ammonium salt,

Samudram – Sea salt,

Audbhidam – Rhea salt, Usa salt, efflorescent salts,

Romakam – Sambhar salt, earthen salt,

Pamsujam – salt prepared from saline earth,

Sisam – lead and

Kshara – alkalis.

Tikta Gana – group of bitter substances:
तिक्तः पटोली त्रायन्ती वालकोशीरचन्दनम्।
भूनिम्बनिम्बकटुकातगरागुरुवत्सकम्॥२८॥
नक्तमालदिवरजनीमुस्तमूर्वाटरूषकम्।
पाठापामार्गकांस्यायोगुडूचीधन्वयासकम्॥२९॥
पञ्चमूलं महद्व्याघ्र्यौ विशालाऽतिविषा वचा।

The group of tikta (bitter) substances comprise of –
Patoli – pointed gourd – Trichosanthes dioica,
Trayanti – Gentiana kurroo,
Valaka – Aporusa lindleyana / Coleus vettiveroides,
Ushira – Vetiveria zizanioides,
Chandanam – sandalwood,
Bhunimba – Andrographis paniculata,
Nimba – Azadirachta indica – neem,
Katuka – Picrorhiza kurroa,
Tagara – Valeriana wallichi, Indian Valerian,
Aguru – Aquilaria agallocha,
Vatsakam – Holarrhena antidysenterica,
Naktamala – Pongamia pinnata,
Dvirajani – the two types of Rajani – Haridra (turmeric) and Daruharidra
(tree turmeric),
Musta – Cyperus rotundus (nut grass),
Murva – Marsdenia tenacissima,
Atarushaka – Adhatoda vasica,
Patha – Cyclea peltata,
Apamarga – Achyranthes aspera – Prickly chaff flower,
Kamsya – bronze,
Ayas – iron,
Guduchi – Tinospora cordifolia,
Dhanvayasakam – Alhagi camelorum,
Panchamoolam maha – Roots of Bilva (Aegle marmelos, Bael root),
Agnimantha (Clerodendrum phlomidis), Shyonaka (Oroxylum indicum),
Patala (Stereospermum suaveolens), Gambhari (Gmelina arborea),
Vyaghryau – Brihati (Solanum indicum) and Kantakari (Solanum
surattense, Solanum xanthocarpum),

Visala – Citrullus colocynthis,
Ativisha – Aconitum heterophyllum and
Vacha – Acorus calamus.

Katu Gana – group of pungent substances:
कटुको हिङ्गुमरिचकृमिजित्पञ्चकोलकम्||३०||
कुठेराद्या हरितकाः पित्तं मूत्रमरुष्करम्|
The group of katu (pungent) substances comprise of –
Hingu – asafoetida,
Maricha – black pepper,
Krmijit pancakolakam – Krimijit (Embelia ribes), Pippali (long pepper), Pippalimula (root of long pepper), Chavya (Piper retrofractum), Chitraka (Plumbago zeylanica), Shunti (ginger)
Kutheradhya haritakah – leafy vegetables such as Kutheraka and others,
Pittam – bile of animals,
Mutra – urine of animals and
Arushkara – Semecarpus anacardium – Marking Nut.

Kashaya Gana – group of astringent substances:
वर्गः कषायः पथ्याऽक्षं शिरीषः खदिरो मधु||३१||
कदम्बोदुम्बरं मुक्ताप्रवालाञ्जनगैरिकम्|
बालं कपित्थं खर्जूरं बिसपद्मोत्पलादि च||३२||
The group of Kashaya (astringent) substances comprise of –
Pathya – Haritaki (Terminalis chebula),
Aksha – Bibhitaki (Terminalia bellirica),
Sirisah – Albizia lebbeck,
Khadira – Acacia catechu,
Madhu – honey,
Kadamba – Neolamarckia cadamba,
Udumbara – Ficus racemosa – cluster fig,
Mukta – pearls,
Pravala – coral,
Anjana – aqueous extract of Berberis aristata,
Gairikam – Purified red ochre,
Balam kapittham – unripe wood apple,
Karjuram – dates,
Bisa – lotus stalk,

Padma – Nelumbium speciosum,

Utpala – Nymphaea stellata etc.

General properties of tastes and exceptions:
Madhura rasa (sweet taste):
मधुरं श्लेष्मलं प्रायो जीर्णाच्छालियवादृते।
मुद्गाद्गोधूमतः क्षौद्रात्सिताया जाङ्गलामिषात्॥३३॥
Generally, substances of sweet taste are sleshmala (increases Kapha) except
Jeerna (more than one year old) grains of
Shali – rice,
Yava – Barley – Hordeum vulgare,
Mudga – green gram,
Godhuma – wheat,
Kshaudra – honey,
Sita – sugar and
Jangala amisha – meat of animals of desert – like land.

Amla rasa (sour taste):
प्रायोऽम्लं पित्तजननं दाडिमामलकादृते।
Generally substances of Amla rasa (sour taste) are pitta jananam (aggravate
Pitta), except Dadima – Pomegranate – Punica granatum and
Amalaka – Indian gooseberry.

Lavana rasa (salty taste):
अपथ्यं लवणं प्रायश्चक्षुषोऽन्यत्र सैन्धवात्॥३४॥
Generally salts are apathyam prayaschakshusho (bad for the eyes / vision)
except Saindhava – Rock Salt.

Tikta and Katu rasa (bitter and pungent tastes):
तिक्तं कटु च भूयिष्ठमवृष्यं वातकोपनम्।
ऋतेऽमृतापटोलीभ्यां शुण्ठीकृष्णारसोनतः॥३५॥
Generally tikta (bitter) and katu (pungent) rasa are avrishyam
(non–aphrodisiacs) and vatakopanam (aggravate Vata) except for
Amrita – Indian Tinospora,
Patoli – pointed gourd – Trichosanthes dioica,
Shunthi – ginger,
Krishna – long pepper and

Rasona – Garlic – Allium sativum.

Kashaya rasa (Astringent taste):
कषायं प्रायशः शीतं स्तम्भनं चाभयां विना|

Substances having kashaya rasa (astringent taste) are usually sheeta (cold in potency) and stambhanam (obstructive) except

Abhaya – Chebulic Myrobalan (fruit rind) – Terminalia chebula.

Tastes, their potencies and qualities:
रसाः कट्वम्ललवणा वीर्येणोष्णा यथोत्तरम्||३६||
तिक्तः कषायो मधुरस्तद्वदेव च शीतलाः|
तिक्तः कटुः कषायश्च रूक्षा बद्धमलास्तथा||३७||
पट्वम्लमधुराः स्निग्धाः सृष्टविण्मूत्रमारुताः|
पटोः कषायस्तस्माच्च मधुरः परमं गुरुः||३८||
लघुरम्लः कटुस्तस्मात्तस्मादपि च तिक्तकः|

Katu (pungent), Amla (sour), Lavana (salt) are of hot potency (Ushna Veerya) each one, more so in their succeeding order; i.e. lavana rasa is the most ushna and katu the least.

Similarly Tikta (bitter), Kashaya (astringent) and Madhura (sweet) are cold in potency, each one more in their succeeding order; i.e. madhura is the most sheeta and tikta the least.

Tikta (bitter), Katu (pungent) and Kashaya (astringent) are dry and cause constipation (each one more so in their succeeding order) i.e. kashaya is the most ruksha and tikta the least.

Patu (salt), Amla (sour), Madhura (sweet) are snigdha (unctuous) and help elimination of vit (faeces), mutra (urine) and maruta (flatus), each one more so in their succeeding order; i.e.

Madhura is the most snigdha and patu (lavana) the least.

Patu (salt), Kashaya (astringent) and Madhura (sweet) are guru (heavy to digest), each one more so in their succeeding order; i.e. madhura is the most guru and patu (lavana) the least.

Amla (sour), Katu (pungent) and Tikta (bitter) are laghu (easy to digest), each one more so in their succeeding order; i.e. tikta is the most laghu and amla the least.

Rasa Samyoga, Sankhya (permutation and combination of tastes, numbers of combination):

Number of rasas (tastes):

संयोगाः सप्तपञ्चाशत्कल्पना तु त्रिषष्टिधा||३९||
रसानां यौगिकत्वेन यथास्थूलं विभज्यते|

The combination (samyoga) of tastes is of 57 types, but the count is again of 63 types (including the 6 rasas individually) on the basis of usage of the tastes and has been classified grossly.

एकैकहीनास्तान् पञ्चदश यान्ति रसा द्विके||४०|

Eliminating 1 rasa (taste) from each combination, the number of combinations of 2 tastes will sum up to 15 types

Combination of 2 tastes = 15 types
1. Madhura + Amla 2. Madhura + Lavana
3. Madhura + Tikta 4. Madhura + Katu
5. Madhura + Kashaya 6. Amla + Lavana
7. Amla + Tikta 8. Amla + Katu
9. Amla + Kashaya 10. Lavana + Tikta
11. Lavana + Katu 13. Lavana + Kashaya
14. Tikta + Katu 15. Tikta + Kashaya

त्रिके स्वादुर्दशाम्लः षट् त्रीन् पटुस्तिक्त एककम्|

In the combination of 3 tastes each, it will be 10 with sweet, 6 with sour, 3 with salt, 1 with bitter (total 20 types in combination of three tastes)

Combination of 3 tastes = 20 types
1. Madhura + Amla + Lavana 2. Madhura + Amla + Tikta
3. Madhura + Amla + Katu 4. Madhura + Amla + Kashaya
5. Madhura + Lavana + Tikta 6. Madhura + Lavana + Katu
7. Madhura + Lavana + Kashaya 8. Madhura + Tikta + Katu
9. Madhura + Tikta + Kashaya 10. Madhura + Katu + Kashaya
11. Amla + Lavana + Tikta 12. Amla + Lavana + Katu
13. Amla + Lavana + Kashaya 14. Amla + Tikta + Katu
15. Amla + Tikta + Kashaya 16. Amla + Katu + Kashaya
17. Lavana + Tikta + Katu 18. Lavana + Tikta + Kashaya
19. Lavana + Katu + Kashaya 20. Tikta + Katu + Kashaya

चतुष्केषु दश स्वादुश्चतुरोऽम्लः पटुः सकृत्||४१||

In the combination of 4 tastes, it will be 10 with sweet, 4 with sour and 1 with salt (total 15 types in combination of 4 tastes together).

Combination of 4 tastes = 15 types
1. Madhura + Amla + Lavana + Tikta 2. Madhura + Amla + Lavana + Katu
3. Madhura + Amla + Lavana + Kashaya 4. Madhura + Amla + + Tikta + Katu
5. Madhura + Amla + Tikta + Kashaya 6. Madhura + Amla + Katu + Kashaya
7. Madhura + Lavana + Tikta + Katu 8. Madhura + Lavana + Tikta + Kashaya
9. Madhura + Lavana + Katu + Kashaya 10. Madhura + Tikta + Katu + Kashaya
11. Amla + Lavana + Tikta + Katu 12. Amla + Lavana + Tikta + Kashaya
13. Amla + Lavana + Katu + Kashaya 14. Amla + Tikta + Katu + Kashaya
15. Lavana + Tikta + Katu + Kashaya

पञ्चकेष्वेकमेवाम्लो मधुरः पञ्च सेवते|
In combination of 5 tastes, it will be only 1 with sour and
5 with sweet (total 6 in combination of fives).
Combination of 5 tastes = 6 types
1. Madhura + Amla + Lavana + Tikta + Katu 2. Madhura + Amla + Lavana + Tikta + Kashaya
3. Madhura + Amla +Lavana +Katu + Kashaya 4. Madhura + Lavana + Tikta + Katu + Kashaya
5. Madhura + Amla + Tikta + Katu + Kashaya 6. Amla + Lavana + Tikta + Katu + Kashaya

द्रव्यमेकं षडास्वादमसंयुक्ताश्च षड्रसाः||४२|
In the combination of 6 tastes, we will get 1 combination.
Each taste taken individually (not in combination with any other taste) will make 6 types, thus forming a total of 63 combinations.

Combination of 6 tastes together – 1 type
1. Madhura + Amla + Lavana + Tikta + Katu + Kashaya

Summary of rasa combinations:
षट् पञ्चकाः, षट् च पृथग्रसाः स्युश्चतुर्दिर्वकौ पञ्चदशप्रकारौ|
भेदास्त्रिका विंशतिरेकमेव द्रव्यं षडास्वादमिति त्रिषष्टिः||४३||
The combination of five rasas is of six types and single rasas constitute six

divisions.

The combinations of four rasas and two rasas are of fifteen types each.

The combinations of three rasas are of twenty types.

The combination of six rasas together constitutes one division.

Thus the total number of combinations is sixty three.

Method of judiciously using the tastes:

ते रसानुरसतो रसभेदास्तारतम्यपरिकल्पनाय च।
सम्भवन्ति गणनां समतीता दोषभेषजवशादुपयोज्याः ॥४४॥

These Rasa (primary tastes) and Anurasas (secondary tastes) in their proportional (more, moderate and less) combinations become innumerable. These are to be selected and used after considering the conditions of the Dosas and drugs.

इति श्री वैद्यपतिसिंहगुप्तसूनु वाग्भटविरचितायां अष्टाङ्गहृदयसंहितायां सूत्रस्थाने रसभेदीयोनाम दशमोऽध्यायः ।

Thus ends the 10th chapter of Ashtangahridaya Samhita Sutrasthana, named Rasabhediya Adhyaya, written by Shrimad Vagbhata, son of Shri Vaidyapati Simhagupta.

11

दोषादिविज्ञानीयमध्यायम् (doshadi vijnaniyam adhyayam)

The 11th chapter of Sutrasthanam of Ashtanga Hridayam is named as Doshadi Vijnaniyam Adhyayam. This chapter explains in detail regarding Tridoshas. The Tridoshas are Vata, Pitta and Kapha. Understanding the concept of Tridosha is the first step towards learning Ayurveda.

अथातो दोषादिविज्ञानीयमध्यायं व्याख्यास्याम: इति ह स्माहुरात्रेयादयो महर्षय: ।
Atreya and other sages pledge that henceforth they will be explaining the chapter named Doshadivijnaniyam.

The chief constituents of the body:
दोषधातुमला मूलं सदा देहस्य
Dosha - Vata, Pitta and Kapha
Dhatu - Body tissues – Rasa, Rakta, Mamsa, Meda, Asthi, Majja and Shukra
Mala - Waste products – Sweda, Mutra and Pureesha
are the roots / chief constituents of the body.

Functions of Normal Vata Dosha:
तं चल:|
उत्साहोच्छ्वासनिश्वासचेष्टावेगप्रवर्तनै:||१||
सम्यग्गत्या च धातूनामक्षाणां पाटवेन च|

अनुगृह्णात्यविकृतः
The non-vitiated (avikrita) vata helps the body by promoting
Utsaha - enthusiasm,
Ucchvasa nisvasa - controlling exhalation and inhalation,
Chesta - regulating all the movements,
Vega pravartanaih - initiating the free flow of body's natural urges,
Samyaggatya ca dhatunam – causing proper nourishment and functions of
the tissues in the body and
Akshanam patavena ca - proper functioning (perception) of sense organs.

Functions of Normal Pitta Dosha:
पित्तं पक्त्यूष्मदर्शनैः||२||
क्षुत्तृड्रुचिप्रभामेधाधीशौर्यतनुमार्दवैः|
In its normal state, Pitta promotes
Paktyi - digestion,
Ushma – generation of body heat,
Darshanaih – vision,
Kshut - hunger,
Trit - thirst,
Ruchi - taste,
Prabha - complexion,
Medha - retention of knowledge,
Dhi - knowledge,
Shourya - courage,
Tanu mardavaih - softness of the body.

Functions of Normal Kapha Dosha:
श्लेष्मा स्थिरत्वस्निग्धत्वसन्धिबन्धक्षमादिभिः||३||
Normal Kapha confers
Sthiratva - stability,
Snigdhatva - lubrication,
Sandhibandha - compactness of the joints of the body,
Kshamadibhi - tolerance power.

Functions of the body tissues – Prakrita Dhatu Karma:
प्रीणनं जीवनं लेपः स्नेहो धारणपूरणे|
गर्भोत्पादश्च धातूनां श्रेष्ठं कर्म क्रमात्स्मृतम्||४||

Prinanam - rasa dhatu (product of digestion and metabolism, digestive juice, nutritive fluid, lymph) provides nourishment,

Jivanam - rakta dhatu (blood) helps in maintenance of life activities,

Lepah - mamsa dhatu (muscle) helps in enveloping,

Sneho - medo dhatu (fat) causes lubrication,

Dharana - asthi dhatu (bone tissue) helps in providing the support to the body,

Purane - majja dhatu (bone marrow) helps in filling the inside of the bones,

Garbhotpadasca – shukra dhatu (reproductive fluid, semen), helps in formation of garbha (fetus), i.e. helps in conception and pregnancy.

Functions of the body waste products – Prakrita Mala Karma:

अवष्टम्भः पुरीषस्य, मूत्रस्य क्लेदवाहनम्|

स्वेदस्य क्लेदविधृतिः

The functions of Mala (body waste) in normalcy are as follows -

Avashtambah purishasya - maintenance of the strength of the body is the chief function of faeces,

Mutrasya kledavahanam - elimination of moisture is the main function of urine,

Svedasya kledavidhrtih - maintaining the moisture is the main function of sweat.

Symptoms of Increased Doshas – Vriddha Dosha Lakshana:
Symptoms of Increased Vata – Vriddha Vata Lakshana:

वृद्धस्तु कुरुतेऽनिलः ॥ ५ ॥

काश्र्यकाष्ण्यर्योष्णकामित्वकम्पानाहशकृद्ग्रहान् ।

बलनिद्रेन्द्रियभ्रंशप्रलापभ्रमदीनताः ॥ ६ ॥

Vata, when increased produces

Karshya – emaciation, derived by the word krusha

Karshnya – black discoloration, derived by the word krishna

Ushna kamitva – desire for hot things,

Kampa – tremors,

Anaha – bloating, distension of the abdomen,

Shakrut graha – constipation,

Bala bhramsha – loss of strength,

Nidra bhramsha – loss of sleep,

Indriya bhramsha – loss of sensory functions,

Pralapa – irrelevant speech,

Bhrama – Delusion, giddiness and

Deenata – timidity (peevishness).

Symptoms of Increased Pitta – Vriddha Pitta Lakshana:

पीतविण्मूत्रनेत्रत्वक्क्षुत्तृइदाहाल्पनिद्रताः ।

पित्तं

Pitta when increased produces

Peeta vinmutra netra tvak - yellowish discoloration of the faeces, urine, eyes and skin,

Kshut - excess of hunger,

Trit - excessive thirst,

Daha - burning sensation and

Alpa nidrata - reduced sleep.

Symptoms of increased of Kapha – Vriddha Kapha Lakshana:

श्लेष्माग्निसदनप्रसेकालस्यगौरवम् ॥ ७ ॥

श्वैत्यशैत्यश्लथाङ्गत्वं श्वासकासातिनिद्रताः ।

Sleshma (Kapha), when increased produces

Agnisadana – weak digestive activity,

Praseka – excess salivation,

Alasya – lassitude,

Gaurava – feeling of heaviness,

Shvaithya – white discoloration,

Shaithya – coldness,

Shlathangatva – looseness of the body parts,

Shwasa – dyspnoea, asthma, COPD,

Kasa – cough and

Atinidrata – excess of sleep.

Symptoms of increased body tissues – Vriddha Dhatu Lakshana:

Symptoms of increased Rasa dhatu – Rasa Dhatu Vriddhi Lakshana:

रसोऽपि श्लेष्मवत्

Rasa dhatu (nutritive fluid, essence of digestion, lymph) when increased, produces the same symptoms as that of increased sleshma (Kapha).

Symptoms of increased Rakta dhatu (blood) – Rakta Dhatu Vriddhi

Lakshana:

रक्तं विसर्पप्लीहविद्रधीन् ॥ ८ ॥
कुष्ठवातास्रपित्तास्रगुल्मोपकुशकामलाः ।
व्यङ्गाग्निनाशसम्मोहरक्तत्वइनेत्रमूत्रताः ॥ ९ ॥

Rakta (blood) when increased produces

Visarpa – Herpes, spreading skin disease,

Pleeha – diseases of the spleen,

Vidradhi – abscesses,

Kushta – skin diseases,

Vatasra – gout,

Pittasra - bleeding disease,

Gulma – abdominal tumours,

Upakusa – a disease of the teeth,

Kamala – jaundice,

Vyanga – discoloured patch on the face,

Agninasha – loss of digestion strength,

Sammoha – Coma, unconsciousness,

Rakta tvak netra mutrata - Red discoloration of the skin, eyes, and urine.

Symptoms of increased Mamsa dhatu (muscle) – Mamsa Dhatu Vriddhi Lakshana:

मांसं गण्डार्बुदग्रन्थिगण्डोरूदरवृद्धिधताः ।
कण्ठादिष्वधिमांसं च

Mamsa (muscle tissue), when increased produces

Ganda arbuda – cervical lymphadenitis, tumours,

Granthi – tumour, cysts,

Gandorudara vriddhi - Increase in size of the cheeks, thighs, and abdomen,

Kantadishu adhimamsam ca - excessive growth of muscles of the neck and other places.

Symptoms of increased Meda dhatu (fat) – Meda Dhatu Vriddhi Lakshana:

तद्वन्मेदस्तथा श्रमम् ॥ १० ॥ अल्पेऽपि चेष्टिते श्वासं स्फिक्स्तनोदरलम्बनम् ।

Medas (fat tissue), when increased produces similar symptoms and in addition, it causes

Shrama - fatigue,

Alpe api cheshtite swasam - difficulty in breathing even after little work,

Sphik stanodaralambanam - drooping of the buttocks, breasts and abdomen.

Symptoms of increased Asthi dhatu (bone) – Asthi Dhatu Vriddhi Lakshana:

अस्थ्यध्यस्थ्यधिदन्तांश्च

Asthi (bone tissue), when increased causes

Adhyasthi - overgrowth of bones and

Adhidanta - extra teeth.

Symptoms of increased Majja dhatu (bone marrow) – Majja Dhatu Vriddhi Lakshana:

मज्जा नेत्राङ्गगौरवम् ॥ ११ ॥ पर्वसु स्थूलमूलानि कुर्यात् कृच्छ्राण्यरूंषि च ।

Majja (marrow), when increased produces

Netra gauravam - heaviness of the eyes,

Anga gauravam – heaviness of the body,

Parvasu sthulamoolani - increase of size of the body joints and

Krichranyarumshi - ulcers which are difficult to cure.

Symptoms of increased Shukra dhatu (semen) – Shukra Dhatu Vriddhi Lakshana:

अतिस्त्रीकामतां वृद्धं शुक्रं शुक्राश्मरीमपि ॥ १२ ॥

Shukra (semen) when increased produces

Ati strikamatam - great sexual desire for the woman and

Shukrashmari - seminal calculi (spermolith).

Symptoms of increased waste products – Vriddha Mala Lakshanas:
Symptoms of increased Shakrt (Pureesha) – Shakrt Vriddhi Lakshana:

कुक्षावाध्मानमाटोपं गौरवं वेदनां शकृत् ।

Shakrit (faeces), when increased causes

Kukshavadhmanam - distension of abdomen,

Atopam - gurgling noise,

Gauravam - feeling of heaviness and

Vedanam – pain in the abdomen.

Symptoms of increased Mutra – Mutra Vriddhi Lakshana:

मूत्रं तु वस्तिनिस्तोदं कृतेऽप्यकृतसञ्ज्ञताम् ॥ १३ ॥

Mutra (urine), when increased produces

V(b)asti nistodam - severe pain in the bladder and

Krte apyakrta samjnatam - feeling of non-elimination even after urination.

Symptoms of increased Sweda – Sweda Vriddhi Lakshana:

स्वेदोऽतिस्वेददौर्गन्ध्यकण्डू

Sweda (sweat) when increased produces

Ati sweda - excess of perspiration,

Daurgandhya - foul smell and

Kandu - itching.

Symptoms of increased Kha Malas (waste substances produced by the nose, eye and ear) – Kha Mala Vriddhi Lakshana:

एवं च लक्षयेत् । दूषिकादीनपि मलान् बाहुल्यगुरुतादिभिः ॥ १४ ॥

The increase of Dushika (excretion of the eyes) and other waste products are to be understood by bahulya (their increased quantity), guruta (heaviness of their sites) and such other symptoms.

Symptoms of decreased Doshas – Ksheena Dosha Lakshana:
Symptoms of decreased Vata – Vata Kshaya Lakshana:

लिङ्गं क्षीणेऽनिलेऽङ्गस्य सादोऽल्पं भाषितेहितम् ।

सञ्ज्ञामोहस्तथा श्लेष्मवृद्ध्युक्तामयसम्भवः ॥ १५ ॥

Decreased Vata produces symptoms like –

Angasada – debility of the body,

Alpam bhashite hitam – the person speaks very little,

Sanjna moha – loss of awareness and consciousness and

Occurrence of all the symptoms of increased Kapha.

Symptoms of decreased Pitta – Pitta Kshaya Lakshana:

पित्ते मन्दोऽनलः शीतं प्रभाहानिः

Decreased Pitta causes

Mando anala – weakness of digestive activity,

Sheetam – coldness and

Prabha hani – loss of lustre / complexion.

Symptoms of decreased Kapha – Kapha Kshaya Lakshana:

कफे भ्रमः । श्लेष्माशयानां शून्यत्वं हृद्द्रवः श्लथसन्धिता ॥ १६ ॥

Decrease of Kapha causes

Bhrama – delusion, dizziness,
Sleshmashayanam shunyatva – emptiness of the organs of Kapha,
Hrudrava –palpitations and
Shlatha sandhita – looseness of the joints.

Symptoms of decrease of Dhatus – Dhatu Kshaya Lakshana:
Symptoms of decreased Rasa Dhatu – Rasa Kshaya Lakshana:
रसे रौक्ष्यं श्रमः शोषो ग्लानिः शब्दासहिष्णुता ।
Decrease of Rasa Dhatu produces
Raukshya - dryness,
Shrama - fatigue,
Shosha - emaciation,
Glani - exhaustion without any work and
Shabda asahishnuta - noise intolerance.

Symptoms of decreased Rakta dhatu – Rakta Kshaya Lakshana:
रक्तेऽम्लशिशिरप्रीतिसिराशैथिल्यरूक्षताः ॥ १७ ॥
Decrease of Rakta produces
Amla shishira preeti - desire for sour and cold things,
Sira shaitilya - loss of tension of blood vessels and
Rukshata - dryness.

Symptoms of decreased Mamsa dhatu – Mamsa Kshaya Lakshana:
मांसेऽक्षग्लानिगण्डस्फिक्शुष्कतासन्धिवेदनाः
Decrease of Mamsa causes
Aksha glani - debility of the sense organs,
Ganda sphik shushkata - emaciation of cheeks, buttocks and
Sandhi vedana - pain in the joints.

Symptoms of decreased Meda dhatu – Meda Kshaya Lakshana:
मेदसि स्वपनं कट्याः प्लीहनो वृद्धिः कृशाङ्गता ॥ १८ ॥
Decrease of Medas causes
Svapanam katyah - loss of sensation in the waist,
Pleehno vriddhi - enlargement of spleen and
Krishangata - emaciation of the body.

Symptoms of decreased Asthi dhatu – Asthi Kshaya Lakshana:

अस्थ्न्यस्थितोदः शदनं दन्तकेशनखादिषु ।

Decrease of Asthi causes

Asthi toda - pain in the joints,

Shadanam danta kesha nakhadishu - falling off of the teeth, hairs, nails etc.

Symptoms of decreased Majja dhatu – Majja Kshaya Lakshana:

अस्थ्नां मज्जानि सौषिर्यं भ्रमस्तिमिरदर्शनम् ॥ १९ ॥

Decrease of Majja causes

Saushiryam - hollowness (of the bones inside),

Bhrama - giddiness and

Timira darshanam - darkness in front of the eyes.

Symptoms of decreased Shukra dhatu – Shukra Kshaya Lakshana:

शुक्रे चिरात् प्रसिच्येत शुक्रं शोणितमेव वा ।

तोदोऽत्यर्थं वृषणयोर्मेढ्रं धूमायतीव च ॥ २० ॥

Decrease of Shukra results in

Chirat prasichyate - delay in ejaculation,

Shukram shonitameva va - ejaculation accompanied with bleeding,

Todo atyartham vrsanayo - severe pain in the testicles and

Medhram dhumayativa ca - a feeling of hot fumes coming out of the penis (urethra).

Symptoms of decreased waste products – Mala Kshaya Lakshana:
Symptoms of decreased Pureesha (faeces) – Pureesha Kshaya Lakshana:

पुरीषे वायुरान्त्राणि सशब्दो वेष्टयन्निव ।

कुक्षौ भ्रमति यात्यूर्ध्वं हृत्पार्श्वे पीडयन् भृशम् ॥ २१ ॥

Decrease of faeces gives rise to

Vayurantrani sashabdo veshtayanniva - gurgling noise in the intestines and bloating.

The vata moves around and travels in the upward direction (urdhvam) in the intestine causing discomfort and pain in the region of the hrit (heart) and parshva (flanks).

Symptoms of decreased Mutra (urine) – Mutra Kshaya Lakshana:

मूत्रेऽल्पं मूत्रयेत् कृच्छ्रादिववर्णं सास्रमेव वा ।

Decrease of urine causes

Alpam mutrayet - scanty urination,

Krichrat - dysuria,
Vivarnam - urine discoloration or
Sasrameva va - hematuria.

Symptoms of decreased Sweda (sweat) – Sweda Kshaya Lakshana:
स्वेदे रोमच्युतिः स्तब्धरोमता स्फुटनं त्वचः ॥ २२ ॥
Decrease of sweat leads to
Roma chyuti - falling of hair,
Stabdha romata - stiffness of hair and
Sphutanam tvacha - cracking of the skin.

Symptoms of decrease of wastes of small quantities – Sukshma Mala Kshaya Lakshana:
मलानामतिसूक्ष्माणां दुर्लक्ष्यं लक्षयेत् क्षयम् ।
स्वमलायनसंशोषतोदशून्यत्वलाघवैः ॥ २३ ॥
Decrease of Malas which are of small quantities are difficult to perceive, it should be inferred by
Samshosha - dryness,
Toda - pricking pain,
Shunyatva - emptiness and
Laghavaih - lightness of Svamalayana (their respective sites of production and elimination).

Method of identifying Kshaya (decrease) and Vriddhi (increase) of Dosha, Dhatu and Mala:
दोषादीनां यथास्वं च विद्याद्वृद्धिक्षयौ भिषक् ।
क्षयेण विपरीतानां गुणानां वर्धनेन च ॥ २४ ॥
वृद्धिं मलानां सङ्गाच्च क्षयं चातिविसर्गतः ।
मलोचितत्वाद्देहस्य क्षयो वृद्धैस्तु पीडनः ॥ २५ ॥
The decrease of Dosha, Dhatu etc can be observed by the increase of opposite qualities.
The increase of Dosha Dhatu etc can be observed by the increase of similar qualities.
The increase of Malas is observed by their non-elimination (too much of waste product accumulation leading to obstruction) and their decrease by too much elimination in little quantities.
Since the body is accustomed to accumulation of waste products in the

intestines and bladder, the decreased formation of waste products is considered to be more troublesome in comparison to its increase.

Ashraya-Ashrayi Sambandha - Relationship between Dosha and Dhatu:

तत्रास्थीनि स्थितो वायुः पित्तं तु स्वेदरक्तयोः ।
श्लेष्मा शेषेषु तेनैषामाश्रयाश्रयिणामिथः ॥ २६ ॥
यदेकस्य तदन्यस्य वर्धनक्षपणौषधम् ।
अस्थिमारुतयोर्नैवं

Tatra asthani sthito vayuh - in the bones reside the Vata

Pittam tu sveda raktayo - Pitta resides in the sweat (sweda) and blood (rakta)

Sleshma sheseshu - kapha (shleshma) resides in the rest of the dhatus (tissues) and malas (waste products, other than those mentioned for Vata and Pitta)

Due to this reason, the doshas and dhatus are related mutually in ashraya ashrayi (abode and resident) relationship.

When one among the ashraya (tissues) and ashrayi (doshas) increases, the other one too increases; similarly if one decreases, the other too decreases.

This can be treated with the help of vardhana (increasing, when there is decrease) and kshapana (decreasing when there is increase).

Asthi marutayor naivam - but the above rule is not applicable in case of asthi (bone) and vata. If vata decreases, then the asthi increases and when vata increases, the asthi decreases.

Cause of increase and decrease of Dosha, their treatment:

प्रायो वृद्धिर्हि तर्पणात् ॥ २७ ॥
श्लेष्मणानुगता तस्मात् सङ्क्षयस्तद्विपर्ययात् ।
वायुनानुगतास्माच्च वृद्धिःक्षयसमुद्भवान् ॥ २८ ॥
विकारान् साधयेच्छीघ्रं क्रमाल्लङ्घनबृंहणैः ।
वायोरन्यत्र तज्जांस्तु तैरेवोत्क्रमयोजितैः ॥ २९ ॥

The increase of Doshas, Dhatus and Mala is usually due to excess nutrition (tarpana), which is followed later on with increase of Kapha.

The decrease of Doshas, Dhatus and Mala is due to kshaya (loss of nutrition) which is followed, later with increase of Vayu (Vata).

Hence, the diseases arising from increase of Dosha and Dhatu should be usually treated quickly by adopting Langhana (therapies causing thinning of the body).

The diseases arising from the decrease of Dosha and Dhatu should be treated with Brimhana therapy (nourishing therapies).

But in the case of Vata, the order is reversed. If Vata is increased, then Brihmana therapy should be adopted and if Vata decreases then Langhana therapy should be adopted.

Specific treatments for diseases due to increase and decrease of Dhatus and Mala:

विशेषाद्रक्तवृद्ध्युत्थान् रक्तसुतिविरेचनैः ।
मांसवृद्धिभवान् रोगान् शस्त्रक्षाराग्निकर्मभिः ॥ ३० ॥

Diseases arising from increase of blood should be treated by

Raktasruti - bloodletting and

Virechana – purgation.

Diseases caused due to increase of muscle tissue should be treated with the help of

Shastrakarma - sharp instruments (surgery),

Ksharakarma – use of caustic alkalis and

Agnikarma - fire cautery.

स्थौल्यकार्श्योपचारेण मेदोजानस्थिसङ्क्षयात् ।
जातान् क्षीरघृतैस्तिक्तसंयुतैर्वस्तिभिस्तथा ॥ ३१ ॥

Diseases caused by increase and decrease of fat (meda) should be treated by therapies indicated for sthoulya (obesity) and karshya (emaciation) respectively.

Diseases caused by decrease of bone tissue should be treated by basti (enema therapy) prepared with ksheera (milk), grita (ghee) and tikta (bitter) drugs.

Treatment for diseases due to increase of Majja (bone marrow) and Shukra (reproductive fliud, semen):

मज्जशुक्रोद्भवान् रोगान् भोजनैः स्वादुतिक्तकैः ।
वृद्धं शुक्रं व्यवायाद्यैर् यच्चान्यच्छुक्रशोषिकम् ॥ ३१+१ ॥

Majja and Shukra Dhatu related disorders should be treated with foods predominant in Svada (sweet) and Tikta (bitter) rasa.

Increase of Shukra Dhatu can by managed by vyavaya (sexual intercourse) or with herbs to dry up excess shukra (Shukra Shoshikam)

Treatment for diseases due to increase and decrease of Purisha (faeces):

विड्वृद्धिधजानतीसारक्रियया विट्क्षयोद्भवान् ।
मेषाजमध्यकुल्माषयवमाषद्वयादिभिः ॥ ३२ ॥

Diseases caused by the increase of faeces should be treated on the lines of atisara (diarrhea).

Diseases caused by decrease of feces should be treated by the use of abdominal viscera of mesha (ram / sheep) or aja (goat), kulmasha (half steamed pulses), yava (barley) and masha dvaya (two varieties of black gram) etc. for food.

Treatment for increase and decrease of Mutra (urine) and decrease of Sweda (sweat):

मूत्रवृद्धिधक्षयोत्थांश्च मेहकृच्छ्रचिकित्सया ।
व्यायामाभ्यञ्जनस्वेदमद्यैः स्वेदक्षयोद्भवान् ॥ ३३ ॥

Increase and decrease of mutra (urine) should be treated by adopting the treatments indicated for meha (urinary disorders, diabetes) and krichra (dysuria) respectively.

Diseases caused due to decrease of sweda (sweat) should be treated by adopting

Vyayama - physical exercises,

Abhyanjana - oil bath (massage),

Sweda - sudation therapies and

Madya - use of wine.

Relation of Kayagni with increase and decrease of Dhatu:

स्वस्थानस्थस्य कायाग्नेरंशा धातुषु संश्रिताः ।
तेषां सादातिदीप्तिभ्यां धातुवृद्धिधक्षयोद्भवः ॥ ३४ ॥
पूर्वो धातुः परं कुर्यादवृद्धः क्षीणश्च तद्विधम् ।

Located (present) in its own seat (place), the kayagni or the fire in the body has portions of itself located in the dhatu (tissues) also.

The decrease and increase of these agnis or fires (located in the tissues) will lead to Dhatu vriddhi (increase of tissues) and dhatu kshaya (decrease of the tissues) respectively.

When the purva dhatu (preceding tissue) gets increased, it also increases the succeeding dhatu (example, if rasa dhatu increases, it subsequently leads to increase of rakta dhatu).

Similarly, when the preceding tissue decreases, it also decreases the succeeding tissue.

Effects of vitiated Doshas – Dushta Dosha Karmani:

दोषा दुष्टा रसैर्धातून् दूषयन्त्युभये मलान् ॥ ३५ ॥

अधो द्वे सप्त शिरसि खानि स्वेदवहानि च ।

मला मलायनानि स्युर्यथास्वं तेष्वतो गदाः ॥ ३६ ॥

The doshas which are vitiated by unmethodical consumption of rasas (tastes) further vitiate the tissues. Later, these two (the vitiated doshas and dhatus) together vitiate the malas (waste products).

The vitiated malas (waste products) in turn vitiate the malayanas (channels of elimination of waste products) among which

Adho dve - two are located in the lower portion of the body (anus and urethra),

Sapta shirasi - seven are located in the head (2 in eyes, 2 in ears, 2 nostrils and 1 mouth) and

Khani svedavahani ca - the channels of sweat are innumerable and located all throughout the body.

From these vitiated channels develop many diseases related to the channels.

Ojas – The essence of the tissues:

ओजस्तु तेजो धातूनां शुक्रान्तानां परं स्मृतम् ।

हृदयस्थमपि व्यापि देहस्थितिनिबन्धनम् ॥ ३७ ॥

स्निग्धं सोमात्मकं शुद्धं ईषल्लोहितपीतकम् ।

यन्नाशे नियतं नाशो यस्मिन् तिष्ठति तिष्ठति ॥ ३८ ॥

निष्पद्यन्ते यतो भावा विविधा देहसंश्रयाः ।

Ojas is the essence of the Dhatus;

It is mainly located in the hridaya (heart). It is present all over the body and regulates health.

Qualities of Ojas –

Snigdha – unctuous, oily,

Somatmaka – watery,

Shuddha – clear,

Ishat Lohita Peetakam – slight reddish yellow in colour;

Loss of Ojas leads to loss of life.

All aspects of health are related to Ojas.

Causes of decrease of Ojas – Ojo Kshaya Karanani:

ओजः क्षीयते कोपक्षुद्ध्यानशोकश्रमादिभिः ॥ ३९ ॥
बिभेति दुर्बलोऽभीक्ष्णं ध्यायति व्यथितेन्द्रियः ।
दुश्छायो दुर्मना रूक्षो भवेत् क्षामश्च तत्क्षये ॥ ४० ॥
जीवनीयौषधक्षीररसाद्यास्तत्र भेषजम् ।

Causes for decrease of Ojas:

Ojas undergoes decrease in quantity by

Kopa - anger,

Kshut - hunger (starvation),

Dhyana - worry,

Shoka - grief,

Shrama - exertion etc.

Symptoms of decrease of Ojas:

The person presents with the following symptoms -

Bibheti - becomes fretful,

Durbalam - debilitated,

Abhikshnam dhyayati - repeatedly worries without any reason,

Vyathitendriyah - feels discomfort in sense organs,

Duhchayo - develops bad complexion,

Durmana - negative thoughts and

Ruksha – dryness.

Treatment for decrease of Ojas:

Use of drugs of Jivaniya group, ksheera (milk), rasa (meat juice) etc.

Increase of Ojas – Ojo Vriddhi:

ओजोविवृद्धौ देहस्य तुष्टिपुष्टिबलोदयः ॥ ४१ ॥

Increase of Ojas brings about

Tushti - contentment,

Pushti - nourishment of the body and

Bala - increase of strength.

Method of food consumption to combat Dosha increase and decrease:

यदन्नं द्वेष्टि यदपि प्रार्थयेताविरोधि तु ।
तत्त्यजन्समश्नञ्च तौ तौ वृद्धिक्षयौ जयेत् ॥ ४२ ॥

The foods that are disliked should be rejected, and the foods which are desired should be consumed, taking care that the foods are avirodhi (not opposite to the qualities of doshas).

The above mentioned 2 measures will control the vriddhi (increase) and kshaya (decrease) of the doshas respectively.

कुर्वते हि रुचिं दोषा विपरीतसमानयोः ।
वृद्धाः क्षीणाश्च भूयिष्ठं लक्षयन्त्यबुधान तत् ॥ ४३ ॥

The doshas which have undergone vriddhi (increase) and ksheena (decrease) will generally produce a desire for foods which are viparita (dissimilar) and samana (similar) in properties to those of the doshas respectively, but the unintelligent person does not recognize them.

Behaviour of doshas when they are increased decreased and balanced:
यथाबलं यथास्वं च दोषावृद्धा वितन्वते ।
रूपाणि जहति क्षीणाः समाः स्वं कर्म कुर्वते ॥ ४४ ॥

The doshas which have undergone vriddha (increase) will produce their respective signs and symptoms according to their strength (less, moderate or severe vitiation),

The ksheena (decreased) doshas do not produce their respective features and

The sama (balanced) doshas will attend to their normal functions.

Reason for protecting the normalcy of Doshas:
य एव देहस्य समा विवृद्ध्यै त एव दोषा विषमावधाय ।
यस्मादतस्ते हितचर्ययैव क्षयादिववृद्धेरिव रक्षणीयाः ॥ ४५ ॥

The very same doshas, which when sama (balanced), are the cause for growth of the body, when vishama (abnormal), will become the cause for vadha (destruction) of the body.

Hence, by adopting suitable measures, the body should be protected from kshaya (decrease) and vivriddhi (increase) of doshas.

इति श्री वैद्यपतिसिंहगुप्तसूनु वाग्भटविरचितायां अष्टाङ्गहृदय संहितायां सूत्रस्थाने
दोषादिविज्ञानीयो नाम एकादशोऽध्यायः ।

Thus ends the 11th chapter of Ashtangahridaya Samhita Sutrasthana, named Doshadi Vijnaneeya Adhyaya, written by Shrimad Vagbhata, son of Shri Vaidyapati Simhagupta.

12

दोषभेदीयाध्यायम् (doshabhediya adhyayam)

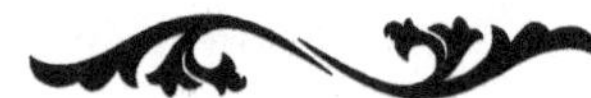

The 12th chapter of Sutrasthanam of Ashtanga Hridayam is named Dosha bhediyaAdhyayam. This chapter explains about the dosha types and location of tridoshas in the body. The classification and functions of each type of tridosha, the causes for their increase or decrease etc are also dealt with in this chapter.

अथातो दोषभेदीयमध्यायं व्याख्यास्याम: इति ह स्माहुरात्रेयादयो महर्षय: ।
Atreya and other sages pledge that they would henceforth be explaining the chapter called Dosha BhediyaAdhyayam (the chapter that deals with the explanation of doshas, their types, imbalance of doshas and the symptoms of their imbalance).

Places of Vata Dosha:
पक्वाशयकटीसक्थिश्रोत्रास्थिस्पर्शनेन्द्रियम्‌|
स्थानं वातस्य, तत्रापि पक्वाधानं विशेषत:॥१॥
The sites of Vata Dosha are –
Pakavasaya – large intestine,
Kati – waist,
Sakthi – hip,
Shrotra – ear,

Asthi – bones,
Sparshanendriya – skin.
Visheshasthana (important / special space) – Pakvashaya – large intestine.

Places of Pitta Dosha:
नाभिरामाशयः स्वेदो लसीका रुधिरं रसः|
दृक् स्पर्शनं च पितस्य, नाभिरत्र विशेषतः||२||
The sites of Pitta Dosha are –
Nabhi – Umbilicus,
Amashaya– stomach and small intestine,
Sweda – sweat,
Lasika– lymph,
Rudhira – blood,
Rasa– plasma,
Druk – eye,
Sparshanam – skin,
Visheshasthana (important / special space) – Nabhi – Umbilicus.

Places of Kapha Dosha:
उरःकण्ठशिरःक्लोमपर्वाण्यामाशयो रसः|
मेदो घ्राणं च जिह्वा च कफस्य, सुत्रामुरः||३||
The sites of Kapha Dosha are –
Ura – Chest,
Kantha – throat,
Shira – head,
Kloma – Pancreas,
Parvani – bone joints,
Amashaya – Stomach and small intestine,
Rasa –plasma,
Meda – fat,
Ghrana – nose and
Jihva – tongue
Visheshasthana (important / special space) – Uras – chest.

Five types of Vayu:
प्राणादिभेदात्पञ्चात्मा वायुः
Vayu (vata) is of 5 types –

Prana Vata
Udana Vata
Vyana Vata
Samana Vata
Apana Vata

Prana Vata – Its sites, functions:

प्राणोऽत्र मूर्धगः|

उरःकण्ठचरो बुद्धिहृदयेन्द्रियचित्तधृक्||४||

ष्ठीवनक्षवथूद्गारनिःश्वासान्नप्रवेशकृत्|

Prana is located in the murdha (head) and moves in the uras (chest) and kanta (throat).
It regulates
Buddhi – will,
Hridaya – heart,
Indriya – sense organs,
Chitta – intellect and
Drik – vision.
It is the cause for
Shteevana – expectoration,
Kshavathu – sneezing,
Udgara – belching,
Niswasa – exhaling / respiration and
Anna pravesha – swallowing of food.

Udana Vata – Its sites, functions:

उरः स्थानमुदानस्य नासानाभिगलांश्चरेत्||५||

वाक्प्रवृत्तिप्रयत्नोर्जाबलवर्णस्मृतिक्रियः|

The uras (chest) is the seat of Udana Vata, it moves in the nasa (nose), nabhi (umbilicus) and gala (throat).
Its functions are
Vakpravritti – initiation of speech,
Prayatana – effort,
Urja – enthusiasm,
Bala – strength,
Varna – colour, complexion and
Smruti – memory.

Vyana Vata – Its sites, functions:

व्यानो हृदि स्थितः कृत्स्नदेहचारी महाजवः||६||

गत्यपक्षेपणोत्क्षेपनिमेषोन्मेषणादिकाः|

प्रायः सर्वाः क्रियास्तस्मिन् प्रतिबद्धाः शरीरिणाम्||७||

Vyana is located in the hridaya (heart), moves all over the body with great speed,

It attends to functions such as

Gati – movement, locomotion,

Apakshepanotkshepa –flexion and extension,

Nimesha unmesha – opening and closing of the eyelids etc.

Generally sarva kriya (all the body activities) are regulated by Vyana Vata.

Samana Vata – Its sites, functions:

समानोऽग्निसमीपस्थः कोष्ठो चरति सर्वतः|

अन्नं गृह्णाति पचति विवेचयति मुञ्चति||८||

Samana Vata is located near the digestive fire (agnisamipastha).

It moves in the Kostha (alimentary tract),

Its functions are –

Annam grhnati – receives the food into stomach,

Pachati – aids in digestion,

Vivechayati – helps in dividing the food into useful part and waste part and

Munchati – excretes the waste part.

Apana Vata – Its sites, functions:

अपानोऽपानगः श्रोणिबस्तिमेढ्रोरुगोचरः|

शुक्रार्तवशकृन्मूत्रगर्भनिष्क्रमणक्रियः||९||

Apana Vata is located in the Apana (large intestine), moves in the shroni (waist), basti (bladder), medhra (genitals) and uru (thighs).

It attends to the functions such as nishkramana (expulsion) of

Shukra – semen / reproductive fluid,

Artava – menstrual blood,

Shakrit – faeces,

Mutra – urine and

Garbha – child birth.

Five types of Pitta:

पित्तं पञ्चात्मकम्
Pitta is of five types –
Pachaka Pitta
Ranjaka Pitta
Sadhaka Pitta
Alochaka Pitta
Bhrajaka Pitta

Pachaka Pitta – Its sites, functions:

तत्र पक्वामाशयमध्यगम्|
पञ्चभूतात्मकत्वेऽपि यत्तैजसगुणोदयात्||१०||
त्यक्तद्रवत्वं पाकादिकर्मणाऽनलशब्दितम्|
पचत्यन्नं विभजते सारकिट्टौ पृथक् तथा||११||
तत्रस्थमेव पित्तानां शेषाणामप्यनुग्रहम्|
करोति बलदानेन पाचकं नाम तत्स्मृतम्||१२||

Pachaka pitta is located between pakvashaya (large intestine) and amashaya (stomach).

It is composed of all the five basic elements (PanchamahaBhuta), is predominant of teja (fire) element and devoid of drava (water) element.

It is called by the term Anala (fire) because of its function of Paka (digestion) and transformation of food materials.

Its functions are –

Pachatiannam – digests the food,

Vibhajate sara kittauprthaktatha – divides it into essence and waste parts,

Karotianugraham – It bestows grace and influence on other types of Pitta by providing bala (strength) to them.

Hence, among all the types of Pitta, Pachaka pitta is the dominant one.

Ranjaka Pitta – Its sites, functions:

आमाशयाश्रयं पित्तं रञ्जकं रसरञ्जनात्|

The Pitta located in the Amashaya (stomach) is known as Ranjaka since it imparts colour (ranjana) to the rasa – the essence part of digestion (and converts it into rakta – blood).

Sadhaka Pitta – Its sites, functions:

बुद्धिमेधाभिमानाद्यैरभिप्रेतार्थसाधनात्||१३|| साधकं हृद्गतं पित्तं

The pitta located in the Hrudaya (heart) is known as Sadhaka Pitta.

It attends to mental functions such as
Buddhi – knowledge,
Medha – intelligence,
Abhimana – self–consciousness / self respect etc,
thereby helping to attain the purpose of life.

Alochaka Pitta – Its sites, functions:
रूपालोचनतः स्मृतम्| दृक्स्थमालोचकं
The Pitta located in the eyes is called Alochaka pitta,
It helps in vision. (Lochana means eyes, vision).

Bhrajaka Pitta – Its sites, functions:
त्वक्स्थं भ्राजकं भ्राजनात्त्वचः||१४||
Brajaka Pitta resides in skin and helps exhibition of colour and complexions.

Five Types of Kapha:
श्लेष्मा तु पञ्चधा
Shleshma (kapha) is of five types –

Avalambaka Kapha
Kledaka Kapha
Bodhaka Kapha
Tarpaka Kapha
Shleshaka Kapha

Avalambaka Kapha – Its sites, functions:
उरःस्थः स त्रिकस्य स्ववीर्यतः|
हृदयस्यान्नवीर्याच्च तत्स्थ एवाम्बुकर्मणा||१५||
कफधाम्नां च शेषाणां यत्करोत्यबलम्बनम्|
अतोऽवलम्बकः श्लेष्मा
Avalambaka Kapha is located in the Uras (chest) and Trika (the meeting place of shoulder, neck and back).
By its swavirya (innate strength) and by the annavirya (power of essence of food), it nourishes the hridaya (heart).
By the virtue of its functions similar to those of water (like lubrication, nourishment etc), Avalambakakapha supports the other sites of kapha and hence is called avalambakashleshma.

(Word meaning of Avalamba is dependent.)

KledakaKapha – sites, functions:

यस्त्वामाशयसंस्थितः||१६||
क्लेदकः सोऽन्नसङ्घातक्लेदनात्

KledakaKapha is located in the Amasaya (stomach). It moistens (kledana) the hard food mass (anna sanghata).

Bodhaka Kapha – It's sites, functions:

रसबोधनात्| बोधको रसनास्थायी

BhodakaKapha is located in rasana (tongue). It helps in taste perception.

TarpakaKapha – Its sites, functions:

शिरःसंस्थोऽक्षतर्पणात्||१७|| तर्पकः

TarpakaKapha is located in the shira (head). It does tarpana (nourishment) of the aksha (sense organs).

Sleshaka Kapha – its sites, functions:

सन्धिसंश्लेषाच्छ्लेषकः सन्धिषु स्थितः|

Shleshakakapha is located in the sandhi (bone joints) and it lubricates and strengthens (samsleshat) the joints (sandhi).

Specific seats of Dosha predominance:

इति प्रायेण दोषाणां स्थानान्यविकृतात्मनाम्||१८||
व्यापिनामपि जानीयात्कर्माणि च पृथक्पृथक्|

Though the non–vitiated doshas are spread out all over the body, the above–mentioned seats should be considered by the physician as the specific seats in which they are predominant.

Qualities that cause Chaya, Kopa and Shamana of Vata:

उष्णेन युक्ता रूक्षाद्या वायोः कुर्वन्ति सञ्चयम्||१९||
शीतेन कोपमुष्णेन शमं स्निग्धादयो गुणाः|

Chaya (mild increase or accumulation) – means increase of dosha in its own place or seat;

Kopa/Prakopa (profound increase or aggravation) – means increase and overflow of doshas from its own place to the other places;

Shama / Prashama (reduction) – means decrease of increased dosha and restoration of normalcy and health.

Ushna (heat) associated with ruksha (dryness) etc qualities of Vata cause sanchaya or chaya of vata;
Sheeta (cold) associated with ruksha (dryness) etc qualities of Vata cause kopa of vata;
Ushna (heat) associated with snigdha (unctuousness) etc qualities (opposite to those of vata) cause shamana of vata.

Qualities that cause chaya, kopa and shamana of Pitta:

शीतेन युक्तास्तीक्ष्णाद्याश्चयं पितस्य कुर्वते॥२०॥
उष्णेन कोपं, मन्दाद्याः शमं शीतोपसंहिताः।

Piercing (strong) and other qualities of pitta (like heat, lightness etc) when associated with sheeta (cold), will cause chaya of pitta;
Piercing (strong) and other qualities of pitta (like heat, dryness, lightness etc) when associated with ushna (heat),will cause kopa of pitta;
Viscous (mild) and other qualities opposite to that of pitta (like stickiness, stability etc) when associated with sheeta (cold) will bring about pitta shamana.

Qualities that cause chaya, kopa and shamana of Kapha:

शीतेन युक्ताः स्निग्धाद्याः कुर्वते श्लेष्मणश्चयम्॥२१॥
उष्णेन कोपं, तेनैव गुणा रूक्षादयः शमम्।

Snigdha (unctuousness) and other Kapha qualities (like heaviness, stickiness, mild etc) when associated with sheeta (cold), causes chaya of shleshma;
Snigdha (unctuousness) and other qualities similar to the qualities of kapha (like heaviness, stickiness, mild etc) when associated with ushna (hot),causes kopa of shleshma;
The same qualities (unctuous etc) when associated with ruksha (dryness) etc qualities (roughness, lightness, movement, clarity etc) cause Shamana of Kapha.

Levels of Dosha Increase and Decrease:

चयो वृद्धिः स्वधाम्न्येव प्रद्वेषो वृद्धिहेतुषु॥२२॥
विपरीतगुणेच्छा च कोपस्तून्मार्गगमिता।
लिङ्गानां दर्शनं स्वेषामस्वास्थ्यं रोगसम्भवः॥२३॥

स्वस्थानस्थस्य समता विकारासम्भवः शमः।

Chaya means slight increase of Dosha in its own place.

It produces

Pradvesha – dislike against the things that would cause further increase of that particular Dosha and

Vipareetagunecha – liking towards substances with qualities opposite to the aggravated dosha.

Kopa is the stage where the doshas increase excessively and overflow into other body channels. It causes the appearance of symptoms of increased Dosha, leading to onset of roga (disease process).

Shama means the state of normalcy of doshas without causing any vikara (disease).

Fluctuations of dosha in different seasons:

चयप्रकोपप्रशमा वायोर्ग्रीष्मादिषु त्रिषु॥२४॥

वर्षादिषु तु पित्तस्य, श्लेष्मणः शिशिरादिषु।

Vata –

Chaya – grishma (summer),

Prakopa – varsha (rainy season) and

Prashama – sharat (autumn)

Pitta –

Chaya – varsha (rainy season),

Prakopa – sharat (autumn) and

Prashama – hemanta (early winter)

Kapha –

Chaya – shishira (winter),

Prakopa – vasanta (spring) and

Prashama – grishma (summer).

Causes for fluctuation of Dosha in different seasons:

चीयते लघुरूक्षाभिरोषधीभिः समीरणः॥२५॥

तद्विधस्तद्विधे देहे कालस्यौष्ण्यान्न कुप्यति।

Vata undergoes chaya (mild increase and accumulation) during summer by the use of plants possessing qualities such as laghu (lightness), ruksha (dryness) etc.

It is especially so in the bodies of persons possessing such qualities.

During grishma (summer), Vata does not undergo a profound increase due to the ushna (heat) of the kala (season).

अद्भिरम्लविपाकाभिरोषधीभिश्च ताद्दशम्||२६||
पित्तं याति चयं कोपं न तु कालस्य शैत्यतः|

Pitta undergoes chaya (mild increase and accumulation) in varsha (rainy) season, because of production of amla viplaka (sour taste at the end of digestion) by the use of such water and foods.

But it does not undergo prakopa (aggravation) in the rainy season, because of shaitya (coldness) of the kala (season).

चीयते स्निग्धशीताभिरुदकौषधिभिः कफः||२७||
तुल्येऽपि काले देहे च स्कन्नत्वान्न प्रकुप्यति|

Kapha undergoes chaya (mild increase and accumulation) in shishira (winter) by the use of water and foods possessing snigdha (oily) and sheeta (cold) properties.

But it does not undergo prakopa (aggravation) because Kapha undergoes skannatva (solidification) due to severe cold of the winter.

Influence of seasonal and food variations on chaya, kopa and prashamana of Doshas:

इति कालस्वभावोऽयमाहारादिवशात्पुनः||२८||
चयादीन् यान्ति सद्योऽपि दोषाः कालेऽपि वा न तु|

The chaya, kopa and shamana of Vata, Pitta and Kapha take place under the influence of kala (seasonal effect) and also due to the effect of ahara (foods consumed).

Apart from this, the doshas may suddenly undergo chaya (increase), prakopa (aggravation) and shamana (pacification)even in the absence of favourable seasons for their increase or decrease.

Sometimes the doshas do not undergo chaya (increase), prakopa (aggravation) and shamana (pacification) in spite of the presence of favourable seasons.

Aggravation of doshas is fast, their decrease is slow:

व्याप्नोति सहसा देहमापादतलमस्तकम्||२९||
निवर्तते तु कुपितो मलोऽल्पाल्पं जलौघवत्|

The vitiated doshas quickly spread throughout the body from foot to head.

But the decrease of doshas and restoration of normalcy takes place very slowly,just like the floods (when flood occurs, the water gushes into the cities very fast, but the reversal process i.e. receding of the flood water is very slow).

Cause of dosha aggravation and disease formation:

नानारूपैरसङ्ख्येयैर्विकारैः कुपिता मलाः||३०||
तापयन्ति तनुं तस्मात्तद्धेत्वाकृतिसाधनम्|
शक्यं नैकैकशो वक्तुमतः सामान्यमुच्यते||३१||

The aggravated doshas trouble the body by causing nanarupa (different forms) and asankhye (innumerable types) of vikara (diseases). Therefore it is not possible to individually explain their causes, symptoms and treatments and so they have been generalized.

Doshas are the main causes for all the diseases:

दोषा एव हि सर्वेषां रोगाणामेककारणम्|
यथा पक्षी परिपतन् सर्वतः सर्वमप्यहः||३२||
छायामत्येति नात्मीयां यथा वा कृत्स्नमप्यदः|
विकारजातं विविधं त्रीन् गुणान्नातिवर्तते||३३||
तथा स्वधातुवैषम्यनिमित्तमपि सर्वदा|
विकारजातं त्रीन्दोषान्

The Doshas alone are always the sole causative factors for all diseases.
Just like a pakshi (bird) which keeps flying everywhere, throughout the day cannot escape from its own chaya (shadow), just like the different species of creation without any exclusions, cannot be separated from the trigunas (i.e. sattva, raja and tama), similarly the diseases in spite of getting manifested due to the disturbance of related tissues (swa dhatu vaishamya) can never be separated from the three Doshas.

Three kinds of causes for Dosha increase:

तेषां कोपे तु कारणम्||३४||
अर्थैरसात्म्यैः संयोगः कालः कर्म च दुष्कृतम्|
हीनातिमिथ्यायोगेन भिद्यते तत्पुनस्त्रिधा||३५|||

The causes for dosha increase are –
Asatmya indriya artha samyoga – wrong (improper) contact of sense organs with their respective sense objects,
Asatmya kala – contamination of seasons (abnormal seasonal variations) and

Asatmya karma – wrong deeds.

This is again of three types –

Hinayoga – less or deficit involvement of sense objects, manifestation of seasons and indulgence in actions,

Atiyoga – excessive involvement of sense objects, manifestation of seasons and indulgence in actions and

Mithyayoga – wrong (erratic, perverted) contact of sense objects, manifestation of seasons and indulgence in actions.

Artha Hinayoga, Atiyoga and Mithya yoga – deficit, excessive and perverted contact of the senses with their sense organs:

हीनोऽर्थनेन्द्रियस्याल्पः संयोगः स्वेन नैव वा|

अतियोगोऽतिसंसर्गः, सूक्ष्मभासुरभैरवम्||३६||

अत्यासन्नातिदूरस्थं विप्रियं विकृतादि च|

यदक्ष्णा वीक्ष्यते रूपं मिथ्यायोगः स दारुणः||३७||

एवमत्युच्चपूत्यादीनिन्द्रियार्थान् यथायथम्|

विद्यात्

Hina yoga (poor association) means insufficient contact or absence of contact of the sense objects (sound, touch, sight, taste and smell) with their corresponding sense organs (ear, skin, eye, tongue and nose respectively).

Atiyoga (over indulgence) means excessive contact of the sense objects with their respective sense organs.

Mithya yoga (wrong indulgence) means perverted union of sense objects with their respective sense organs like –

Gazing at the objects which are sukshma (very minute), bhasura (very bright) and bhairavam (frightful),

looking at objects which are atyasanna (very near) or atidoora (very far), objects which are vipriyam (disliked) and vikrita (abnormal) etc.

All these constitute Mithyayoga which are harmful.

Similarly, listening to atyucha (loud sounds), poothyadi (perceiving foul smells) and other perverted perceptions of sense organs should be likewise understood as examples of Mithya yoga.

Kala Hinayoga, Atiyoga and Mithyayoga – Its deficit, excessive and perverted manifestation:

कालस्तु शीतोष्णवर्षाभेदात्त्रिधा मतः||३८||

स हीनो हीनशीतादिरतियोगोऽतिलक्षणः|

मिथ्यायोगस्तु निर्दिष्टो विपरीतस्वलक्षणः।

Seasons are of three kinds i.e. sheeta (cold), ushna (hot) and varsha (rainy),
Hina yoga of kala (deficit manifestation of season) is
less cold in winter,
less heat in summer and
less rain in rainy season.
Atiyoga of kala (excessive manifestation of season) is
more cold in winter,
more heat in summer and
more rain in the rainy season.
Mithyayoga of kala (perverted manifestation of season) is marked by manifestation of qualities opposite to the natural ones of the season, like rain in summer, heat in winter, cold in rainy season or summer etc.

Karma Hinayoga, Atiyoga and Mithyayoga – deficit, excessive and perverted indulgence in actions:

कायवाक्चित्तभेदेन कर्मापि विभजेत्त्रिधा।
कायादिकर्मणो हीना प्रवृत्तिर्हीनसंज्ञकः॥४०॥
अतियोगोऽतिवृत्तिस्तु, वेगोदीरणधारणम्।
विषमाङ्गक्रियारम्भपतनस्खलनादिकम्॥४१॥
भाषणं सामिभुक्तस्य रागद्वेषभयादि च।
कर्म प्राणातिपातादि दशधा यच्च निन्दितम्॥४२॥
मिथ्यायोगः समस्तोऽसाविह वाऽमुत्र वा कृतम्।

Karma (actions) are also classified into three types i.e.
kaya (physical, pertaining to body activities),
vak (speech, pertaining to speaking activities) and
chitta (mental, pertaining to mind activities).
Hina yoga of karma (deficit actions) is indulgence in very less physical activity, very less speaking and very less thought process.
Atiyoga of karma (excessive actions) is indulgence in excessive physical activities, excessive speaking and thinking.
Mithyayoga of kayika karma (perverted physical activities) includes –
forceful expulsion and suppression of natural urges,
improper postures (doing activities with weird body postures),
and activities like abrupt falling, abrupt jumping etc
Mithyayoga of vachika karma (perverted speech action) includes –
Speaking too much while taking food or immediately after food.

Mithyayoga of manasika karma (perverted mind actions) includes – harbouring of desires, hatred, fear etc.

Committing the ten forbidden heinous actions in the present world or the world hereafter etc constitutes Mithyayoga of Karma.

Manifestation of diseases pertaining to viscera, tissues and vital organs:

निदानमेतद्दोषाणां, कुपितास्तेन नैकधा||४३||

कुर्वन्ति विविधान् व्याधीन् शाखाकोष्ठास्थिसन्धिषु|

These are the causes for the increase of Doshas. The doshas thus increased, produce many kinds of diseases, involving the shaka (tissues), koshta (viscera), asthi (bones) and sandhi (joints).

Bahi Koshta / Bahi (bahya) Rogamarga – The external pathway of diseases:

शाखा रक्तादयस्त्वक् च बाह्यरोगायनं हि तत्||४४||

तदाश्रया मषव्यङ्गगगण्डालज्यर्बुदादयः|

बहिर्भागाश्च दुर्नामगुल्मशोफादयो गदाः||४५||

Rakta (blood) and others tissues (muscles, bone, fat, bone marrow and sex related secretions) and twak (skin) constitute the BahyaRogamarga – external pathway of diseases.

It is related with diseases such as

Masha – moles,

Vyanga – discoloured patches on face,

Gandalaji– goitre, glandular ulcer on the face,

Arbuda – malignant tumours,

and externally manifested (bahirbhagascha)

Durnama – haemorrhoids,

Gulma – abdominal tumour,

Shophadi – swelling and other external diseases.

Anta Koshta / Anta Rogamarga – The internal pathway of diseases:

अन्तःकोष्ठो महास्रोत आमपक्वाशयाश्रयः|

तत्स्थानाः च्छद्र्यतीसारकासश्वासोदरज्वराः||४६||

अन्तर्भागं च शोफार्शोगुल्मवीसर्पविद्रधि|

Amashaya (stomach and small intestine), Pakvashaya (large intestine) along with the entire gastro intestinal tract is called Mahasrota (the big channel). This constitutes the Anta Koshta.

Diseases which affect this path are –
Chardi – vomiting,
Atisara – diarrhoea,
Kasa – cough,
Swasa – dyspnoea,
Udara – enlargement of the abdomen,
Jwara – fever,
and internally manifested (antarbhagam)
Shopha – oedema,
Arshas – haemorrhoids,
Gulma – abdominal tumours,
Visarpa – herpes, spreading skin diseases and
Vidradhi – abscess etc.

Madhyama Koshta / Madhyama Rogamarga – The middle pathway of diseases:

शिरोहृदयबस्त्यादिमर्माण्यस्थ्नां च सन्धयः||४७||
तन्निबद्धाः शिरास्नायुकण्डराद्याश्च मध्यमः|
रोगमार्गः स्थितास्तत्र यक्ष्मपक्षवधार्दिताः||४८||
मूर्धादिरोगाः सन्ध्यस्थित्रिकशूलग्रहादयः|

Shira – head,
Hridaya – heart,
Bastyadimarmani – urinary bladder and such other vital organs,
Asthnam sandhi – joints of bones,
Sira – blood vessels,
Snayu – tendons,
Kandara – ligaments etc
constitute the Madhyama rogamarga.
From it arise,
Yakshma – tuberculosis,
Pakshavadha – hemiplegia,
Ardita – facial paralysis,
Murdhadiroga – diseases of the head and other organs,
Shoola (pain), graha (stiffness) of sandhi (joints), asthi (bones), trika (sacral region) etc.

Symptoms of increase of Vata:

स्रंसव्यासव्यधस्वापसादरुक्तोदभेदनम्||४९||
सङ्गाङ्गभङ्गसङ्कोचवर्तहर्षणतर्षणम्|
कम्पपारुष्यसौषिर्यशोषस्पन्दनवेष्टनम्||५०||
स्तम्भः कषायरसता वर्णः श्यावोऽरुणोऽपि वा|
कर्माणि वायोः

The following are the abnormal signs and symptoms of increased Vata –
Sramsa – drooping down (ptosis),
Vyasa – dilation,
Vyadha – cutting pain,
Swapa – loss of sensation,
Sada – weakness, loss of function,
Ruk – pain,
Toda – continuous pain,
Bhedanam – splitting pain,
Sanga – constriction,
Angabhanga – body ache,
Sankocha – shrinking of the organ, reduction in size,
Varta – twisting,
Harshana – tingling sensation,
Tarshana – thirst,
Kampa – tremors,
Parushya – roughness,
Saushirya – feeling of emptiness,
Shosha – dryness,
Spandana – pulsating pain,
Veshtana – rigidity, as if tied,
Sthambha – stiffness,
Kashaya rasata – astringent taste in mouth,
ShyavaAruna Varna – appearance of blue or crimson discoloration.

Symptoms of increase of Pitta:
पित्तस्य दाहरागोष्ममपाकिताः||५१||
स्वेदः क्लेदः स्रुतिः कोथः सदनं मूर्च्छनं मदः|
कटुकाम्लौ रसौ वर्णः पाण्डुरारुणवर्जितः||५२||
The following are the symptoms of increased Pitta –
Daha – burning sensation,
Raga – reddish discoloration,

Ushmapakita – heat, increase in temperature, formation of pus, ulcers,

Sveda – sweating,

Kleda – excessive moistness,

Sruti – inflammation with pus / oozing / secretions,

Kotha – putrefaction– decomposition,

Sadana – debility,

Murchana – fainting,

Mada– toxicity,

Katuka Amla Rasa – pungent and sour taste in the mouth,

Varna panduarunavarjitaha – appearance of colours other than yellowish white and crimson.

Symptoms of increase of Kapha:

श्लेष्मणः स्नेहकाठिन्यकण्डूशीतत्वगौरवम्|

बन्धोपलेपस्तैमित्यशोफापक्त्यतिनिद्रताः||५३||

वर्णः श्वेतो रसौ स्वादुलवणौ चिरकारिता|

The following are the symptoms of Kapha increase –

Sneha – unctuousness, oiliness,

Katinya – hardness,

Kandu – itching,

Sheetatva – coldness,

Gaurava – heaviness,

Bandha – obstruction,

Upalepa – coating, as if tied with a wet cloth,

Staimitya – stiffness, loss of movement,

Shopha – inflammation,

Apakti – indigestion,

Atinidrata – excessive sleep,

Shveta varna – white discolouration,

Svadulavana rasa – sweet, salt taste in mouth,

Chirakarita – delay in all activities.

इत्यशेषमयव्यापि यदुक्तं दोषलक्षणम्||५४||

दर्शनाद्यैरवहितस्तत्सम्यगुपलक्षयेत्|

व्याध्यवस्थाविभागज्ञः पश्यन्नार्तान् प्रतिक्षणम्||५५||

Thus, the above said symptoms of all the doshas should be properly learnt by darshana (inspection) and other measures of examination of the patient by a physician who is attentive, who knows the different stages of diseases,after observing the patients every moment.

अभ्यासात्प्राप्यते दृष्टिः कर्मसिद्धिप्रकाशिनी|
रत्नादिसदसज्ज्ञानं न शास्त्रादेव जायते||५६||

By abhyasa (constant practice), the karmasiddhi (practical knowledge and experience) is gained, which would reflect in the success of treatment just like the knowledge of identifying ratna (gems, gold, precious stones etc) will not be obtained just by theoretical knowledge.

Three kinds of diseases based on the cause:
दृष्टापचारजः कश्चित्कश्चित्पूर्वापराधजः|
तत्सङ्कराद्भवत्यन्यो व्याधिरेवं त्रिधा स्मृतः||५७||

The diseases are said to be of three types,

Kaschitdrishtapacharajah – some are due to misdeeds done in the present life,

Kaschitpoorvaparadhaja –some occur due to the misdeeds done previously (in previous life)

Tatsankaradbhavatyanyo – and some manifest due to combination of both the above said factors.

यथानिदानं दोषोत्थः कर्मजो हेतुभिर्विना|
महारम्भोऽल्पके हेतावातङ्को दोषकर्मजः||५८||

Doshaja vyadhis (drishtapacharaja) are those diseases which get manifested due to the doshas (which are aggravated due to the causative factors which vitiate them).

Karmaja vyadhis (purvaparadhaja, adrushtaja) are those diseases which get manifested without the involvement of any causative factors.

Dosha karmaja vyadhis are diseases which get manifested with severe and profound symptoms in spite of minimum vitiating factors (caused due to mixed factors i.e. causative factors of a disease and misdeeds done previously).

विपक्षशीलनात्पूर्वः कर्मजः कर्मसङ्क्षयात्|
गच्छत्युभयजन्मा तु दोषकर्मक्षयात्क्षयम्||५९||

Doshaja vyadhis get cured by indulgence in food, activities and medicines which have opposite qualities to the causes of the disease.

Karmaja vyadhis get cured after the termination of the effects of acts or misdeeds done in previous lives.

Dosha–karmaja diseases get cured after the mitigation of doshas along with nullifying the effects of misdeeds done in previous life.

Swatantra (independent/primary) and Paratantra (dependent/secondary) types of diseases:

द्विधा स्वपरतन्त्रत्वाद्व्याधयोऽन्त्याः पुनर्द्विधा।

Diseases are again of two types; they are

Swatantra (independent / primary) and

Paratantra (dependent / secondary) diseases.

The second type of disease (paratantra) is again of two types.

Classification of Paratantra (dependent/secondary) Roga:

पूर्वजाः पुर्वरूपाख्या, जाताः पश्चादुपद्रवाः||६०||

Purvajavyadhis are also called as purvarupas (premonitory symptoms which manifest before the manifestation of the actual disease) and

Paschatjatavyadhis are manifested after the formation of the disease and are also called upadravas (complications of a disease).

Definition of Swatantra or primary disease:

यथास्वजन्मोपशयाः स्वतन्त्राः स्पष्टलक्षणाः।

Swatantra vyadhi (independent, primary disease) are those which have

Svajanma – their own specific causes, due to which they get manifested,

Svaupashaya – their own comforting remedies which when administered will cure those diseases and

Spashtalakshana – clearly manifested signs and symptoms which are specific to those diseases.

Definition of Paratantra or secondary disease:

विपरीतास्ततोऽन्ये तु

Paratantravyadhi (secondary disease) are those that will have opposite features as that of Swatantra vyadhi (primary disease).

Swatantra and Paratantra Doshas:

विद्यादेवं मलानपि||६१||
तांल्लक्षयेदवहितो विकुर्वाणान् प्रतिज्वरम्।

Similarly, the doshas will also have swatantra (independent, primary) and paratantra (dependent, secondary) types of manifestation.

An attentive physician should understand this by observation with presence of mind.

Treatment of Paratantravyadhis and doshas:

तेषां प्रधानप्रशमे प्रशमोऽशाम्यतस्तथा||६२||

पश्चाच्चिकित्सेत्पूर्णं वा बलवन्तमुपद्रवम्|

व्याधिक्लिष्टशरीरस्य पीडाकरतरो हि सः||६३||

Paratantra (secondary) diseases subside when the pradhana or swatantra (primary disease) disease is pacified.

The paratantra (secondary) diseases which do not get subsided in spite of the treatment of primary disease should be treated independently after the treatment of the primary disease, considering it as an independent disease.

Immediate treatment should be administered if the upadrava (complications) are very powerful because these complications will cause more trouble to the body which is already debilitated by the disease.

विकारनामाकुशलो न जिह्रीयात् कदाचन|

न हि सर्वविकाराणां नामतोऽस्ति ध्रुवा स्थितिः||६४||

The physician who does not know the nama (names) of all the diseases should never feel shy about it, because all the diseases do not have a definitive and fixed name.

Factors to be considered to treat diseases:

स एव कुपितो दोषः समुत्थानविशेषतः|

स्थानान्तराणि च प्राप्य विकारान् कुरुते बहून्||६५||

तस्मादि्वकारप्रकृतीरधिष्ठानान्तराणि च|

बुद्ध्वा हेतुविशेषांश्च शीघ्रं कुर्यादुपक्रमम्||६६||

The very same vitiated dosha (doshas), depending upon the nature of their causative factors,on reaching the different parts of the body, will produce many vikara (diseases),

Therefore, the upakrama (treatment) of the disease should be done quickly, after knowing the

Vikara prakriti – main doshas causing the disease,

Adhishtana antarani – various parts of the body in which the vitiated doshas have caused the disease and

Hetu vishesha – specific causes for vitiation of doshas.

Factors to observe in the patient:
दूष्यं देशं बलं कालमनलं प्रकृतिं वयः|
सत्त्वं सात्म्यं तथाऽऽहारमवस्थाश्च पृथग्विधाः||६७||
सूक्ष्मसूक्ष्माः समीक्ष्यैषां दोषौषधनिरूपणे|
यो वर्तते चिकित्सायां न स स्खलति जातुचित्||६८||
The physician should minutely examine and determine –
Dushya – the Dhatus and Malas involved in a diseases,
Desha – the area of the body where disease is manifested, the living place of
the patient,
Bala – strength of the patient,
Kala– season, how old is the disease, age of the person etc.,
Anala– digestive power of the patient,
Prakriti– body constitution,
Vayas– age of the patient and disease,
Satva– mind, tolerance capacity of the patient,
Satmya– The food and activities to which the patient is accustomed to,
Ahara– food habits and
Avastha– stages of the disease.
The physician should watch for the above factors and then should decide
on the aggravated Dosha and its appropriate treatment. Such a doctor will
never commit mistakes in treatment.

Guru Vyadhi and Laghu Vyadhi (strong and weak disease):
गुर्वल्पव्याधिसंस्थानं सत्त्वदेहबलाबलात्|
दृश्यतेऽप्यन्यथाकारं तस्मिन्ननवहितो भवेत्||६९||
Depending on the bala (strength) and abala (weakness) of the satva (mind)
and deha (body), the symptoms of guru vyadhi (strong disease) and alpa
vyadhi (weak disease) may appear in a contrasting way, hence the physician
should be very attentive.

गुरुं लघुमिति व्याधिं कल्पयंस्तु भिषग्ब्रुवः|
अल्पदोषाकलनया पथ्ये विप्रतिपद्यते||७०||
An unintelligent physician who diagnoses a guru vyadhi (severe, grievous
disease) as a laghuvyadhi (weak, mild disease) goes wrong in treatment
because he considers the doshas to be alpa (less quantity of dosha

aggravation) in a grievous disease (in which there is actually severe aggravation of doshas).

Effect of wrongly diagnosing grievous disease as mild disease and vice versa:

ततोऽऽल्पमल्पवीर्यं वा गुरुव्याधौ प्रयोजितम्|
उदीरयेतरां रोगान् संशोधनमयोगतः||७१||
शोधनं त्वतियोगेन विपरीतं विपर्यये|
क्षिणुयान्न मलानेव केवलं वपुरस्यति||७२||

Thus, when medicines in less quantity (alpam) and less potency (alpaveeryam) are administered in guru vyadhi (severe disease), it will lead to worsening of disease because of ayogasamshodhanam (deficit, ineffective cleansing).

In the opposite condition i.e. in a feeble or weak disease, if medicines and treatment in more quantity and more potency are administered,they will not only destroy the morbid doshas, but will also cause excessive destruction of the body because of atiyogenashodhanam (excessive cleansing).

Right approach of a determined physician towards comprehensive treatment:

अतोऽभियुक्तः सततं सर्वमालोच्य सर्वथा|
तथा युञ्जीत भैषज्यमारोग्याय यथा ध्रुवम्||७३||

Hence, the physician who is constantly engaged and committed towards learning the science should determine the exact condition of all the factors (involved in the causation of a disease) and analyze everything in all ways and at all times and later should administer the treatment as needed for the sake of proper health.

Number of permutations and combinations of Doshas – Dosha Samyoga Samkhya:

वक्ष्यन्तेऽतःपरं दोषा वृद्धिक्षयविभेदतः|

After this, we are going to explain the permutations and combinations of dosha vriddhi (increase) and kshaya (decrease).

Permutations and combinations of Doshas:

पृथक् त्रीन् विद्धि संसर्गस्त्रिधा तत्र तु तान्नव||७४||

त्रीनेव समया वृद्ध्या षडेकस्यातिशायने।
त्रयोदश समस्तेषु षड् द्व्येकातिशयेन तु ॥७५॥
एकं तुल्याधिकैः षट् च तारतम्यविकल्पनात्।
पञ्चविंशतिमित्येवं वृद्धैः क्षीणैश्च तावतः ॥७६॥
(In the below explanation,
vriddhi = increase,
vriddhitara = more or moderate increase,
vriddhitama = severe increase)
Considering the vriddhi (increase) of Doshas, they are –
Eka Dosha Vriddhi (Single dosha increase) is of 3 types:
– Vata Vriddhi
– Pitta Vriddhi
– KaphaVriddhi

Samsarga, Dvi Dosha Vriddhi (two dosha increase) is of 9 types:

a. 3 types of increase in equal proportions –
– Vata–pitta vriddhi
– Vata–kaphavriddhi
– Pitta–kaphavriddhi

b. 6 types with preponderance of one dosha –
– Vata vriddhi–Pitta vriddhitaram
– Pitta vriddhi–Vata vriddhitaram
– Kaphavriddhi–Pitta vriddhitaram
– Pitta vriddhi–Kaphavriddhitaram
– Kaphavriddhi–Vata vridhhitaram
– Vata vriddhi–Kaphavriddhitaram

Sannipata, Tri Dosha Vriddhi (three dosha increase) is of 13 types:
a. 6 types with preponderance of any one dosha –
– Vata vriddhi–Pitta KaphaAtivriddhi
– Pitta vriddhi–Vata KaphaAtivridddhi
– Kaphavriddhi–Vata Pitta Ativriddhi
– Vata Ativriddhi–Pitta KaphaVriddhi
– Pitta Ativriddhi–Vata KaphaVriddhi
– KaphaAtivriddhi–Vata Pitta Vriddhi

b. 1 type with preponderance of all three doshas –
– Vata–Pitta–KaphaVriddhi

c. 6 types by disproportionate subdivisions –
– Vata vriddhi–Pitta vriddhitara–Kaphavriddhitama
– Vata vriddhi–Kaphavriddhitara–Kaphavriddhitama
– Pitta vriddhi–Kaphavriddhitara–Vata vriddhitama
– Pitta vriddhi–Vata vriddhitara–Kaphavriddhitama
– Kaphavriddhi–Vata vriddhitara–Pitta vriddhitama
– Kaphavriddhi–Pitta vriddhitara–Vata vriddhitama

Thus, the vriddhi of doshas is only of 25 types. Similarly the decrease of doshas is also of 25 types.

Other types of combinations of doshas:
एकैकवृद्धिसमताक्षयैः षट् ते पुनश्च षट्।
एकक्षयद्वन्द्ववृद्ध्या सविपर्ययया॑पि ते ॥७७॥
भेदा द्विषष्टिर्निर्दिष्टाः त्रिषष्टः स्वास्थ्यकारणम् ।
(In the below explanation –
vriddhi = increase,
sama = normalcy,
kshaya = decrease)

Increase, normalcy and decrease of one dosha each is of 6 types, they are –

– Vata vriddhi–Pitta sama–Kapha kshaya
– Pitta vriddhi–Vata sama–Kapha kshaya
– Kaphavriddhi–Pitta sama–Vata kshaya
– Kaphavriddhi–Vata sama–Pitta kshaya
– Vata vriddhi–Kaphasama–Pitta kshaya
– Pitta vriddhi–Kaphasama–Vata kshaya

In the combination of one dosha decrease and two dosha increase, and two dosha decrease and one dosha increase, they are once again of 6 types.

Decrease of 1 dosha and increase of two doshas is of 3 types, they are –

– Vata kshaya–Pitta Kapha vriddhi
– Pitta kshaya–Vata Kapha vriddhi
– Kaphakshaya–Vata Pitta vriddhi

Decrease of 2 doshas and increase of 1 dosha is of 3 types, they are –
– Vata Pitta kshaya–Kaphavriddhi
– Vata Kaphakshaya–Pitta vriddhi
– Pitta Kaphakshaya–Vata vriddhi

Thus 62 types of combination of dosha increase and decrease have been explained.

The 63rd is the condition where all the three doshas are in equilibrium, which is called as the state of health.

Permutations and combinations of doshas and dhatus are innumerable:

संसर्गादिरसरुधिरादिभिस्तथैषां दोषांस्तु क्षयसमताविवृद्धिभेदैः |
आनन्त्यं तरतमयोगतश्च यातान् जानीयादवहितमानसो यथास्वम्॥७८॥

Different levels of decrease, normalcy and increase of doshas when associated with rasa, rakta and other tissues, can result in innumerable permutations and combinations.

The physician should understand them by their features with anattentive mind.

इति श्रीवैद्यपतिसिंहगुप्तसूनुवाग्भटविरचितायां अष्टाङ्गहृदयसंहितायां सूत्रस्थाने दोषभेदीयो नाम द्वादशोऽध्यायः ॥

Thus ends the 12th chapter of Ashtangahridaya Samhita Sutrasthana, named DoshabhediyaAdhyaya, written by Shrimad Vagbhata, son of Shri VaidyapatiSimhagupta.

13
दोषोपक्रमणीयमध्यायम्‌ (doshopakramaniyam adhyayam)

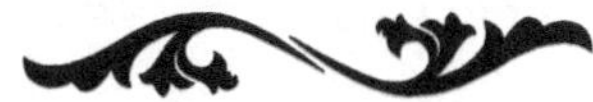

The 13th chapter of Sutrasthanam of Ashtanga Hridayam is Doshopakramaniyam Adhyayam. This chapter explains treatment options to combat dosha imbalance. The concept of ama, the way in which the doshas combine with ama to produce disease symptoms and the ways of treating these conditions, time of administration of medicines based on the disease are also explained in this chapter.

अथातो दोषोपक्रमणीयमध्यायं व्याख्यास्यामः इति ह स्माहुरात्रेयादयो महर्षयः ।
Atreya and other sages pledge that they will henceforth explain the chapter named Doshopakramaniyam (pertaining to treatment of Dosha imbalance).

Treatment for increased Vata – Vriddha Vata Chikitsa:
वातस्योपक्रमः स्नेहः स्वेदः संशोधनं मृदु ।
स्वाद्वम्ललवणोष्णानि भोज्यान्यभ्यङ्गमर्दनम्‌ ॥ १ ॥
वेष्टनं त्रासनं सेको मद्यं पैष्टिकगौडिकम्‌ ।
स्निग्धोष्णा वस्तयो वस्तिनियमः सुखशीलता ॥ २ ॥
दीपनैः पाचनैः सिद्धाः स्नेहाश्चानेकयोनयः ।
विशेषान्मेद्यपिशित रसतैलानुवासनम्‌ ॥ ३ ॥
The treatment for increased Vata includes -
Sneha – oleation,

Sveda – sudation,

Mrudu Samshodhana – mild purification procedures,

Svadu Amla Lavana Bhojya – foods which are of sweet, sour and salt taste,

Ushna Bhojya – foods that are hot,

Abhyanga – oil massage,

Mardana – mild massage,

Veshtana – binding / bandaging with cloth,

Trasana – frightening,

Seka – pouring of herbal decoctions / oils on the affected part,

Paishtika Goudika Madya – wine prepared from corn flour and jaggery (molasses),

Snigdha Ushna Basti – enema therapy which is unctuous, enema prepared with drugs of hot potency,

Bastiniyama – habitual use of enema,

Sukhasheelata – comforting the patient,

Deepana Pachana Siddha Sneha – medicated fats prepared with drugs causing increase of hunger and improving digestion,

Medya Pishita rasa – intake of meat and meat soup which is nourishing,

Taila – use of oil,

Anuvasana – oil enema.

Treatment for increased Pitta – Vriddha Pitta Chikitsa:

पित्तस्य सर्पिषः पानं स्वादुशीतैर्विरेचनम् ।

स्वादुतिक्तकषायाणि भोजनान्यौषधानि च ॥ ४ ॥

सुगन्धिशीतहृद्यानां गन्धानामुपसेवनम् ।

कण्ठेगुणानां हाराणां मणीनामुरसा धृतिः ॥ ५ ॥

कर्पूरचन्दनोशीरैरनुलेपः क्षणे क्षणे ।

प्रदोषश्चन्द्रमाः सौधं हारि गीतं हिमोऽनिलः ॥ ६ ॥

अयन्त्रणसुखं मित्रं पुत्रः सन्दिग्धमुग्धवाक् ।

छन्दानुवर्तिनो दाराः प्रियाः शीलविभूषिताः ॥ ७ ॥

शीताम्बुधारागर्भाणि गृहाण्युद्यानदीर्घिकाः ।

सुतीर्थविपुलस्वच्छ सलिलाशयसैकते ॥ ८ ॥

साम्भोजजलतीरान्ते कायमाने द्रुमाकुले ।

सौम्या भावाः पयः सर्पिर्विरेकश्च विशेषतः ॥ ९ ॥

The treatment for increased Pitta includes -

Sarpi paana – drinking of Ghrita (ghee),

Svadu, sheeta virechana – purgation therapy with drugs of sweet taste and cold potency,

Svadu, tikta kashayani bhojanani aushadhani - Intake of foods and drugs having sweet, bitter and astringent tastes,

Sugandhi gandhanam upasevanam - Inhaling of fumes from herbs that are sheeta (coolant) and hridya (pleasant and cordial),

Anulepa - Anointing the body with karpura (camphor), chandana (sandalwood paste), ushira (vetiver) paste, very frequently.

Pradosha chandrama saudham - Residing on terraces lit by moonlight in the evenings,

Hari gitam - enjoying pleasant music and

Himo anila - soft cold breeze,

Ayantranam sukham mitram - company of friends who do not restrain him / her,

Putra sandigdhamugdhavak - of sons who speak cordially and with innocence.

Spending time with dara (wife), who is obedient, pleasing and virtuous;

Residing in griha (houses) equipped with sheetambu dhara (fountains emitting cooled water), parks and ponds,

Spending time in houses near water reservoirs having clean water, sand, lotus, flowers, and trees, with a calm mind;

Consuming paya (milk), sarpi (ghee) and

Virechana - Purgation therapy.

Treatment for increased Kapha – Vriddha Kapha Chikitsa:

श्लेष्मणो विधिना युक्तं तीक्ष्णं वमनरेचनम् ।
अन्नं रूक्षाल्पतीक्ष्णोष्णं कटुतिक्तकषायकम् ॥ १० ॥
दीर्घकालस्थितं मद्यं रतिप्रीतिः प्रजागरः ।
अनेकरूपो व्यायामश्चिन्ता रूक्षं विमर्दनम् ॥ ११ ॥
विशेषाद्वमनं यूषः क्षौद्रं मेदोघ्नमौषधम् ।
धूमोपवासगण्डूषा निःसुखत्वं सुखाय च ॥ १२ ॥

The treatment for increased Kapha includes -

Teekshna Vamana Virechana – Strong emesis and purgation,

Annam ruksha - Consuming food which are dry,

Alpa - Consuming food in limited quantity,

Consuming food that have Teekshna (strong, penetrating), Ushna (hot),

Katu tikta kashayakam - pungent, bitter and astringent taste,

Deerga kala sthitam madyam - old wine,

Ratipreeti – sexual activity,

Prajagarah - keeping awake at night,

Aneka roopo vyayama - exercises of different kinds,

Chinta - Worry,

Ruksham vimardanam - dry massage of the body,

Vamana – emesis therapy,

Yusha - drinking of soups prepared using grains,

Kshaudra - Use of honey,

Medognam aushadham - Therapies and medicines that reduce fat,

Dhuma - Inhalation of medicinal smoke,

Upavasa - Fasting,

Gandusha – Gargling,

Nishukhatvam - Facing difficulties.

Treatment for simultaneous increase of two doshas (samsarga) and three doshas (sannipata):

उपक्रमः पृथग्दोषान् योऽयमुद्दिश्य कीर्तितः ।

संसर्गसन्निपातेषु तं यथास्वं विकल्पयेत् ॥ १३ ॥

ग्रैष्मः प्रायो मरुत्पित्ते वासन्तः कफमारुते ।

मरुतो योगवाहित्वात् कफपित्ते तु शारदः ॥ १४ ॥

The different treatment prescribed for each Dosha individually, may be combined appropriately in conditions of combinations of two Doshas (samsarga) or three Doshas (sannipata).

Generally the treatment for the combination of Vata and Pitta is similar to the regimen of Grishma (summer).

For Kapha and Vata combination, the treatment is similar to the regimen of Vasanta (spring) because Maruta (Vata) is Yogavahi (it means, Vata, when associated with Pitta, boosts Pitta Dosha, when it is associated with Kapha, it boosts Kapha Dosha).

For the combination of Kapha and Pitta the treatment shall be similar to the regimen of Sarad (autumn).

Dosha Treatment as per level of aggravation:

चय एव जयेद्दोषं कुपितं त्वविरोधयन् ।

सर्वकोपो बलीयांसं शेषदोषाविरोधतः ॥ १५ ॥

The Doshas should be treated properly when they are in Chaya stage (stage of mild increase / accumulation) only.

In their stage of Kopa (Dosha aggravation), they should be vanquished without interfering with another Dosha.

When there is sarvakopa (simultaneous increase of all the three Doshas), the most aggravated Dosha should be controlled first, without opposing the remaining Doshas.

Shuddha Chikitsa - pure treatment:

प्रयोगः शमयेद्व्याधिं योऽन्यमन्यमुदीरयेत् ।
नासौ विशुद्धः शुद्धस्तु शमयेद्यो न कोपयेत् ॥ १६ ॥

The treatment which cures one disease but gives rise to another disease is not a pure treatment.

A pure treatment is that which cures one disease but does not give rise to another.

Movement of Doshas from Koshta (digestive tract) to Shakha (tissues):

व्यायामादूष्मणस्तैक्ष्ण्यादहिताचरणादपि ।
कोष्ठाच्छाखास्थिमर्माणि द्रुतत्वान्मारुतस्य च ॥ १७ ॥

By the effect of

Vyayama - exercise,

Ushmana: taikshnyat - increase of body heat,

Ahita charanat - unhealthy activities and

Drutatvat marutasya - due to quick movement of Vata,

the increased Doshas move out of the Kostha (gastrointestinal tract) to the Shakha (tissues), Asthi (bones) and Marmas (vital organs and vulnerable points).

Movement of Doshas from Shakha (tissues) to Koshta (digestive tract):

दोषा यान्ति तथा तेभ्यः स्रोतोमुखविशोधनात् ।
वृद्ध्यभिष्यन्दनात् पाकात् कोष्ठं वायोश्च निग्रहात् ॥ १८ ॥
तत्रस्थाश्च विलम्बेरन् भूयो हेतुप्रतीक्षिणः ।
ते कालादिबलं लब्ध्वा कुप्यन्तान्याश्रयेष्वपि ॥ १९ ॥

Doshas move from body channels and tissues to the gastrointestinal tract, by the effect of

Shrotomukha vishodhanat - purification, clearing and widening of the minute body channels,

Vriddhi - by further increase of Doshas,

Abhishandanat - by liquefaction,

Pakat - by maturity,

Vayoscha nigrahat - by balancing and controlling Vata.

When Doshas move from one place to another, they remain there for some time, waiting for an exciting factor. After deriving strength by kala (season) etc, they get further aggravated and move to other places as well.

Native (Sthayi) and foreign (Agantu) doshas:

तत्रान्यस्थानसंस्थेषु तदीयामबलेषु तु ।

कुर्याच्चिकित्सां स्वामेव बलेनान्याभिभाविषु ॥ २० ॥

आगन्तुं शमयेद्दोषं स्थानिनं प्रतिकृत्य वा ।

For the abala (weak) doshas which have travelled into anyasthana (the sites of other doshas), treatment should be done for the local dosha (sthanika or sthayi dosha).

In case of doshas which have the capacity to dominate i.e. for strong doshas which have travelled into other sites, treatment for these strong doshas should be administered.

The foreign (agantu) dosha should be treated either after treating the native dosha (sthanika) or even otherwise.

Tiryak gata dosha (obliquely placed doshas):

प्रायस्तिर्यग्गता दोषाः क्लेशयन्त्यातुरांश्चिरम् ॥ २१ ॥

कुर्यान्न तेषु त्वरया देहाग्निबलवित् क्रियाम् ।

शमयेत् तान् प्रयोगेण सुखं वा कोष्ठमानयेत् ॥ २२ ॥

ज्ञात्वा कोष्ठप्रपन्नांश्च यथासन्नं विनिर्हरेत् ।

The tiryak gata doshas cause troubles to the atura (patient) for a long time (chira),

In these conditions, the physician knowing the deha bala (strength of the body) and agni bala (digestive activity) should not do the treatment in a hurry.

They should be mitigated with stipulated palliative treatment (shamana) or should be brought into the koshta (alimentary tract) without causing much trouble.

After knowing that the doshas have come into the alimentary tract, they should be expelled out by the nearby route (through mouth in the form of emesis - vamana or by anal route, by purgation - virechana).

Sama dosha lakshanas – Symptoms of doshas associated with ama:

स्रोतोरोधबलभ्रंशगौरवानिलमूढताः ॥ २३ ॥
आलस्यापक्तिनिष्ठीव मलसङ्गारुचिक्लमाः ।
लिङ्गं मलानां सामानां निरामाणां विपर्ययः ॥ २४ ॥

When imbalanced Doshas get associated with Ama (factor of indigestion), it is called as Sama Dosha. (Sa ama Dosha, Sa means 'with').

The features that are seen due to Sama Dosha are -

Srotorodha - Obstruction of the channels, pores,

Balabhramsha – loss of strength,

Gaurava – feeling of heaviness of the body,

Anila Moodata – inactivity of Anila (vata),

Alasya – laziness, lassitude,

Apakti – loss of digestive power,

Nishteeva – Person spits saliva frequently, more of expectoration,

Malasanga – constipation or low frequency of urination leading to accumulation of wastes,

Aruchi – anorexia,

Klama – exhaustion.

The features of Nirama Doshas (Doshas not mixed up with the Ama) are opposite to the above symptoms.

Features of Nirama Doshas (Doshas not associated with Ama):
विण्मूत्रनखदन्तत्वक्चक्षुषां पीतता भवेत् ।
रक्तत्वमथ कृष्णत्वं पृष्ठास्थिकटिसन्धिरुक् ॥ २४१+१ ॥
शिरोरुक् जायते तीव्रा निद्रा विरसता मुखे ।
क्वचिच्च श्वयथुर्गात्रे ज्वरातीसारहर्षणम् ॥ २४१+२ ॥

The symptoms of Doshas not associated with Ama are -

Peetatvam (yellowish), raktatvam (reddish) or krishnatvam (bluish black) discolouration of vit (faeces), mutra (urine), nakha (nails), danta (teeth), tvak (skin) and chakshu (eyes),

Prishta asthi kati sandhi ruk – Pain in the hip, bones, low back and joints

Teevra shiroruk – severe headache,

Nidra – sleep,

Virasata mukhe – odd taste in mouth,

Shvayathu gatre – oedema,

Jwara – fever,

Atisara – diarrhoea,

Harshanam – horripilation.

Definition of Ama and its formation:

ऊष्मणोऽल्पबलत्वेन धातुमाद्यमपाचितम् ।
दुष्टमामाशयगतं रसमामं प्रचक्षते ॥ २५ ॥

Due to lack of digestion strength (ushmano alpa bala), the adya dhatu (first dhatu i.e. Rasa Dhatu) does not form well, it remains in raw (apachitam) state. It gets vitiated (dushtam), stays in the Amashaya (stomach and intestines) itself, and becomes 'Ama'.

अन्ये दोषेभ्य: एवातिदुष्टेभ्योऽन्योऽन्यमूर्छनात् ।
कोद्रवेभ्यो विषस्येव वदन्त्यामस्य सम्भवम् ॥ २६ ॥

Other authors opine that just like visha (poison) develops in stored Kodrava (kodo millet), the mixing of greatly increased doshas with one another leads to the formation of Ama.

Definition of Sama:

आमेन तेन सम्पृक्ता दोषा दूष्याश्च दूषिताः ।
सामा इत्युपदिश्यन्ते ये च रोगास्तदुद्भवाः ॥ २७ ॥

The vitiated doshas and dushyas (dhatus and malas, i.e. tissues and excreta) when mixed or associated with ama, are called Sama (mixed with or associated with ama).
The diseases originating from these Sama doshas are called as Sama rogas.

Saama Vata Lakshana:

वायुः सामो विबन्धाग्निसादस्तम्भान्त्रकूजनैः ।
वेदनाशोफनिस्तोदैः क्रमशोऽङ्गानि पीडयन् ॥ २७+१ ॥
विचरेद् युगपच्चापि गृह्णाति कुपितो भृशम् ।
स्नेहाद्यैर्वृद्धिमायाति सूर्यमेघोदये निशि ॥ २७+२ ॥

The symptoms of Vata associated with Ama are as follows -
Vibhanda – obstruction to the passage of Vata,
Agnisada – loss of digestive power,
Stambha – stiffness,
Antrakujana – gurgling sound in the abdomen,
Vedana – pain,
Shopha – oedema,
Nisthoda – pricking type of pain,
Kramasho angani peedayan – gradual increase of body ache.

The symptoms increase by administering oils and fats (Sneha), during sunrise (Surya Udaya), when there are clouds in the sky (Meghodaya) and at night (Nishi).

Nirama Vata Lakshana:

निरामो विशदो रूक्षो निर्विबन्धोऽल्पवेदनः ।
विपरीतगुणैः शान्तिं स्निग्धैर्याति विशेषतः ॥ २७+३ ॥

The symptoms of Vata not associated with Ama are as follows -

Vishada – clarity,

Ruksha – dryness,

Nirvibandha – no obstruction to the path of Vata, no constipation, easy bowel movements,

Alpa vedana – mild pain,

Viparita gunaih shanti – opposite qualities provide relief,

Snigdhairyati visheshatah – especially snigdha guna (unctuousness) provides relief.

Saama Pitta Lakshana:

दुर्गन्धि हरितं श्यावं पित्तमम्लं घनं गुरु ।
अम्लीकाकण्ठहृद्दाहकरं सामं विनिर्दिशेत् ॥ २७+४ ॥

The sypmtoms of Pitta associated with Ama are as follows -

Durghandi – foul odour,

Haritam – greenish discolouration,

Shyavam – bluish discolouration,

Amlam – sour taste,

Ganam – thick,

Guru – heavy,

Amlika – sour belching,

Kanta hrit dahakaram – burning sensation in throat, chest region.

Nirama Pitta Lakshana:

आताम्रपीतमत्युष्णं रसे कटुकमस्थिरम् ।
पक्वं विगन्धि विज्ञेयं रुचिपक्तिबलप्रदम् ॥ २७+५ ॥

The symptoms of Pitta not associated with Ama are as follows -

Atamram – coppery coloured,

Peetam – yellowish,

Atyushnam – very hot,

Rase katukam – pungent taste,

Asthiram – unstable,

vigandhi – no bad smell,

Ruchi pakti balapradam – improves taste, digestion and strength.

Saama Kapha Lakshana:

आविलस्तन्तुलः स्त्यानः कण्ठदेशेऽवतिष्ठते ।
सामो बलासो दुर्गन्धिः क्षुदुद्गारविघातकृत् ॥ २७+६ ॥

The symptoms of Kapha associated with Ama are as follows -

Avilam – turbid,

Tantulam – thread like,

Styana – stagnant,

Kanta deshe avathishtathe – lodged in the throat,

Durghandi – foul odour,

Kshud udgara vighatakrit - lack of hunger and belching.

Nirama Kapha Lakshana:

फेनवान् पिण्डितः पाण्डुर्निःसारोऽगन्ध एव च ।
पक्वः स एव विज्ञेयश्छेदवान् वक्त्रशुद्धिधदः ॥ २७+७ ॥

The symptoms of Kapha not associated with Ama are as follows -

Phenavan – Kapha or saliva or sputum will be frothy

Pinditah – in a bolus shape

Pandu – pale coloured

Nisaro – not thick

Agandha – without smell

Chedavan – in small pieces

Vaktrashuddhitah – clarity of mouth.

Treatment of Saama Doshas (Doshas associated with Ama):

सर्वदेहप्रविसृतान् सामान् दोषान् न निर्हरेत् ।
लीनान् धातुष्वनुत्क्लिष्टान् फलादामाद्रसानिव ॥ २८ ॥
आश्रयस्य हि नाशाय ते स्युर्दुर्निर्हरत्वतः ।

The Sama Doshas which are

Sarva deha pravisrtan - spread all over the body,

Leenan dhatushu - which are stagnated (leena) in the Dhatus and

Anutklishtan - which are not moving out of their places of accumulation,

should not be forced out (na nirharet) by purification therapies like emesis, purgation etc.

Just as attempts of extracting juice from an unripe fruit (ama phala) leads to its destruction (nasha), the dwelling place (ashraya) itself will get destroyed if Doshas are tried to be expelled along with Ama.

Ama Chikitsa Sutra:

पाचनै: दीपनैः स्नेहैस्तान् स्वेदैश्च परिष्कृतान् ॥ २९ ॥

शोधयेच्छोधनैः काले यथासन्नं यथाबलम् ।

Sama Doshas should be treated

- first with drugs which are pachana (digestive) and deepana (which increase hunger),

- next with snehana (oleation) and svedana (sudation) therapies and

- finally they should be expelled out with Shodhana therapies- emesis, purgation at the proper time, and in accordance with the strength of the patient.

Passages from which the doshas are eliminated:

हन्त्याशु युक्तं वक्त्रेण द्रव्यमामाशयान् मलान् ॥ ३० ॥

घ्राणेन चोर्ध्वजत्रूत्थान् पक्वाधानाद्गुदेन तु ।

Medicines administered through the vaktra (mouth), expels out the doshas from stomach and small intestines (amashaya).

Medicines administered through the grana (nose) will expel the doshas from the urdhvajatru (parts above the shoulder i.e. head and neck),

Medicines administered through the guda (anus) will expel out the doshas from the pakvashaya (large intestine).

उत्क्लिष्टानध ऊर्ध्वं वा न चामान् वहतः स्वयम् ॥ ३१ ॥

धारयेदौषधैर्दोषान् विधृतास्ते हि रोगदाः ।

Greatly vitiated (utklishta) ama doshas going out of the body on their own accord, either in adha (downward) or urdhva (upward) routes should not be stopped by aushada (medicines), because, when stopped forcibly, the sama doshas produce diseases.

Conditions for ignoring and removing the ama doshas:

प्रवृत्तान् प्रागतो दोषानुपेक्षेत हिताशिनः ॥ ३२ ॥

विबन्धान् पाचनैस्तैस्तैः पाचयेन्निर्हरेत वा ।

Therefore in patients who are hitashina (habituated to consuming compatible foods), the sama doshas which are going out should be ignored in the early stages, the doshas which are vibandha (not getting expelled or getting expelled in small quantities) should be treated with pachana aushadas (medicines which promote digestion) or expelled out by administration of purification therapies as per the situational demand.

Time and proper seasons for eliminating Doshas out of the body:

श्रावणे कार्तिके चैत्रे मासि साधारणे क्रमात् ॥ ३३ ॥

ग्रीष्मवर्षाहिमचितान् वाय्वादीनाशु निर्हरेत् ।

Vata - undergoes chaya (mild increase) in Greeshma (summer) – should be expelled from the body in the months of Shravana (July-August),

Pitta – undergoes chaya in Varsha (rainy season) – expelled from the body in the months of Karthika (Oct-Nov),

Kapha – undergoes chaya in Shishira (winter) - expelled from the body in the months of Chaitra (March-April).

These are the sadharana kala (seasons in which the doshas do not undergo severe vitiation) for these doshas (vata, pitta and kapha) respectively.

Rules for elimination of doshas in healthy people:

अत्युष्णवर्षशीता हि ग्रीष्मवर्षाहिमागमाः ॥ ३४ ॥

सन्धौ साधारणे तेषां दुष्टान् दोषान् विशोधयेत् । स्वस्थवृत्तमभिप्रेत्य

Greeshma (summer), varsha (rainy season) and hemanta (winter) seasons will have too much heat, rain and cold respectively.

Therefore these vitiated doshas should be cleared out in the period between these seasons (like the period between summer and rain, rainy and winter, and winter and summer) and this is applicable when cleansing is done as part of a healthy regime.

Rules for elimination of Doshas in diseases:

व्याधौ व्याधिवशेन तु ॥ ३५ ॥

कृत्वा शीतोष्णवृष्टीनां प्रतीकारं यथायथम् ।

प्रयोजयेत् क्रियां प्राप्तां क्रियाकालं न हापयेत् ॥ ३६ ॥

In diseased conditions, the cleansing should be done as and when the diseases are manifested after having overcome the effects of cold, hot and rainy seasons suitably (according to season). Kriya (treatments) should be administered according to the manifested kriyakala (appropriate time for giving treatment, planned according to the successive stages of dosha aggravation and disease formation) without allowing further progression of disease.

Time of administration of medicines - Aushadha Sevana Kala:

युञ्ज्यादनन्नमन्नादौ मध्येऽन्ते कवलान्तरे ।
ग्रासे ग्रासे मुहुः सान्नं सामुद्गं निशि चौषधम् ॥ ३७ ॥

Medicines should be administered,

1. Ananna – on empty stomach,
2. Annadau – just before food or at the beginning of food intake,
3. Anna Madhye – During / in between food intake,
4. Anna ante – at the end of food intake,
5. Kavalantare – in between morsels,
6. Grase Grase – With each morsel,
7. Muhu: – Repeatedly, many a times a day,
8. Sa annam – Mixed with food,
9. Samudgam – before and after food,
10. Nishi – at night, bed time.

कफोद्रेके गदेऽनन्नं बलिनो रोगरोगिणोः ।

Ananna - Medicines should be administered anannam (on empty stomach) in

Kaphodreke gada - diseases arising from increase of Kapha,
Balino roga - in severe diseases and
Balino rogi - in diseases occurring in strong persons.

अन्नादौ विगुणेऽपाने समाने मध्य इष्यते ॥ ३८ ॥

Annadau Medicines should be administered just before food (annadau) when apana vayu is disturbed.

Anna Madya Medicines should be administered between food intake or during food intake (anna madhya) when samana vayu is disturbed.

व्यानेऽन्ते प्रातराशस्य सायमाशस्य चोत्तरे ।

Annanta Medicines should be administered at the end of morning meals (ante pratarashasya) when Vyana vayu is disturbed.

Medicines should be administered at the end of dinner (ante sayamashasya) when Udana vayu is disturbed.

ग्रासग्रासान्तयोः प्राणे प्रदुष्टे मातरिश्वनि ॥ ३९ ॥

Grasantara - Medicines should be administered in between morsels (grasa grasantayo) when Prana Vayu is disturbed.

मुहुर्मुहुर्विषच्छर्दिहिध्मा तृट्श्वासकासिषु ।

Muhurmuhu - Medicines should be repeatedly administered many times in a day (muhurmuhu), in diseases caused by

Visha - poison,

Chardi - vomiting,

Hidhma - hiccough,

Trit - thirst,

Swasa - dyspnoea and

Kasa – cough.

योज्यं सभोज्यं भैषज्यं भोज्यैश्चित्रैररोचके ॥ ४० ॥

Sa Bhojya - Medicines should be administered mixed with different kinds of foods (yojyam sabhojyam) in anorexia (arochaka).

कम्पाक्षेपकहिध्मासु सामुद्गं लघुभोजिनाम् ।

Samudga - Medicines should be administered before and after food (samudgam), in

Laghubhojitam - those who consume light food,

Kampa - in conditions of tremors,

Akshepaka - convulsions,

Hidhma – hiccough.

ऊर्ध्वजत्रुविकारेषु स्वप्नकाले प्रशस्यते ॥ ४१ ॥

Svapna kala (night) - Medicines should be administered at bedtime (swapnakala), in those who are suffering from diseases affecting head and neck (urdhvajatru vikara).

इति श्री वैद्यपतिसिंहगुप्तसूनु वाग्भटविरचितायां अष्टाङ्गहृदयसंहितायां सूत्रस्थाने दोषोपक्रमणीयो नाम त्रयोदशोऽध्यायः ॥

Thus ends the 13th chapter of Ashtangahridaya Samhita Sutrasthana, named Doshopakramaniya Adhyaya, written by Shrimad Vagbhata, son of Shri Vaidyapati Simhagupta.

14

दि्वविधोपक्रमणीयमध्यायम् (dvividhopakramaniyam adhyayam)

Dvividha means two types. Upakrama means treatment. The two main types of treatments namely nourishing (bulk promoting) and depleting (lightening) treatments will be explored in detail in this chapter, hence the name – Dvividha Upakramaneeyam Adhyayam.

अथातो दि्वविधोपक्रमणीयमध्यायं व्याख्यास्याम: इति ह स्माहुरात्रेयादयो महर्षय: ।
Atreya and other sages pledge that they would henceforth be explaining the chapter named Dvividhopakramaneeyamadhyayam.

Two types of treatment:
उपक्रम्यस्य हि द्वित्वादि्द्वधैवोपक्रमो मत:।
एक: सन्तर्पणस्तत्र दि्वतीयश्चापतर्पण:।१।
Since the diseases (upakramya) are mainly of two types (sama and nirama), the treatment (upakrama) is also of two types.
1. Santarpana (nourishing therapy)
2. Apatarpana (reduction therapy)

बृंहणो लङ्घनश्चेति तत्पर्यायावुदाहृतौ।

बृंहणं यद्बृहत्वाय लङ्घनं लाघवाय यत्||२||

Brimhana (bulk promoting therapy) and Langhana (lightening therapy) are the synonyms of Santarpana and Apatarpana respectively.

Brimhana is that which makes the body stout and fat (brihatvaya)

Langhana is that which makes the body light and thin (laghavaya).

Mahabhuta composition of brimhana and langhana treatments:

देहस्य भवतः प्रायो भौमापमितरच्च ते |

Among these two therapies, generally Brimhana treatment is predominant with bhauma (Earth element) and ap (water element) whereas

Langhana is predominantly made up of the other elements (i.e. fire, air and ether elements).

स्नेहनं रूक्षणं कर्म स्वेदनं स्तम्भनं च यत्||३||

भूतानां तदपि द्वैध्यादिद्वतयं नातिवर्तते|

The karma (functions) which are considered of 4 types namely

Snehana (oleation),

Rukshana (imparting dryness),

Swedana (sweating therapy, sudation) and

Stambhana (withholding, obstructing, and constipating)

are also not apart from these two types of treatment (brimhana and langhana) because the bhutas (five elements of nature) which make up the above karmas (functions) are also distributed among brimhana and langhana.

Types of Langhana or lightening treatments:

शोधनं शमनं चेति द्विधा तत्रापि लङ्घनम्||४||

Langhana (lightening treatments) is of two types –

Shodhana (purification procedures i.e. Panchakarma treatments) and

Shamana (palliative treatments).

Meaning, types of Shodhana:

यदीरयेद्वहिर्दोषान् पञ्चधा शोधनं च तत्|

निरूहो वमनं कायशिरोरेकोऽस्रविसुतिः||५||

That which forcibly expels the vitiated doshas out of the body is called Shodhana.

Shodhana is of five kinds, they are –

Niruha – decoction enema,
Vamanam – emesis, vomiting therapy,
Kaya reka – virechana, purgation of the body,
Shiro reka –nasya, nasal instillation of the medicines,
Asravisruti – raktamokshana, bloodletting.

Shamana Therapy: Meaning, types
न शोधयति यद्दोषान् समान्नोदीरयत्यपि‍।
समीकरोति विषमान् शमनं तच्च सप्तधा॥६॥
पाचनं दीपनं क्षुत्तृड्व्यायामातपमारुताः।

Shamana (palliative treatment) is that which
Na shodhayati – does not expel the increased Doshas out of the body,
Samannodirayatyapi – it does not increase the normal Dosha,
Sameekasotivishaman – but brings the abnormal Doshas back to normalcy.

Shamana is of 7 types –
Pachana – digestive, carminatives,
Deepana – hunger producing, stomachic,
Kshut – withstanding hunger, avoidance of food, fasting,
Trut – withstanding thirst, avoiding liquid food intake,
Vyayama– physical activity,
Aatapa– exposure to sunlight and
Maruta– exposure to the breeze.

बृंहणं शमनं त्वेव वायोः पित्तानिलस्य च॥७॥

Brimhana (stoutening therapies) are also a form of shamana (palliative treatment) since they pacify the aggravated vata and vata–pitta.

Brimhaneeya – Persons indicated for stoutening (nourishing) therapies:
बृंहयेद्व्याधिभैषज्यमद्यस्त्रीशोककर्शितान्।
भाराध्वोरःक्षतक्षीणरूक्षदुर्बलवातलान्॥८॥
गर्भिणीसूतिकाबालवृद्धान् ग्रीष्मेऽपरानपि।

Brimhana– stoutening therapy should be given to persons who are
Vyadhi karshita – emaciated by diseases,
Bhaishajya Karshita – emaciated by medicines / therapies,
Madya Karshita – emaciated by alcohol,
StriKarshita – Emaciated by excess sexual activity,

Shoka karshita – Emaciated by grief,

Bhara – who carries heavy loads frequently,

Adhva – who has travelled a long distance,

Urakshata – person with chest injury,

Kshatakseena – who is debilitated due to injury,

Ruksha – who has excess dryness,

Durbala – debilitated,

Vatala – Person with Vata body type,

Garbhini – pregnant,

Sutika –the women who has delivered,

Bala – children,

Vruddha – the aged and

Greeshme – in the month of summer, even the other people, who are not indicated above should be given brihmana (nourishing therapy).

Methods to administer Brihmana:

मांसक्षीरसितासर्पिर्मधुरस्निग्धबस्तिभिः॥९॥
स्वप्नशय्यासुखाभ्यङ्गस्नाननिर्वृतिहर्षणैः।

Brihmana can be administered by the use of

Mamsa – meat,

Ksheera – milk,

Sita – sugar,

Sarpi – ghee,

Madhura snigdhavasti – enema prepared using sweet substances and fats,

Swapna – sleep,

Shayyasukha – comfortable bed,

Abhyanga – oil massage,

Snana – bath,

Nivritti – comforts, rest and

Harshana – happiness of the mind.

Langhaneeya – Persons indicated for lightening therapies:

मेहामदोषातिस्निग्धज्वरोरुस्तम्भकुष्ठिनः॥१०॥
विसर्पविद्राधिप्लीहशिरःकण्ठाक्षिरोगिणः।
स्थूलांश्च लङ्घयेन्नित्यं शिशिरे त्वपरानपि॥११॥

Langhana (lightening therapy) should be done in the following conditions –
Meha – diabetics, urinary disorders,

Amadosha – persons suffering from Ama,
Atisnigdha – who has undergone excess oleation treatment,
Jvara – fever,
Urustambha – stiffness of the thighs,
Kushta – skin diseases,
Visarpa – herpes,
Vidradhi – abscess,
Pleeha – diseases of spleen,
Shira, KantaAkshiroga – diseases of head, throat, and eyes,
Sthula –obese,
In Shishira (winter), even the other people who are not indicated for langhana above should be subjected to it.

Indications for Langhana therapy by means of Shodhana (panchakarma):

तत्र संशोधनैः स्थौल्यबलपित्तकफाधिकान्।
आमदोषज्वरच्छर्दिरतीसारहृदामयैः ॥१२॥
विबन्धगौरवोद्गारहृल्लासादिभिरातुरान्।

The patients should be treated with langhana (lightening therapies) administered in the form of shodhana (panchakarma, cleansing therapies) in the below mentioned conditions –
Sthoulya – those who are very obese,
Bala – strong,
Pitta kaphadhikan – having predominance of Pitta and Kapha,
Ama dosha – those suffering from Amadosha,
Jwara – fever,
Chardi – vomiting,
Atisara – diarrhoea ,
Hridamaya – heart diseases,
Vibandha – constipation,
Gaurava – feeling of heaviness,
Udgara – excess of belching,
Hrillasa – nausea, etc.

Indications for Langhana therapy by means of pachana (digestives) and deepana (carminatives):

मध्यस्थौल्यादिकान् प्रायः पूर्वं पाचनदीपनैः ॥१३॥

Generally in obesity (sthoulya) and other conditions having moderate (madhya) strength and in patients having moderate strength, langhana should be initially administered in the form of pachana (digestives) and deepana (appetite or hunger producing medicines) and later should be subjected to shodhana (purification treatments).

Indications for Langhana therapy by means of kshut–trishnanigraha (control of hunger and thirst):

एभिरेवामयैरार्तान् हीनस्थौल्यबलादिकान्। क्षुत्तृष्णानिग्रहैः

In patients suffering from the same diseases like sthoulya etc. explained above having less (heena) strength and in patients having less strength, langhana (lightening therapies) should be administered in the form of kshut–trishnanigraha (forcible control of hunger and thirst).

Indications for Langhana therapy by means of samirana–atapa–ayasa (exposure to breeze, sunlight and exercise):

दोषैस्त्वार्तान् मध्यबलैर्दृढान्॥१४॥

समीरणातपायासैः किमुताल्पबलैर्नरान्।

For strong patients who have vitiated doshas of moderate strength, langhana should be administered in the form of

Samirana (exposure to wind or breeze),

Atapa (heat of the Sun) and

Ayasa (exercise).

For patients with less strength and when the vitiated doshas also have less strength, langana in the form of samirana, atapa and ayasa is recommended.

Rules for implementing nourishing and lightening therapies:

न बृंहयेल्लङ्घनीयान् बृंह्यांस्तु मृदु लङ्घयेत्॥१५॥

युक्त्या वा देशकालादिबलतस्तानुपाचरेत्।

Those who are indicated for lightening therapy (langhana) should not be administered bulk promoting therapy (brihmana).

For those who are indicated for bulk promoting therapy (brihmana), lightening treatments (langhana) can be given in a milder (mridu) form.

Or skilfully both lightening (langhana) and bulk promoting (brihmana) therapies can be given together, after having considered the nature of habitat (desha), season (kala), strength (bala) and other factors in the patient.

Benefits of Brimhana therapy:

बृंहिते स्याद्बलं पुष्टिस्तत्साध्यामयसङ्क्षयः||१६||

In those who have undergone brimhana (stoutening therapy),

Bala – strength is obtained,

Pushti – body is nourished properly, and

Tat sadhya amaya samkshayah – diseases which are curable by that therapy are cured.

Benefits of Langhana therapy:

विमलेन्द्रियता सर्गो मलानां लाघवं रुचिः|

क्षुतृट्सहोदयः शुद्धहृदयोद्गारकण्ठता||१७||

व्याधिमार्दवमुत्साहस्तन्द्रानाशश्च लङ्घिते|

In those who have undergone langhana (lightening therapies), the below mentioned benefits are obtained –

Vimalendriyata – keenness and clarity of sense organs,

Sargomalanam – timely and proper expulsion of wastes (doshas and excreta),

Laghavam – feeling of lightness of the body,

Ruchi – good taste perception,

Kshuttritsahodayaha – appearance of hunger and thirst together,

Shuddhahridaya – feeling of purity in the chest region (heart),

Shuddha udgarakantatha – clear belching and clear throat,

Vyadhimardavam – softening of the diseases (decreased severity of diseases),

Utsaha – energy and enthusiasm and

Tandranasha – loss of stupor, laziness.

Excessive use of stoutening and thinning therapies:

अनपेक्षितमात्रादिसेविते कुरुतस्तु ते||१८||

अतिस्थौल्यातिकाश्र्यादीन्, वक्ष्यन्ते च सौषधाः|

रूपं तैरेव च ज्ञेयमतिबृंहितलङ्घिते||१९||

These therapies (brimhana and langhana) when taken in excess will cause atisthoulya (profound obesity) and atikarshya (profound emaciation) etc. They will be enumerated now along with their treatment.

The same symptoms should be considered as the symptoms of excessive stoutening (atibrihmana) and excessive lightening (atilanghana) therapies respectively.

Symptoms of AtiBrimhana or excessive administration of stoutening therapy:

अतिस्थौल्यापचीमेहज्वरोदरभगन्दरान्‌।

काससन्न्यासकृच्छ्रामकुष्ठादीनतिदारुणान्‌॥२०॥

Excess of Brimhana therapy produces

Atisthaulya – profound obesity,

Apachi – scrofula,

Meha – Diabetes, urinary disorders,

Jvara – fever,

Udara – enlargement of abdomen,

Bhagandara – fistula–in–ano,

Kasa – cough,

Sanyasa – loss of consciousness,

Mutrakruchra – dysuria,

Ama– disorders due to poor digestive activities,

Kushta–skin diseases which are very dreadful.

Treatment for disorders manifested due to Ati brihmana (excessive administration of stoutening therapies):

तत्र मेदोऽनिलश्लेष्मनाशनं सर्वमीष्यते। कुलत्थजूर्नश्यामाकयवमुद्गमधूदकम्॥२१॥

मस्तुदण्डाहतारिष्टचिन्ताशोधनजागरम्। मधुना त्रिफलां लिह्याद्गुडूचीमभयां धनम्॥२२॥

रसाञ्जनस्य महतः पञ्चमूलस्य गुग्गुलोः। शिलाजतुप्रयोगश्च साग्निमन्थरसो हितः॥२३॥

विडङ्गं नागरं क्षारः काललोहरजो मध। यवामलकचूर्णं च योगोऽस्थौल्यदोषजित्॥२४॥

Treatment for Atibrihmana includes –

Treatments which reduce Medas– fat, Anila– Vata and Kapha are desirable;

Use of Kulattha – horse gram – Dolichos biflorus,

Jurna – a cereal,

Shyamaka – millet,

Yava – Barley – Hordeum vulgare,

Mudga – green gram – Averrhoa carambola,

Madhudakam – Honey mixed with water,

Mastu – whey,

Dandahatam – variety of buttermilk,

Arishta – fermented beverages,

Chinta – Indulgence Brin worry, stressful activities,

Shodhana – Purification therapies,
Jagaram – avoidance of sleep,

Either Triphala, Guduci, Abhaya (Haritaki) or Ghana (musta), should be licked with honey daily;
Either Rasanjana, Brihat Pancamula (Agnimantha, Shyonaka, Gambhari, Patala, Bilva), Guggulu – along with the fresh juice of Agnimantha is suitable;
Powder of Vidanga, Nagara (Ginger), Kshara (Yavakshara) and kala loha raja (iron filing) or powder of Yava (Barley) and Amla along with honey should be licked daily.

व्योषकट्वीवराशिग्रुविडङ्गातिविषास्थिराः।
हिङ्गुसौवर्चलाजाजीयवानीधान्यचित्रकाः॥२५॥
निशे बृहत्यौ हपुषा पाठा मूलं च केम्बुकात्। एषां चूर्णं मधु घृतं तैलं च सदृशांशकम्॥२६॥
सक्तुभिः षोडशगुणैर्युक्तं पीतं निहन्ति तत्। अतिस्थौल्यादिकान् सर्वान् रोगानान्यांश्च तदि्द्वधान्॥२७॥
हृद्रोगकामलाश्विव्रश्वासकासगलग्रहान्। बुद्धिमेधास्मृतिकरं सन्नस्याग्नेश्च दीपनम्॥२८॥

Powders of
Vyosha– Trikatu – pepper, long pepper and ginger,
Katvi – Elettaria cardamomum,
Vara – Triphala,
Shigru – drum stick,
Vidanga – False black pepper – Embeliaribes,
Ativisha – Aconitum heterophyllum,
Sthira – Desmodium gangeticum,
Hingu – Asafoetida,
Sauvarcala – black salt
Ajaji – Cuminum cyminum,
Yavani – Trachyspermum ammi,
Dhanya – Coriandrum sativum,
Chitraka – Plumbago zeylanicum,
The two Nisa – turmeric and tree turmeric,
The two Brihati– brihati and kantakari,
Hapusa – Sphaeranthus indicus,
Root of Patha – Cycleapeltata and

Kebuka – Brassica oleraceae,
should be mixed with Madhu (honey), Gritam (ghee) and Tailam (oil) in equal proportions and sixteen parts of saktu (corn flour).
This mixture cures diseases due to atiyoga of Brihmana like atisthoulya etc. mentioned earlier and even others of similar nature such as
Hridroga – heart diseases, Kamala – jaundice, Shvitra – leucoderma, Swasa – dyspnoea,
Kasa – cough, Gala graha – obstruction in the throat etc.
It improves
Buddhi – power of thinking,
Medha – intelligence,
Smriti – memory and
Sannasyaagneschadeepanam – kindles the weakened digestive fire.

Symptoms of Ati Langhana (excessive administration of lightening therapy):

अतिकार्श्यं भ्रमः कासस्तृष्णाधिक्यमरोचकः।
स्नेहाग्निनिद्रादृक्श्रोत्रशुक्रौजःक्षुत्स्वरक्षयः॥२९॥
बस्तिहृन्मूर्धजङ्घोरुत्रिकपार्श्वरुजा ज्वरः।
प्रलापोध्वानिलग्लानिच्छर्दिपर्वास्थिभेदनम्॥३०॥
वर्चोमूत्रग्रहाद्याश्च जायन्तेऽतिविलङ्घनात्।

Atilanghana (excessive weight loss therapy) causes –
Atikarshyam – profound emaciation,
Bhrama – delusion, dizziness,
Kasa – cough,
Trushnadhikyam – severe thirst,
Arochaka – anorexia;
It causes loss / decrease of –
Sneha – moistness,
Agni – digestive power,
Nidra – sleep,
Drik – vision,
Srotra – hearing,
Shukra – semen,
Ojas – essence of tissues,
Kshut – hunger and
Svara – voice;

It causes ruja (pain) in the
Vasti – urinary bladder,
Hrid – heart,
Murdha – head,
Janga – calves,
Uru – thighs,
Trika – upper shoulders and
Parshva – flanks;
Jwara – fever,
Pralapa – delirium,
Urdhvaanila – belching,
Glani – exhaustion,
Chardi – vomiting,
Parvasthi bhedanam – cutting pain in the joints and bones;
Vit mutradi graham – non–elimination of faeces, urine etc.,
arise from the excess of Langhana.

Emaciation is better than Obesity:
कार्श्यमेव वरं स्थौल्यात् न हि स्थूलस्य भेषजम्||३१||
बृंहणं लङ्घनं वाऽलमतिमेदोऽग्निवातजित्|
मधुरस्निग्धसौहित्यैर्यत्सौख्येन च नश्यति||३२||
कृशिमा स्थविमास्त्यन्तविपरीतनिषेवणैः|
Emaciation (karshya) is better than obesity (sthoulya).
There is no treatment for the obese, because brihmana (stoutening therapies) or langana (thinning therapies) are incapable of vanquishing atimeda (excess of fat), atyagni (excessive digestive activity) or excessive vata.
Emaciation gets cured by use of madhura (sweet) and snigdha (unctuous) foods and comfortable living;
Obesity gets cured by the use of foods and activities which are atyanta viparita (extremely opposite) to those mentioned above, that too when used in maximum quantity (ati nishevana).

Treatment principles of emaciation:
योजयेद्बृंहणं तत्र सर्वं पानान्नभेषजम्||३३||
अचिन्तया हर्षणेन ध्रुवं सन्तर्पणेन च|
स्वप्नप्रसङ्गाच्च कृशो वराह इव पुष्यति||३४||

न हि मांससमं किञ्चिदन्यद्देहबृहत्त्वकृत्|
मांसादमांसं मांसेन सम्भृतत्वादिवशेषतः||३५||

In emaciation, all sorts of pana (liquids), anna (foods) and bheshaja (drugs) which are brihmana (stoutening) should be adopted.

Achintya – by absence of worry,

Harshana – by happiness,

Dhruvam santarpanena ca – more use of nutritious food and

Svapna prasanga cha – more of sleep,

the emaciated person becomes stout like a varaha (pig).

There is nothing equivalent to mamsa (meat) to cause dehabrihatva (stoutness of the body), especially so the meat of meat eating animals, for they get nourished by meat itself.

Foods that are good for obese and thin people:
गुरु चातर्पणं स्थूले विपरीतं हितं कृशे|
यवगोधूममुभयोस्तद्योग्याहितकल्पनम्||३६||

Foods which are guru (heavy) and apatarpana (non–nutritious) are ideal for sthula (obese), whereas the opposites are ideal for the krisha (emaciated), i.e. foods which are light and nutritious.

Yava (barley) and godhuma (wheat) should be used in both these conditions considering them as beneficial foods respectively (yava being heavy and non–nutritious is good for obese people while godhuma being light and nutritious is beneficial for emaciated people).

Brimhana and langhana are the only two important forms of treatments:
दोषगत्याऽतिरिच्यन्ते ग्राहिभेद्यादिभेदतः|
उपक्रमा न ते द्वित्वादिभिन्ना अपि गदा इव||३७||

Though the states of doshas are innumerable, and the types of treatments are also innumerable, like grahi (withholding, constipating), bhedi (purgatives) etc.,still the treatments do not surpass these two kinds i.e.brimhana (stoutening) and langhana (thinning), as the diseases, though innumerable fall into two kinds only i.e. sama and nirama (with ama and without ama).

इति श्रीवैद्यपतिसिंहगुप्तसूनुश्रीमद्वाग्भटविरचितायामष्टाङ्गहृदयसंहितायां सूत्रस्थाने
द्विविधोपक्रमणीयो नाम चतुर्दशोऽध्यायः||१४||

Thus ends the 14th chapter of Ashtangahridaya Samhita Sutrasthana, named

Dvividhopakramaniyo Adhyaya, written by Shrimad Vagbhata, son of Shri VaidyapatiSimhagupta.

वैद्य जनार्धन वि हेब्बार्

15

शोधनादिगणसङ्ग्रहमध्यायम् (shodhanadi gana sangraham adhyayam)

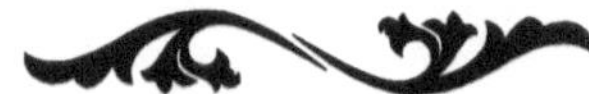

The 15th chapter of Sutrasthanam of Ashtanga Hridayam is named as Shodhanadi Gana Sangraham Adhyayam. This chapter deals with various groups (gana) of herbs that are used in cleansing therapies i.e. Panchakarma treatments. The chapter also gives a list of other groups of herbs which are used in preparing Ayurvedic medicines for various purposes and benefits.

अथातो शोधनादिगणसङ्ग्रहमध्यायं व्याख्यास्याम: इति ह स्माहुरात्रेयादयो महर्षय:॥
Atreya and other sages pledge that henceforth they will be explaining the chapter named Shodhanadi ganasangraham (pertaining to the group of herbs used in Panchakarma or purification treatments).

Chardana Gana — Group of Emetics:
मदनमधुकलम्बानिम्बबिम्बीविशाला त्रपुसकुटजमूर्वादेवदालीकृमिघ्नम्।
विदुलदहनचित्राः कोशवत्यौ करञ्जः कणलवणवचैलासर्षपाश्छर्दनानि॥१॥
Madana – Randia spinosa,
Madhuka – Licorice – Glycyrrhiza glabra,
Lamba – bitter bottle gourd – Labgenaria siceraria,
Nimba – neem – Azadirachta indica,
Bimbi – ivy gourd – Coccinia grandis,
Vishala – bitter apple – Citrullus colocynthis,

"

Trapusha – common cucumber – Cucumis sativus,
Kutaja – conessi – Holarrhenaantidysenterica,
Murva – Chonemorpha fragrans,
Devadali – Luffa echinata,
Krimighna – Vidanga – Embeliaribes,
Vidula – Salix caprea,
Dahana – leadwort – Plumbago zeylanica,
Chitra – Merremiaemarginata,
The two Kosavati – Dhamarghava – Luffa cylindrica, Rajakoshataki – Luffa acutangula,
Karanja – Indian beech – Pongamia pinnata,
Kana – long pepper – Piper longum,
Lavana – Salt,
Vacha – sweet flag – Acorus calamus,
Ela – cardamom – Elettaria cardamomum and
Sarhsapa – mustard – Brassica juncea
form the group known as ChardanaGana (group of emetics).

Virechana Gana – group of purgatives:
निकुम्भकुम्भत्रिफलागवाक्षी सुक्शङ्खिनीनीलिनितिल्वकानि|
शम्याककम्पिल्लकहेमदुग्धा दुग्धं च मूत्रं च विरेचनानि||२||
Nikumbha – Baliospermum montanum,
Kumbha – Indian jalap – Operculina turpethum,
Triphala – Haritaki – Terminalia chebula, Vibhitaki – Terminalia bellirica,
Amalaki – Emblica officinalis,
Gavakshi – bitter apple – Citrullus colocynthis,
Snuk – Snuhi – common milk hedge – Euphorbia neriifolia,
Shankhini – Clitoria ternatea,
Nilini – Indian indigo – Indigofera tinctoria,
Tilvaka – Symplocos cochinchinensis,
Samyaka – purging fistula – Cassia fistula,
Kampillaka – Mallotus philippinensis,
Hemadugdha – Mexican poppy – Argemone mexicana,
Dugdha – milk and
Mutra – urine
form the group known as VirechanaGana (group of purgatives).

NiruhanaGana– group of drugs for decoction enema:
मदनकुटजकुष्ठदेवदाली मधुकवचादशमूलदारुरास्नाः।
यवमिशिकृतवेधनं कुलत्था मधु लवणं त्रिवृता निरूहणानि॥३॥
Madana – Emetic nut – Randia spinosa,
Kutaja – conessi – Holarrhena antidysenterica,
Kustha – costus – Saussurea lappa,
Devadali – Luffa echinata,
Madhuka – Liquorice – Glycyrrhiza glabra,
Vacha – sweet flag – Acorus calamus,
Dashamoola – group of 10 roots,
Daru – Devadaru – Cedrus deodara,
Rasna – Alpinia galanga,
Yava – barley – Hordeum vulgare,
Mishi – garden dil – Anethum sowa,
Kritavedhanam – ribbed gourd – Luffa acutangula,
Kulattha – Horse gram – Dolichos biflorus,
Madhu – Honey,
Lavana – salt and
Trivrit – Indian jalap – Operculina turpethum
form the group of drugs known as Niruhana Gana.

NaavanaGana– group of Drugs for nasal medication:
वेल्लापामार्गव्योषदार्वीसुराला बीजं शैरीषं बाहतं शैग्रवं च।
सारो माधूकः सैन्धवं ताक्ष्र्यशैलं त्रुट्यौ पृथ्वीका शोधयन्त्युत्तमाङ्गम्॥४॥
Vella – Embelia ribes,
Apamarga – prickly chaff flower plant – Achyranthes aspera,
Vyosha – Pippali – long pepper, Maricha – black pepper and Shunti – ginger,
Darvi – Berberis aristata,
Surala – Resin or gum of Vateria indica / Shorearobusta,
Beejam shaireesham – seeds of Albizia lebbeck,
Barhatam – seed of Solanum indicum,
Shaigravam – seeds of drumsticks – Moringa oleifera,
Saro madhuka – extract or essence of the flowers of Madhuca longifolia,
Saindhavam – rock salt,
Tarkshyashailam – solidified extract of Berberis aristata,
Trutyau – small and big cardamom varieties – Elettaria cardamomum, Amomum subulatum and

Prithvika – Hingupatri – Ferulajaeschkeana, Gardenia gummifera
Form the group of drugs for Navana (nasal medication).

Vataghna Gana – group of herbs which balance Vata:
भद्रदारु नतं कुष्ठं दशमूलं बलाद्वयम्।
वायुं वीरतरादिश्च विदार्यादिश्च नाशयेत्॥५॥
Bhadradaru – Deodar – Cedrus deodara,
Natham – Indian valerian – Valerianawallichii,
Kushtam – costus – Saussurealappa,
Dashamoola – group of 10 roots,
Baladvayam – two varieties of Bala – Bala – Sida cordifolia and Atibala –
Abutilon indicum,
Virataradi group of herbs,
Vidaryadi group of herbs,
form the group of herbs which balance vata (Vataghnagana).

Pittaghna Gana – group of herbs which balance Pitta:
दूर्वाऽनन्ता निम्बवासाऽऽत्मगुप्ता गुन्द्राऽभीरुः शीतपाकी प्रियङ्गुः।
न्यग्रोधादिः पद्मकादिः स्थिरे द्वे पद्मं वन्यं सारिवादिश्च पित्तम्॥६॥
Durva – conch grass– Cynodon dactylon,
Ananta – Hemidesmus indicus,
Nimba – Neem – Azadirachta indica,
Vasa – Adhatoda vasica,
Atmagupta – common cowitch – Mucuna pruriens,
Gundra – Cyperus rotundus,
Abhiru – Crotalaria verrucosa / Asparagus racemosus,
Sheetapaki – Abrus precatorius,
Priyangu – Callicarpa macrophylla,
Nyagrodhadi group of herbs,
Padmakadi group of herbs,
Two varieties of Sthira – Shalaparni – Desmodiumgangeticum and
Prishniparni – Urariapicta,
Padmam – Prunus cerasoides,
Vanyam – Oroxylum indicum,
Sarivadi group of herbs,
Form the group of herbs that balance Pitta (Pittagnagana).

Kaphaghna Gana – group of herbs which balance Kapha:

आरग्वधादिरर्कादिर्मुष्ककाद्योऽसनादिकः।
सुरसादिः समुस्तादिर्वत्सकादिर्बलासजित्॥७॥

Aragwadadi group of herbs, Arkadi group of herbs,

Muskakadi group of herbs, Asanadi group of herbs,

Surasadi group of herbs, Mustadi group of herbs and

Vatsakadi group of herbs

Form the group of herbs that balance Balasa / Kapha (Kaphagnagana).

JeevaniyaGana – Jeevaniya group of herbs:

जीवन्ती काकोल्यौ मेदे द्वे मुद्गमाषपर्ण्यौ च।
ऋषभकजीवकमधुकं चेति गणो जीवनीयाख्यः॥८॥

Jeevanti – Leptadeniareticulata,

Two types of Kakoli – Kakoli – Roscoeaprocera, Kshirakakoli – Lilium polphyllum,

Two types of Meda – Meda – Polygonatum cirrhifolium, Mahameda – Polygonatum verticillatum,

Mudgaparni – Phaseolus trilobus,

Mashaparni – Teramnus labialis,

Rishabhaka – Malaxis acuminata, Microstylis wallichii,

Jivaka – Microstylis musifera,

Madhukam – licorice – Glycyrrhiza glabra etc

form the group of herbs called Jivaniya Gana.

VidaryadiGana – Vidaryadi group of herbs:

विदारिपञ्चाङ्गुलवृश्चिकाली वृश्चीवदेवाह्वयशूर्पपर्ण्यः।
कण्डूकरी जीवनह्रस्वसंज्ञे द्वे पञ्चके गोपसुता त्रिपादी॥९॥

Vidari – Pueraria tuberosa,

Panchangula – castor – Ricinus communis,

Vrischikali – Tragia involucrata,

Vrischiva – small variety of Boerhavia diffusa,

Devahvaya – deodar – Cedrus deodara,

Shurpaparni – Mudgaparni – Phaseolus trilobus, Mashaparni – Teramnus labialis,

Kandukari – Mucuna pruriens,

Jivana panchamoola – Abhiru – Asperagus racemosus, Vira – Coccinia grandis, Jivanti – Holostemma adakodein, Jivaka – Microstylis wallichi,

Rishabhaka – Microstylis muscifera,
Hrisva panchamoola – Brihati – Solanum anguivi, Kantakari – Solanum xanthocarpum, Gokshura – Tribulus terrestris, Prishniparni – Desmodiumgangeticum, Salaparni – Pseudarthriaviscida,
Gopasuta – Hemidesmus indicus and
Tripadi – Adiantum lunulatum
Form the group of herbs known as VidaryadiGana.

Benefits of Vidaryadi Gana:
विदार्यादिरयं हृद्यो बृंहणो वातपित्तहा।
शोषगुल्माङ्गमर्दोर्ध्वश्वासकासहरो गणः॥१०॥
The Vidaryadi group of herbs are
Hridya – good to the heart,
Brihmana – stoutening,
Vatapittaha – mitigate vata and pitta,
It cures
Shosha – emaciation,
Gulma – abdominal tumors,
Angamarda – bodyache,
Urdhva swasa – wheezing (breathlessness)
Kasa – cough.

SarivadiGana – Sarivadi group of herbs:
सारिवोशीरकाश्मर्यमधूकशिशिरद्वयम्।
यष्टी परूषकं हन्ति दाहपित्तास्रतृड्ज्वरान्॥११॥
Sariva – Hemidesmus indicus,
Ushira – Vetiveria zizanioides,
Kashmarya – Gmelina arborea,
Madhuka – Madhuca longifolia,
Shishiradvayam – Chandana – sandalwood – Santalum album and
Raktachandana – red sandalwood – Pterocarpus santalinus,
Yashti – Licorice – Glycyrrhiza glabra and
Parushakam – Grewia asiatica
form the group of drugs known as Sarivadigana.
It cures
Daha – burning sensation,
Pittasra – bleeding disorders,

Trit – excessive thirst and
Jwara – fever.

PadmakadiGana – Padmakadi group of herbs:

पद्मकपुण्ड्रौ वृद्धिधतुगद्र्ध्दः शृङ्ग्यमृता दश जीवनसंज्ञाः।
स्तन्यकरा घ्नन्तीरणपित्तं प्रीणनजीवनबृंहणवृष्याः॥१२॥

Padmaka – Prunus cerasoides,
Pundra – Nymphaea lotus,
Vriddhi – Habenaria intermedia,
Tuga – Bambusaarundinacea,
Riddhi – Sphaeranthus indicus,
Shringi – Pistacia integerrima,
Amrita – Tinospora cordifolia and
Dasha jivana sajna – 10 herbs of Jivantyadi group of herbs
are the herbs that form Padmakadigana, which is
Stanyakara – increases production of breast milk,
Gnantiranapittam – balance vata and pitta,
Prinana – nourishing,
Jivana – enlivening,
Brihmana – stoutening and
Vrishya – aphrodisiac.

ParushakadiGana – Parushakadi group of herbs:

परूषकं वरा द्राक्षा कट्फलं कतकात् फलम्। राजाह्वं दाडिमं शाकं तृण्मूत्रामयवातजित्॥१३॥

Parushaka – Grewia asiatica,
Vara – Triphala
Draksha – Vitis vinifera,
Katphalam – Myrica nagi,
Kataka phalam – Strychnos potatorum,
Rajahvam – Mimonsops hexen, Pterospermum acerifolium, Cassia fistula,
Dadimam – Punica granatum –pomegranate and
Shakam – Tectona grandis
are the group of herbs known as Parushakadigana.
It cures
Trit – thirst,
Mutramaya – urinary disorders and
Vatajit – mitigate Vata.

Anjanadi Gana – Anjanadi group of herbs:

अञ्जनं फलिनी मांसी पद्मोत्पलरसाञ्जनम्| सैलामधुकनागाह्वं
विषान्तर्दाहपित्तनुत्||१४||

Anjana –Collyrium,

Phalni – Priyangu – Callicarpa macrophylla,

Mamsi – Nardostachysjatamansi,

Padma – lotus – Nelumbo nucifera,

Utpala – water lily – Nymphaeanauchalii,

Rasanjanam – aqueous extract of Berberis aristata,

Ela – cardamom – Elettaria cardamomum,

Madhuka – licorice – Glycyrrhiza glabra,

Nagahvam – Messua ferrea,

form the group of herbs known as Anjanadigana.

It cures

Visha – diseases due to poison,

Antardaha – burning sensation inside the body and

Pittanut – balances pitta.

Patoladi Gana – Patoladi group of herbs:

पटोलकटुरोहिणीचन्दनं मधुस्रवगुडूचिपाठान्वितम्|
निहन्ति कफपित्तकुष्ठज्वरान् विषं वमिमरोचकं कामलाम्||१५||

Patola – Trichosanthes anguina,

Katurohini – Picrorhizakurroa,

Chandanam – sandalwood – Santalum album,

Madhusrava – Marsdeniatenacissima,

Guduchi – Tinospora cordifolia,

Patha – Cissampelos pareira,

form the group of herbs known as Patoladigana.

They cure

Nihanti kapha pitta – balance kapha and pitta,

Kushta – skin diseases,

Jwara – fevers,

Visha – poison,

Vami – vomiting,

Arochaka – anorexia and

Kamala – jaundice.

Guduchyadi Gana – Guduchyadi group of herbs:

गुडूचीपद्मकारिष्टधान्यकारक्तचन्दनम्‌|
पित्तश्लेष्मज्वरच्छर्दिदाहतृष्णाघ्नमग्निकृत्‌||१६||

Guduchi – Tinospora cordifolia,

Padmaka – Prunus cerasoides,

Arishta – neem – Azadirachta indica,

Dhanyaka – coriander – Coriandrum sativum,

Raktachandanam – red sandalwood – Pterocarpus santalinus

form the group of herbs known as Guduchyadi gana.

They cure

Pitta sleshma – mitigate pitta and kapha,

Jwara – fever,

Chardi – vomiting,

Daha – burning sensation,

Trishna – thirst and

Agnikrit – improves digestion.

Aragwadhadi Gana – Aragwadhadi group of herbs:

आरग्वधेन्द्रयवपाटलिकाकतिक्ता निम्बामृतामधुरसासुववृक्षपाठाः|
भूनिम्बसैर्यक्रपतोलकरञ्जयुग्म सप्तच्छदाग्निसुषवीफलबाणघोण्टाः||१७||

Aragvadha – Cassia fistula,

Indrayava – seeds of Holarrhena antidysenterica,

Patali – Stereospermum suaveolens,

Kakatikta – Trichosanthes tricuspidata, Pongamia pinnata, Clerodendrum serratum,

Nimba – neem – Azadirachta indica,

Amrita – Tinospora cordifolia,

Madhurasa – Marsdenia tenacissima,

Sruvavriksha – Flacourtia indica,

Patha – Cissampelos pareira,

Bhunimba – Andrographis paniculata,

Sairyaka – Strobilanthes ciliates,

Patola – Trichosanthes anguina,

Karanja yugma – Chirabilva – Holoptelia integrifolia and Naktamala – Pongamia pinnata,

Saptachada – Alstonia scholaris,

Agni – Plumbago zeylanica,
Sushavi – bitter gourd – Momordica charantia,
Phala – emetic nut – Randia dumetorum,
Bana – Barleria stringosa,
Gonta – a variety of Acacia catechu
constitute the Aragwadhadi group of herbs.

Benefits of AragwadhadiGana:

आरग्वधादिर्जयति छर्दिकुष्ठविषज्वरान्| कफं कण्डूं प्रमेहं च दुष्टव्रणविशोधनः||१८||

Drugs of Aragwadhadigana cures –
Chardi – vomiting,
Kushta – skin diseases,
Visha – poison,
Jwara – fevers,
Kapham – mitigate kapha,
Kandu – itching,
Prameha – diabetes, and
Dushta vrana vishodhanam – cleanses bad wounds.

Asanadi Gana – Asanadi group of herbs:

असनतिनिशभूर्जश्वेतवाहप्रकीर्याः खदिरकदरभण्डीशिंशिपामेषशृङ्ग्यः|
त्रिहिमतलपलाशा जोङ्गकः शाकशालौ क्रमुकधवकलिङ्गच्छापकर्णाश्वकर्णाः||१९||

Asana – Pterocarpus marsupium,
Tinisha – Ogeiniadalbergiodes,
Bhurja – Betula utilis,
Swatavaha – Arjuna – Terminalia arjuna,
Prakirya – Caesalpinia bonducella,
Khadira – Acacia catechu,
Kadara – white variety of Acacia catechu,
Bhandi – Albizia lebbeck,
Shimshipa – Dalbergia sissoo,
Meshashringi – Gymnemasylvestre,
Trihima – 3 types of sandalwood – Malayaja – Santalum album, Raktachandana – Pterocarpus santalinus, Daru haridra – Cosciniumfenestratum,
Tala – Toddy palm,
Palasha – Grewia asiatica,

Jongaka – Agaru – Aquilaria agallocha,
Shaka – Tectona grandis,
Shala – Shorea robusta,
Kramuka – Areca catechu,
Dhava – Anogeissus latifolia,
Kalinga – Holarrhena antidysenterica,
Chagakarna – Acacia leucophloea,
Ashvakarna – Dipterocarpus turbinatus
Form the group of herbs known as AsanadiGana.

Benefits of Asanadi Gana:

असनादिर्विजयते शिवत्रकुष्ठकफक्रिमीन्| पाण्डुरोगं प्रमेहं च मेदोदोषनिबर्हणः||२०||

Asanadigana cures
Switra – leucoderma,
Kushta – skin diseases,
Kapha – mitigates kapha,
Krimi – intestinal worms,
Panduroga – anaemia,
Prameha – diabetes and
Medo dosha – diseases of fat accumulation.

VarunadiGana – Varunadi group of herbs:

वरुणसैर्यकयुग्मशतावरी दहनमोरटबिल्वविषाणिकाः|

द्विबृहतीद्विकरञ्जजयाद्वयं बहलपल्लवदर्भरुजाकराः||२१||

Varuna – Crataeva nurvala,
Sairyakayugma – two types of sairyaka –Strobilanthes ciliates,
Shatavari – Asparagus racemosus,
Dahana – Plumbago zeylanica,
Morata – Marsdenia tenacissima,
Bilva – Aegle marmelos,
Vishanika – Pistacia integerrima,
Dvibrihati – Brihati – Solanum indicum and Kantakari – Solanum xanthocarpum,
Dvikaranja – Karanja – Pongamia pinnata and Putikaranja – Caesalpinia bonducella,
Jayadvayam – Tarkari – Clerodendrumphlomidis and Haritaki – Terminalia chebula,

Bahalapallava – drumstick – Moringa oleifera,
Darbha – Desmostachya bipinnata,
Rujakara – Semecarpus anacardium
form the group of herbs known as Varunadi Gana.

Benefits of Varunadi Gana:
वरुणादिः कफं मेदो मन्दाग्नित्वं नियच्छति|
आढ्यवातं शिरःशूलं गुल्मं चान्तः सविद्रधिम्||२२||
Varunadi Gana cures
Kapha – mitigates kapha disorders,
Meda – mitigates diseases due to fat accumulation,
Mandagnitvam – dyspepsia,
Adhyavata– rigidity of the thighs,
Shirashoola – headaches,
Gulma – tumours and
Antarvidradhi – abscess inside the abdomen.

Ushakadi Gana – Ushakadi group of herbs:
ऊषकस्तुत्थकं   हिङ्गु   कासीसद्वयसैन्धवम्| सशिलाजतु
कृच्छ्राश्मगुल्ममेदःकफापहम्||२३||
Ushaka – alkaline sand,
Thuttakam – copper sulphate,
Hingu – Ferula narthex, asafoetida,
Kasisadvaya – purified ferrous sulphate,
Saindhavam – Rock salt,
Shilajatu – Asphaltum,
constitute Ushakadi Gana, which cures
Krichra –dysuria,
Ashma – urinary calculus,
Gulma –abdominal tumours,
Meda kaphapaham – destroys fat and kapha.

Virataradi Gana – Virataradi group of herbs:
वेल्लन्तरारणिकबूकवृषाश्मभेद गोकण्टकेत्कटसहाचरबाणाकाशाः|
वृक्षादनीनलकुशद्वयगुण्ठगुन्द्रा भल्लूकमोरटकुरण्टकरम्भपार्थाः||२४||
Vellantara – Dichrostachys cinerea,
Aranika – Clerodendrum phlomidis,

Buka – Sesbania grandiflora,
Vrisha – Adhatoda vasica,
Ashmabheda – Bergenia ligulata,
Gokantaka – Tribulus terrestris,
Itkata – Saccharum munja,
Sahachara – Strobilanthes heynianus,
Bana – Barleria prionitis, bearing blue flowers,
Kasha – Saccharum spontaneum,
Vrikshadani – Pothos scandens, Loranthus falcatus,
Nala – Lobelia nicotianifolia,
Kushadvaya – two varieties of Desmostachya bipinnata,
Gunta – Cordia dichotoma,
Gundra – Cyperus rotendus,
Bhalluka – Oroxylumrotendus,
Morata – Chonemorpha fragrans,
Kuranta – Pergularia daemia,
Karambha – Pandanus latifolia,
Partha – Terminalia arjuna
Constitute the group of herbs called Virataradi Gana.

Benefits of Virataradi Gana:
वर्गो वीरतराद्योऽयं हन्ति वातकृतान् गदान्| अश्मरीशर्करामूत्रकृच्छ्राघातरुजाहरः||२५||
Virataradi group cures
Vatakritagada – diseases produced by Vata,
Ashmari – urinary stones and
Sharkara – Urinary gravel,
Mutrakrichra – Dysuria,
Mutraghata – retention of urine and
Ruja – pain.

RodhradiGana – Rodhradi group of herbs:
रोध्रशाबरकरोध्रपलाशा जिङ्गिणीसरलकट्फलयुक्ताः|
कुत्सिताम्बकदलीगतशोकाः सैलवालुपरिपेलवमोचाः||२६||
Rodhra – Symplocos racemosa,
Shambarakarodhra – white variety of Symplocos racemosa,
Palasha – Butea monosperma,
Jingini – Bombax ceiba, black variety of Silk cotton tree,

Sarala – Pinus roxburghii,
Katphala – Myrica nagi,
Yuktah – Pluchea lanceolata,
Kutsitanga –Kadamba – Neolamarckia cadamba,
Kadali –plantain – Musa paradisiaca,
Gatashoka – Saraca asoka,
Elavalu – Brunus cerasus,
Paripelava – Oroxylum indicum,
Mocha – Boswellia serrata
Constitute Rodhradi Gana.

Benefits of Rodhradi Gana:
एष रोध्रादिको नाम मेदः कफहरो गणः| योनिदोषहरः स्तम्भी वर्ण्यो विषविनाशनः||२७||
This group known as Rodhradika, cures diseases of
MedaKapha – fat and Kapha,
Yoni dosha – disorders of vagina,
Stambhi – produces obstruction to movements of Dosas and Malas,
Varnya – improves complexion and
Vishavinashana – destroys poison.

ArkadiGana – Arkadi group of herbs:
अर्कालर्कौ नागदन्ती विशल्या भाङ्र्गी रास्ना वृश्चिकाली प्रकीर्या|
प्रत्यक्पुष्पी पीततैलोदकीर्या श्वेतायुग्मं तापसानां च वृक्षः||२८||
Arka – Calotropis gigantea,
Alarka – variety of Calotropis gigantea,
Nagadanti – Croton oblongifolius,
Vishalya – Baliospermum montanum,
Bharngi – Clerodendrum serratum,
Rasna – Pluchea lanceolata,
Vrishchikali – Gymnema sylvestre,
Prakirya – Pongamia pinnata,
Pratyakpushpi – Achyranthes aspera,
Pitataila – Kakadani – Cardiospermum halicacabum,
Jyotishmati – Celastruspaniculatus,
Udakirya – Caesalpinia bonducella,
Swetayugmam – Sweta – Albizia lebbeck and Mahasweta – Albizia procera,
Tapasana ca vriksha – tree of Balanites aegyptiaca

constitute Arkadi Gana.

Benefits of Arkadi Gana:
अयमर्कादिको वर्गः कफमेदोविषापहः| कृमिकुष्ठप्रशमनो विशेषाद्व्रणशोधनः||२९||
Arkadi Gana mitigates
Kapha,
Meda – fat,
Visha – poison,
Krimi –worms,
Kushta – skin diseases and
Visheshat vrana shodana – especially cleanses the ulcers.

Surasadi Gana – Surasadi group of herbs:
सुरसयुगफणिज्जं कालमाला विडङ्गं खरबुसवृषकर्णीकट्फलं कासमर्दः|
क्षवकसरसिभाङ्गीकार्मुकाः काकमाची कुलहलविषमुष्टीभूस्तृणो भूतकेशी||३०||
Surasayuga – Sacred basil – Ocimum tenuiflorum and holy basil – Ocimum
sanctum,
Phanijam – Camphor basil – Ocimum kilimandscharicum,
Kalamala – Ocimum basilicum, Orthosiphon pallidus,
Vidangam – Embelia ribes,
Kharabusa – Origanum majorana,
Vrishakarni – Merremia emarginata,
Katphala – Myrica nagi,
Kasamarda – Cassia occidentalis,
Kshavaka – Centipeda minima,
Sarasi – Acacia concinna,
Bharngi – Clerodendrum serratum,
Karmuka – Bambusa bambos,
Kakamachi – Solanum nigrum,
Kulahala – Sphaeranthus indicus,
Vishamushti – Strychnos nux vomica, Ageratum conyzoides,
Bhustrina – Cymbopogon citratus,
Bhutakeshi – Nardostachy sjatamansi
constitute the herbs ofSurasadi Gana.

Benefits of Surasadi Gana:
सुरसादिर्गणः श्लेष्ममेदःकृमिनिषूदनः| प्रतिश्यायारुचिश्वासकासघ्नो व्रणशोधनः||३१||

Surasadi Gana mitigates

Sleshma – kapha,

Meda – fat,

Krimi – worms,

Pratishyaya – common cold,

Aruchi – anorexia,

Swasa – dyspnoea,

Kasa – cough and

Vranashodhana – cleanses the wounds.

MuskakadiGana – Muskakadi group of herbs:

मुष्ककस्नुग्वराद्वीपिपलाशधवशिंशिपाः| गुल्ममेहाश्मरीपाण्डुमेदोर्शःकफशुक्रजित्||३२||

Mushkaka –Schrebera swietenioides,

Snuhi – Euphorbia neriifolia,

Vara – Triphala

Dvipi – Plumbago zeylanica,

Palasha – Butea monosperma,

Dhava – Anogeissus latifolia,

Shimshipa – Dalbergio sissoo

constitute the herbs of Mushkakadi Gana.

They mitigate

Gulma – abdominal tumours,

Meha – diabetes (urinary disorders),

Ashmari – urinary calculi,

Pandu – anaemia,

Meda – excess fat,

Arsha – piles,

Kapha – balances kapha and

Shukrajit – cures disorders of semen.

VatsakadiGana – Vatsakadi group of herbs:

वत्सकमूर्वाभाङ्गीकटुका मरीचं घुणप्रिया च गण्डीरम्|

एला पाठाडजाजीकट्वङ्गफलाजमोदसिद्धार्थवचाः||३३||

जीरकहिङ्गुविडङ्गं पशुगन्धा पञ्चकोलकं हन्ति|

चलकफमेदःपीनसगुल्मज्वरशूलदुर्नाम्नः||३४||

Vatsaka – Holarrhenaantidysenterica,

Murva – Marsdeniatenacissima,

Bharngi – Clerodendrumserratum,

Katuka – Picrorhizakurroa,

Maricham – black pepper,

Ghunapriya – Aconitum heterophyllum,

Gandiram – Euphorbia neriifolia,

Ela – Cardamom – Elettaria cardamomum,

Patha – Cissampelos pareira,

Ajaji – cumin seeds – Foeniculum vulgare,

Katvangaphala – fruit of Oroxylum indicum, Ailanthus excels,

Ajamoda– celery – Tachyspermumroxburghianum,

Siddhartha – mustard – Brassica juncea,

Vacha – Acorus calamus,

Jiraka – cumin – Cuminum cyminum,

Hingu – asafoetida

Vidanga – Embelia ribes,

Pashugandha – Cleome gynandra,

Panchakolam – Pippali, Pippali moola, Chavya, Chitraka and Nagara (ginger),

constitute VatsakadiGana.

This group of drugs cure

Disorders of Vata, Kapha and medas (fat),

Pinasa – rhinitis,

Gulma – abdominal tumour,

Jwara – fever,

Shoola – colic and

Durnamna – Haemorrhoids.

Vacha Haridradi Gana – Vacha Haridradi group of herbs:

वचाजलददेवाह्वनागरातिविषाभयाः। हरिद्राद्वययष्ट्याह्वकलशीकुटजोद्भवाः॥३५॥

Vacha – sweet flag – Acorus calamus,

Jalada – Cyperus rotundus,

Devahva – Cedrus deodara,

Nagara – dry ginger – Zingiber officinale,

Ativisha – Aconitum heterophyllum,

Abhaya – Terminalia chebula,

Haridradvaya – Haridra – Curcuma longa and Daruharidra – Berberis aristata / Coscinium fenestratum,

Yashtyahva – Licorice – Glycyrrhiza glabra,

Kalashi – Urariapicta,
Kutajodbhava – Seeds of Holarrhena antidysenterica
Constitute the herbs of Vacha Haridradi Gana.

Benefits of Vacha Haridradi Gana:
वचाहरिद्रादिगणावामातीसारनाशनौ|
मेदःकफाढ्यपवनस्तन्यदोषनिबर्हणौ||३६||
VachaharidradiGana cures
Amatisara – acute diarrhoea (that is caused by accumulations of Ama),
Medakapha – diseases due to fat accumulation and Kapha,
Adhyapavana– stiffness of the thighs and
Stanya dosha – disorders caused by breast milk.

Priyangu–AmbasthadiGana – Priyangu–Ambasthadi group of herbs:
प्रियङ्गुपुष्पाञ्जनयुग्मपद्माः पद्माद्रजो योजनवल्ल्यनन्ता|
मानद्रुमो मोचरसः समङ्गा पुन्नागशीतं मदनीयहेतुः||३७||
अम्बष्ठा मधुकं नमस्करी नन्दीवृक्षपलाशकच्छुराः|
रोध्रं धातकिबिल्वपेशिके कट्वङ्गः कमलोद्भवं रजः||३८||
Priyangu – Callicarpa macrophylla,
Pushpa – zinc oxide,
Anjanayugma – two types of collyrium, srotoanjana and rasanjana,
Padma – Lotus – Clerodendron serratum,
Padmadrajo – stamens of lotus flower,
Yojanavalli – Rubia cordifolia,
Ananta – Hemidesmus indicus,
Manadruma – Salmaliamalabarica,
Mocharasa – Resin of silk cotton tree – Bombax ceiba,
Samanga – Mimosa pudica / Rubia cordifolia,
Punnaga – Calophyllum inophyllum,
Sheetam – sandalwood – Santalum album,
Madaneeyahetu – Woodfordia fruticosa,
Ambashta – Cissampelos pareira,
Madhukam – licorice – Glycyrrhiza glabra,
Namaskari – Mimosa pudica,
Nandivriksha – Ficus retusa,
Palasha – Butea monosperma,
Kacchura – Alhagi camelorum,

Rodhram – Symplocos racemosa,
Dhataki – Woodfordia fruticosa,
Bilvapeshike – Fruit pulp of Aegle marmelos,
Katvanga – Oroxylum indicum,
Kamalodbhava raja – stamens of lotus flower
constitute the group known as Priyangu–AmbasthadiGana.

Benefits of Priyangu–AmbasthadiGana:
गणौ प्रियङ्ग्वम्बष्ठादी पक्वातीसारनाशनौ|
सन्धानीयौ हितौ पित्ते व्रणानामपि रोपणौ||३९||
Priyangu–AmbasthadiGana cures
Pakvatisara – chronic diarrhoea,
Sandhaniya – heals fractures,
Hitaupitte – good for pitta and
Vranaropana – heals ulcers.

MustadiGana – Mustadi group of herbs:
मुस्तावचाग्निद्विनिशादिद्वितिक्ता भल्लातपाठात्रिफलाविषाख्याः|
कुष्ठं त्रुटी हैमवती च योनि स्तन्यामयघ्ना मलपाचनाश्च||४०||
Musta – Cyperus rotundus,
Vacha – Acorus calamus,
Agni – Plumbago zeylanica,
Dvinisha – Turmeric – Curcuma longa and Daruharidra – Berberis aristata,
Dvitikta – Katurohini – Picrorhiza kurroa and Kiratatikta – Trichosanthes tricuspidata,
Bhallata – Semecarpus anacardium,
Patha – Cissampelos pareira,
Triphala
Vishakhya – Aconitum heterophyllum,
Kushtam – Saussurealappa,
Truti – Cardamom – Elettaria cardamomum,
Haimavati – white variety of Acorus calamus
are the herbs belonging to the group of MustadiGana.
They cure
Yoni amaya – diseases of vagina,
Stanyaamaya – diseases due to breast milk and
Malapachana – prepares and processes the doshas.

NyagrodhadiGana – Nyagrodhadi group of herbs:
न्यग्रोधपिप्पलसदाफलरोध्रयुग्मं जम्बूद्वयार्जुनकपीतनसोमवल्काः।
प्लक्षाम्रवञ्जुलपियालपलाशनन्दी कोलीकदम्बविरलामधुकं मधूकम्॥४१॥
Nyagrodha – Ficus benghalensis,
Pippala – Ficus religiosa,
Sadaphala – Ficus racemosa,
Rodhrayugmam – Rodhra – Symplocos cochinchinensis and Sweta rodhra – Symplocos laurina,
Jambudvaya – Syzygium cumini and Eugenia jambolana,
Arjuna – Terminalia arjuna,
Kapitana – Spondias pinnata,
Somavalka – Myrica nagi,
Plaksha – Ficus lacor,
Amra – mango – Mangifera indica,
Vanjula – Salix capria, Saracaasoca,
Piyala – Buchananialanzan,
Palasha – Butea monosperma,
Nandi – Ficus arnottiana,
Koli – Ziziphus jujube,
Kadamba – Anthocephalus cadamba,
Virala – Diospyros melanoxylon,
Madhukam – licorice – Glycyrrhiza glabra,
Madhukam – Madhuca indica,
Constitute the herbs belonging to NyagrodhadiGana.

Benefits of NyagrodhadiGana:
न्यग्रोधादिर्गणो व्रण्यः सङ्ग्राही भग्नसाधनः।
मेदःपित्तास्रतृड्दाहयोनिरोगनिबर्हणः॥४२॥
NyagrodhadiGana is good for
Vrana – wounds/ ulcers,
Sangrahi – cause constipation,
Bhagnasadhana – unites fractures,
It cures
Meda – fat accumulation,
Pittasra – bleeding disease,
Trit – thirst,

Daha – burning sensation and

Yoniroga – diseases of the vagina.

EladiGana – Eladi group of herbs:

एलायुग्मतुरुष्ककुष्ठफलिनीमांसीजलध्यामकं
स्पृक्काचोरकचोचपत्रतगरस्थौणेयजातीरसाः|
शुक्तिव्याघ्रनखोऽमराह्वमगुरुः   श्रीवासकः   कुङ्कुमं   चण्डागुग्गुलुदेवधूपखपुराः
पुन्नागनागाह्वयम्||४३||

Elayugma – Sukshma ela – Elettaria cardamomum and Sthula ela – Amomum subulatum,

Turushka – Hydnocarpus laurifolia,

Kushta – Saussurea lappa,

Phalini – Callicarpa macrophylla,

Mamsi – Nardostachys jatamansi,

Jala – Coleus zeylanicus / Coleus vettiveroides,

Dhyamakam – Cymbopogon martini,

Sprikka – Anisomeles malabarica,

Choraka – Angelica archagelica,

Chocha – Cinnamomum zeylanicum,

Patra – Cinnamomum tamala,

Tagara – Valeriana wallichii,

Sthauneya – Taxus baccata,

Jatirasa – Commiphor amyrrha,

Shukti – Ostrea edulis,

Vyaghra nakha – Capparis sepiaria,

Amarahvam – Cedrus deodara,

Aguru – Aquilaria agallocha,

Shrivasaka – Pinus longifolia,

Kumkumam – Saffron – Crocus sativus,

Chanda – Angelica glauca,

Guggulu – Commiphora mukul,

Devadhoopa – Shorea robusta,

Khapura – Boswellia serrata,

Punnaga – Calophyllum inophyllum,

Nagahvayam – Messua ferrea

constitute the herbs of EladiGana.

Benefits of Eladi Gana:
एलादिको वातकफौ विषं च विनियच्छति।
वर्णप्रसादनः कण्डूपिटिकाकोठनाशनः॥४४॥
Eladi Gana cures disorders of Vata, Kapha and Visha (poison),
Varna prasadana – improves complexion,
Kandu pitika kota nashana – cures itching, abscesses and pustules.

ShyamadiGana – Shyamadi group of herbs:
श्यामादन्तीद्रवन्तीक्रमुककुटरणा शङ्खिनीचर्मसाह्वा स्वर्णक्षीरीगवाक्षी शिखरिरजनक
च्छिन्नरोहाकरञ्जाः।
बस्तान्त्री व्याधिघातो बहलबहुरस स्तीक्ष्णवृक्षात् फलानि श्यामाद्यो हन्ति गुल्मं
विषमरुचिकफौ
हृद्रुजं मूत्रकृच्छ्रम्॥४५॥
Shyama – Operculina turpethum,
Danti – Baliospermum montanum,
Dravanti – Croton tiglium,
Kramuka – Betel nut,
Kutarana – Operculina turpethum,
Shankhini – Convolvulus pluricaulis,
Charmasahva – Acacia sinuata,
Svarnaksheeri – Argemone mexicana,
Gavakshi – Streblus aspera,
Shikhari – Achyranthes aspera,
Rajanaka – Mallotus philippeinensis,
Chinnaroha – Tinospora cordifolia,
Karanja – Pongamia pinnata,
Bastantri – Argyreia nervosa,
Vyadhighata – Cassia fistula,
Bahala – Moringa oleifera,
Bahurasa – Zanthoxylum alatum,
Tikshnavrikshat phalani – Salvadora persica
constitute Shyamadi Gana.
It cures
Gulma – abdominal tumours,
Visha – poison,
Aruchi – anorexia,
Kapha – vitiation of kapha,

Hridruja – heart diseases and
Mutrakrichram – dysuria.

Including and excluding herbs from the above said 33 group of herbs:
त्रयस्त्रिंशदिति प्रोक्ता वर्गास्तेषु त्वलाभतः।
युञ्ज्यात्तद्विधमन्यच्च द्रव्यं जह्यादयौगिकम्॥४६॥
Thus, thirty three groups of herbs have been described.
Among these drugs if some of the herbs are not available, they shall be
substituted with other herbs having identical properties, and the herbs that
are inappropriate to the group may be rejected.

Utility of the groups of herbs in different forms:
एते वर्गा दोषदूष्याद्यपेक्ष्य कल्कक्काथस्नेहलेहादियुक्ताः।
पाने नस्येऽन्वासनेऽन्तर्बहिर्वा लेपाभ्यङ्गैर्घ्नन्ति रोगान् सुकृच्छ्रान्॥४७॥
These herbs when administered in the form of
Kalka – wet paste,
Kwatha – decoctions,
Sneha – medicated fats (oleation),
Leha – linctus etc;
internally in the form of
Paana – drinking,
Nasya – nasal medication,
Anuvasana – unctuous enema;
and externally for
Lepa – topical application,
Abyanga – oil massage etc;
after having considered the doshas and dushyas (tissues), cure even the
most difficult diseases (krichraroga).

इति श्रीवैद्यपतिसिंहगुप्तसूनुश्रीमद्वाग्भटविरचितायामष्टाङ्गहृदयसंहितायां सूत्रस्थाने
शोधनादिगणसङ्ग्रहो नाम पञ्चदशोऽध्यायः॥१५॥
Thus ends the 15th chapter of Ashtangahridaya Samhita Sutrasthana, named
Shodhanadi gana sangrahamAdhyayam, written by Shrimad Vagbhata, son
of Shri VaidyapatiSimhagupta.

16

स्नेहविधिमध्यायम् (snehavidhim adhyayam)

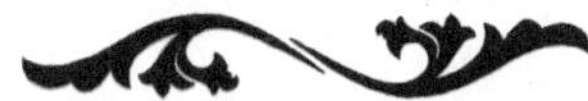

The 16th chapter of Sutrasthanam of Ashtanga Hridayam is named as Sneha Vidhim Adhyaya. This chapter deals with Snehana or oleation procedure. Here we are explaining in detail about the procedure of Snehana, treatment by drinking fat, which is administered just before performing emesis (Vamana) Panchakarma therapy.

अथातो स्नेहविधिमध्यायं व्याख्यास्यामः इति ह स्माहुरात्रेयादयो महर्षयः॥

Atreya and other sages pledge that henceforth they will be explaining the chapter named Sneha Vidhim (pertaining to the group of herbs used in Panchakarma or purification treatments).

Sneha dravya guna:

गुरुशीतसरस्निग्धमन्दसूक्ष्ममृदुद्रवम्।
औषधं स्नेहनं प्रायो, विपरीतं विरूक्षणम्॥१॥

Qualities of oil and fats - Snehana Dravya Guna –

The Snehana substances – used for oleation therapy have the following qualities -

Guru – heaviness

Sheeta – cold

Sara – easily moving, mobility, spreading

Snigdha – unctuous, oily

Manda – mild,

Sookshma – minute

Mrudu – soft

Dravam – liquid

The substances used for imparting dryness to the body (Rookshana) are of opposite qualities to the above-mentioned.

Sneha dravyas:

सर्पिर्मज्जा वसा तैलं स्नेहेषु प्रवरं मतम्‌|

तत्रापि चोत्तमं सर्पिः संस्कारस्यानुवर्तनात्‌||२||

माधुर्यादविदाहित्त्वाज्जन्मादयेव च शीलनात्‌|

Oleating substances – Sneha Dravyah –

Sarpi (ghee, clarified butter),

Majja (bone marrow),

Vasa – muscle fat and

Taila (oil) – are considered best among oleating substances;

Among these, Ghee is the best because it is –

Madhura – sweet in taste

Avidahi – it does not cause burning sensation

Janmadyevasheelanat – it is congenial to the body since birth.

पित्तघ्नास्ते यथापूर्वमितरघ्ना यथोत्तरम्‌||३||

Among them, Ghee is the most efficient for Pitta balance and Taila is the least efficient for the same.

घृतात्तैलं गुरु वसा तैलान्मज्जा ततोऽपि च|

When compared between the four, ghee is very light to digest. Oil is heavier (hard to digest) than ghee, muscle-fat is heavier than oil, marrow is heavier than all.

द्वाभ्यां त्रिभिश्चतुर्भिस्तैर्यमकस्त्रिवृतो महान्‌||४||

Mixture of two oleating substances is called **Yamaka**.

Mixture of three is called as **Trivrit** and

All four combined is called as **Mahasneha**.

Snehana yogya - person suitable for Snehana:

स्वेदसंशोध्यमद्यस्त्रीव्यायामासक्तचिन्तकाः|
वृद्धबालाबलकृशा रूक्षाः क्षीणास्रेतसः||५||
वातार्तस्यन्दतिमिरदारुणप्रतिबोधिनः|

Snehyah – persons suitable for oleation :-

People who require Snehana therapy are -

Svedya, Samshodhya – Those who are to be administered sudation and purification therapies,

Madya, Stree, Vyayamaasakta – who indulge more in wine, women and exercise;

Chintaka – who think too much,

Vruddha – the aged,

Bala – the children,

Abala – the debilitated,

Krusha – the emaciated, fatigue;

Ruksha – who are dry,

Ksheenaasraretas – Depleted blood and semen,

Vatarta – who are suffering from diseases of Vata,

Timira – ophthalmia, blindness,

who suffer from chronic disorder

Snehana Ayogya:

स्नेह्याः न त्वतिमन्दाग्नितीक्ष्णाग्निस्थूलदुर्बलाः||६||
ऊरुस्तम्भातिसाराऽऽमगलरोगगरोदरैः|
मूर्च्छाच्छर्द्यरुचिश्लेष्मतृष्णामद्यैश्च पीडिताः||७||
अपप्रसूता युक्ते च नस्ये बस्तौ विरेचने|

Asnehya – persons unsuitable for oleation :-

Patients who should not be given Snehana therapy are -

Atimandagni – Those who have very weak digestion power

Teekshnagni -or very strong digestive power

Sthula – obsese

Durbala – very weak

Urustambha – stiffness of thighs

Atisara – diarrhoea, dysentery

Amaroga – indigestion, Ama condition, altered metabolism

Galaroga – diseases of throat

Gararoga – chronic poisoning

Murcha – fainting, loss of consciousness

Chardi – Vomiting

Aruchi – anorexia

Shleshmaroga – diseases of Kapha imbalance

Trushnaroga – excessive thirst

Madyapeedita – chronic alcoholic

Apaprasuta – lady who has undergone abortion

Nasya, Basti Virechana – people who are to be given nasal medication, enema and purgative therapies.

Ghrita Ayogya

तत्र धीस्मृतिमेधादिकाङ्क्षिणां शस्यते घृतम्||८||

Ghrita (ghee) is best suited for those who desire improvement of intelligence, memory, intelligence etc.

Taila yogya:

ग्रन्थिनाडीकृमिश्लेष्ममेदोमारुतरोगिषु|

तैलं लाघवदाढर्यार्थिक्रूरकोष्ठेषु देहिषु||९||

Taila (oil) is suited in diseases like

Granthi – tumour,

Nadiroga – sinus ulcer

Krumiroga – worm infestation

Shleshmaroga – diseases of Kapha imbalance

Medoroga – obesity

Marutaroga – Diseases due to imbalance of Vata

for those who desire thinning and sturdiness of the body, and who have hard bowel movements.

Vasa Majja yogya:

वातातपाध्वभारस्त्रीव्यायामक्षीणधातुषु|

रूक्षक्लेशक्षमात्यग्निवातावृतपथेषु च||१०||

शेषौ वसा तु सन्ध्यस्थिमर्मकोष्ठरुजासु च|

तथा दग्धाहतभ्रष्टयोनिकर्णशिरोरुजि||११||

Vasa and Majja - Muscle-fat and marrow are suited for persons

Vatatapa – who are depleted of their tissues from exposure to breeze, sunlight, long distance walk, carrying heavy load, women (sexual activity) and physical activities;

Ruksha – who are dry, who withstand strain, who have very strong digestive activity, and in whom Vata is obstructed in its normal pathways.

Vasa – Muscle-fat is suited for pain of the joints, bones, vital organs and abdominal viscera; so also for pain of burns, assault by weapons, displacement of vagina (prolapsed), earache, and headache.

तैल प्रावृषि, वर्षान्ते सर्पिरन्यौ तु माधवे ।

Oil is ideal for use during Pravrit – first rainy season, ghee during end of Varsa i.e., Sharat- autumn and the others during Madhava i.e. Vasantha – spring.

Snehayogya kala - Ideal time for Snehana:

ऋतौ साधारणे स्नेहः शस्तोऽह्नि विमले रवौ||१२||

तैलं त्वरायां शीतेऽपि घर्मेऽपि च घृतं निशि|

निश्येव पित्ते पवने संसर्गे पित्तवत्यपि||१३||

निश्यन्यथा वातकफाद्रोगाः स्युः पित्ततो दिवा|

During temperate seasons use of oleating materials should be done during day time and when the sun is clear.

Oil may be used in emergencies even in cold season and ghee, even in summer and even at night. 13a.

In diseases produced by increased Pitta and Vata and in their combination with predominance of Pitta – ghee should be used only at nights – during summer.

Otherwise, diseases due to Vata and Kapha arise if fats are used at nights and diseases of Pitta if used during day.

Sneha bheda:

युक्त्याऽवचारयेत्स्नेहं भक्ष्याद्यन्नेन बस्तिभिः||१४||

नस्याभ्यञ्जनगण्डूषमूर्धकर्णाक्षितर्पणैः|

Fats should be used properly either mixed with chewable and other kinds of foods or in the form of enemas, nasal drops, anointing over the body, holding in the mouth, putting over the head, into the ears and eyes.

रसभेदैककत्वाभ्यां चतुःषष्टिर्विचारणाः||१५||

स्नेहस्यान्याभिभूतत्वादल्पत्वाच्च क्रमात्स्मृताः|

By its use with substances of different tastes and separately, without admixture, it will be sixty four number of recipes.

Sneha Vicharana – use of fat mixed with foods is poor – mild in effect because of its mingling with other materials and also because of lesser quantity.

यथोक्तहेत्वभावाच्च नाच्छपेयो विचारणा ॥ १६ ॥
स्नेहस्य कल्पः स श्रेष्ठः स्नेहकर्माशुसाधनात् ।

Acchapeya of Sneha – means consuming the oils / fats without mixing with food.

Sneha Vicharana means – consuming after mixing with food items.

Acchapeya method of administering fats is considered best as it serves the function of fats and lubrication quickly.

Acchapana matra – dose of fats for drinking:

द्वाभ्यां चतुर्भिरष्टाभिर्यामैर्जीर्यन्ति याः क्रमात्॥१७॥
ह्रस्वमध्योत्तमा मात्रास्तास्ताभ्यश्च ह्रसीयसीम्।
कल्पयेद्वीक्ष्य दोषादीन् प्रागेव तु ह्रसीयसीम्॥१८॥

The dose of fats depends upon the digestive activity of the patient.

The heenamatra (least dose) is the one, which digests in 2 yaama (1 yaama = 3 hours)

The medium dose (Madhyama matra) is the one, which undergoes digestion in 3 yama (9 hours)

The high dose (Uttamamatra) is the one, which undergoes digestion in 4 yama (12 hours).

Hraseeyasi matra – the minimum quantity should be administered in the beginning after considering the condition of Dosha etc.

The Hraseeyasi matra is the very little quantity of sneha, which is given to the patient, just to judge the digestive strength. After judging the digestion power, the right dose of the fat is decided.

Snehapanavidhi – procedure of drinking fat:

ह्यस्तने जीर्ण एवान्ने स्नेहोऽच्छः शुद्धये बहुः।
शमनः क्षुद्वतोऽनन्नो मध्यमात्रश्च शस्यते॥१९॥

For **Shodhana** – As a preparation procedure to Panchakarma therapy, Acchasneha – drinking of fat alone should be soon after digestion of previous food and in maximum dose.

For **Shamana** – For mitigation of Doshas, for palliating a disease, fats should be consumed when the person is hungry and without food – fasting and in medium dose.

For Brimhana:

बृंहणो रसमद्यायैः सभक्तोऽल्पः

For weight gain treatment, it should be given mixed with meat soup, wine etc. and consumed along with food, in small quantities – minimum dose.

हितः स च|

बालवृद्धपिपासार्तस्नेहद्विण्मद्यशीलिषु||२०||

स्त्रीस्नेहनित्यमन्दाग्निसुखितक्लेशभीरुषु|

मृदुकोष्ठाल्पदोषेषु काले चोष्णे कृशेषु च||२१||

This kind of mild oleation is suitable to children, the aged, those suffering from thirst, those who have aversion to fat, who indulge in wine, women and fatty foods daily, who have poor digestive ability, who lead happy life, who are afraid of troubles, who are of soft bowel, who have little quantity of – increase of Doshas; during hot season and for the emaciated.

प्राङ्मध्योत्तरभक्तोऽसावधोमध्योर्ध्व-देहजान्|

व्याधीञ्जयेद्बलं कुर्यादङ्गानां च यथाक्रमम्||२२||

If fats are used before food, it is useful in the treatment of diseases affecting the lower part of the body. It strengthens the upper part of the body.

If fats are used during the food intake, it is useful in the treatment of diseases affecting the middle part of the body. It strengthens the middle part of the body.

If fats are used after the food intake, it is useful in treating the diseases of the upper part of the body. It strengthens the lower part of the body.

Care after drinking fats – Sneha upachara:

वार्युष्णमच्छेऽनु पिबेत् स्नेहे तत्सुखपक्तये|

आस्योपलेपशुद्ध्यै च, तौवरारुष्करे न तु||२३||

जीर्णाजीर्णविशङ्कायां पुनरुष्णोदकं पिबेत्|

तेनोद्गारविशुद्धिः स्यात्ततश्च लघुता रुचिः||२४||

After Acchapana – (drinking of fat alone), warm water should be consumed.

It helps in digestion and clears the mouth coating.

But while taking Tuvarakataila or Arushkarataila (very hot in nature), cold water is preferred.

In case of doubts regarding digestion of the fat, warm water should be consumed again;

Purification, clear belching, feeling of lightness in the body and desire for food – these 3 symptoms suggest that the fat has been completely digested.

भोज्योऽन्नं मात्रया पास्यन् श्वः पिबन् पीतवानपि।
द्रवोष्णमनभिष्यन्दि नातिस्निग्धमसङ्करम्॥२५॥

Diet during fat consumption – Foods which are liquid (drava), warm (Ushna), not producing excess moisture inside (anabhishyandi), not very oily (na ati snigdha) and not a mixture of many food materials, should be consumed by the patient in limited quantity.

Regimen after oleation -

उष्णोदकोपचारी स्याद्ब्रह्मचारी क्षपाशयः।
न वेगरोधी व्यायामक्रोधशोकहिमातपान्॥२६॥
प्रवातयानयानाध्वभाष्यात्यासन संस्थितीः।
नीचात्युच्चोपधानाहः स्वप्नधूमरजांसि च॥२७॥
यान्यहानि पिबेत्तानि तावन्त्यन्यान्यपि त्यजेत्।

Ushnodakopachari – The person should use warm water only for all his activities.

Brahmachari – Should maintain celibacy.

Kshapashaya – He should eat only when hungry.

Na vegarodhi – should not suppress natural urges, not indulge in exercise, anger, grief, exposure to cold, sunlight, breeze, riding on animals, travelling in vehicles, walking long distance, too much of speaking, remaining in uncomfortable positions for long time, keeping very low or very high pillow under the head, sleeping during day, contact with smoke and dust; on the days of drinking fats and for same number of days afterwards also.

सर्वकर्मस्वयं प्रायो व्याधिक्षीणेषु च क्रमः॥२८॥

This regimen is the same generally for all purification therapies such as emesis, purgation, enema etc. and also for those debilitated by diseases.

उपचारस्तु शमने कार्यः स्नेहे विरिक्तवत्।

In case of Shamana Sneha – palliative oleation therapy, the regimen as suggested for the person who has undergone purgation therapy – vide chapter 18 should be adopted. 29a.

Acchapana Kala – duration of fat drinking:

त्र्यहमच्छं मृदौ कोष्ठे क्रूरे सप्तदिनं पिबेत्||२९||

सम्यक्स्निग्धोऽथवा यावदतः सात्म्यी भवेत्परम्|

Acchapana – drinking fat alone should be done for

three days for – persons of soft bowels (Mrudukoshta),

for seven days for persons of hard bowels (Krurakoshta) or till the symptoms of good oleation appear.

After that period it – fat becomes accustomed to the patient and does not give the desired effect.

SnigdhaLakshana – signs of oleation :

वातानुलोम्यं दीप्तोऽग्निर्वर्चः स्निग्धमसंहतम्||३०||

स्नेहोद्वेगः क्लमः सम्यक्स्निग्धे, रूक्षे विपर्ययः|

अतिस्निग्धे तु पाण्डुत्वं घ्राणवक्त्रगुदस्रवाः||३१||

Vatanulomana – Downward movement of Vata,

Deeptoagni – keen digestive activity,

Vachahasnigdhamasamhatam – faeces becoming fatty and non formed, not solid,

Snehodvega – aversion to fat,

Klama – exhaustion

– are the signs of proper lubrication;

opposite of these are the signs of dryness.

Appearance of pallor – yellowish white discoloration and secretions from the nose, mouth and rectum are the signs of excess lubrication.

Sneha Vyapat Laksana – bad effects of improper oleation:

अमात्रयाऽहितो काले मिथ्याहारविहारतः|

स्नेहः करोति शोफार्शस्तन्द्रास्तम्भविसंज्ञताः||३२||

कण्डूकुष्ठज्वरोत्क्लेशशूलानाहभ्रमादिकान्|

Fat drinking in improper dose, unsuitable kind, improper time, indulging in improper foods and activities produces dropsy, haemorrhoids, stupor, rigidity – loss of movement, loss of sensation / unconsciousness, itching, skin diseases, fever, nausea, pain in the abdomen, flatulence, dizziness etc. 32 – 33a.

Snehavyapat Chikitsa – treatment of bad effects:

क्षुत्तृष्णोल्लेखनस्वेदरूक्षपानान्नभेषजम्||३३||

तक्रारिष्टखलोद्दालयवश्यामाककोद्रवम्।
पिप्पलीत्रिफलाक्षौद्रपथ्यागोमूत्रगुग्गुलु ॥३४॥
यथास्वं प्रतिरोगं च स्नेहव्यापदि साधनम्।

Kshut, Trushna – Producing hunger, thirst,

Ulleka, sveda – vomiting and perspiration,

administering foods, drinks and medicines which are dry (cause dryness), use of Takrarista (fermented medicine from buttermilk), Khala – menu prepared from curds, Uddala, Yava (barley), Shyamaka, Kodrava, Pippali (long pepper), Triphala, Ksaudra (honey), Pathya (haritaki), Gomutra – cow urine, Guggulu and such others – foods, drugs etc. prescribed for each disease are the methods of treating the diseases due to improper Snehana therapy.

Virukshana – therapy to cause dryness:

विरूक्षणे लङ्घनवत्कृतातिकृतलक्षणम् ॥३५॥

The features of proper and excess Viruksana – dryness are the same as those of proper and excess of Langhana – methods of making the body thin.

Regimen of Panchakarma followed after Snehana:

स्निग्धद्रवोष्णधन्वोत्थरसभुक् स्वेदमाचरेत्।
स्निग्धस्त्र्यहं स्थितः कुर्यादि्वरेकं, वमनं पुनः ॥३६॥
एकाहं दिनमन्यच्च कफमुत्क्लेश्य तत्करैः।

The patient should drink juice of meat of animals of desert – like regions, mixed with fats, made liquid – thin and warm, then undergo sudation therapy; after three days of such regimen, he should be administered purgation therapy, after a lapse of one day, Kapha should be increased by using things – food, drugs etc. which cause its increase and then emesis – therapy should be administered.

मांसला मेदुरा भूरिश्लेष्माणो विषमाग्नयः ॥३७॥
स्नेहोचिताश्च ये स्नेह्यास्तान् पूर्व रूक्षयेततः।
संस्नेह्य शोधयेदेवं स्नेहव्यापन्न जायते ॥३८॥
अलं मलानीरयितुं स्नेहश्चासात्म्यतां गतः।

Persons who are muscular, fatty, having Kapha imbalance, and erratic type of digestive activity, who are accustomed to fats and who need oleation therapy, should be made to become dry first – by use of foods, drugs etc. and then administered oleation therapy followed with purification therapies. By this procedure complications of oleation will not arise. This method is enough to excite the vitiated Dosha to be eliminated.

Sadyasneha Yoga – recipes for immediate oleation:

बालवृद्धादिषु स्नेहपरिहारासहिष्णुषु||३९||
योगानिमाननुद्वेगान् सद्यःस्नेहान् प्रयोजयेत्|

For children, the aged etc., for those who cannot withstand the discomforts or avoidance of things prohibited during oleation therapy, can be administered the following recipes which are Sadyasneha – immediate oleation/ lubrication and which are non-harming.

प्राज्यमांसरसास्तेषु, पेया वा स्नेहभर्जिता||४०||
तिलचूर्णश्च सस्नेहफाणितः, कृशरा तथा|
क्षीरपेया घृताढ्योष्णा, दध्नो वा सगुडः सरः||४१||
पेया च पञ्चप्रसृता स्नेहैस्तण्डुलपञ्चमैः|
सप्तैते स्नेहनाः सद्यः, स्नेहाश्च लवणोल्बणाः||४२||

Juice of meat prepared from more quantity of meat,

Peya – gruels, fried with more quantity of fats,

powder of Tila mixed with fat and half boiled molasses (Phanita),

Krisara – rice cooked along with green gram, mixed with the same things as above,

Ksheerapeya – gruel prepared from milk, mixed with more quantity of ghee – butter fat and made warm;

Dadhi Sara – yoghurt water, whey from curds mixed with Guda (jaggery),

Pancha prasruta Peya – thin gruel prepared from one Prasruta each of ghee, sesame oil, muscle fat, marrow and rice (tandula).

These seven recipes are Sadyassneha – fat recipes which produce immediate oleation.

तद्ध्यभिष्यन्द्यरूक्षं च सूक्ष्ममुष्णं व्यवायि च|

And also fats mixed with more amount of salt are Sadyasneha because salt is

Abhisyandhi (causes exudation in the tissues),

Arooksha – does not cause dryness,

Suksma – capable of entering into minute pores,

Ushna – hot in potency and

Vyavayi spreads all over the body first and later undergoes transformation.

गुडानूपामिषक्षीरतिलमाषसुरादधि||४३||
कुष्ठशोफप्रमेहेषु स्नेहार्थं न प्रकल्पयेत्|

Contra indication for certain substances in certain diseases – For the purpose of Sadyasnehana, Jaggery, meat of birds of marshy lands, milk, sesame seed, black gram, Sura – beer and Dadhi – curds, yogurt should not be used for purposes of oleation in skin diseases (kushta), inflammatory conditions (Shopha) and diabetes (Prameha) because these substances may worsen the disease.

त्रिफलापिप्पलीपथ्यागुग्गुल्वादिविपाचितान्||४४||
स्नेहान् यथास्वमेतेषां योजयेदविकारिणः|

In these conditions, fats boiled with Triphala, Pippali, Pathya, Guggulu, etc., should be used as found suitable, which will not produce abnormalities.

क्षीणानां त्वामयैरग्निदेहसन्धुक्षणक्षमान्||४५||

For those who are debilitated by diseases, fats which are capable of increasing the strength of the body and of the digestive activity should be made use of for oleation therapy.

Snehapana Phala – benefits of drinking fats:
दीप्तान्तराग्निः परिशुद्धकोष्ठः प्रत्यग्र धातुर्बलवर्णयुक्तः |
दृढेन्द्रियो मन्दजरः शतायुः स्नेहोपसेवी पुरूषः प्रदिष्टः || ४६ ||

He, who has very keen digestive activity, clean alimentary tract, well developed/strong tissues, physical strength, colour – complexion and powerful sense faculties, who is slow in getting old and who lives for a hundred years is the person who is habituated to oleation. In other words these are the benefits of oleation therapy if adopted often.

इति श्रीवैद्यपतिसिंहगुप्तसूनुश्रीमद्वाग्भटविरचितायामष्टाङ्गहृदयसंहितायां सूत्रस्थाने स्नेहविधिर्नाम षोडशोऽध्यायः||१५||

Thus ends the chapter named Snehavidhi, the sixteenth in Sutrasthana of Astangahrdayam.

17

स्वेदविधिमध्यायम् (svedavidhim adhyayam)

The 17th chapter of Sutrasthanam of Ashtanga Hridayam is named as Sveda Vidhim Adhyaya. We are explaining Swedana procedure in this chapter. Swedana refers to sweating or sweating therapy. The term sweda means sweat. The patient is made to sweat on purpose. Usually this procedure is done after doing the oleation therapy (Snehakarma), that we studied in the last chapter.

अथातो स्ने स्वेदविधिमध्यायं व्याख्यास्याम: इति ह स्माहुरात्रेयादयो महर्षय:॥
Atreya and other sages pledge that henceforth they will be explaining the chapter named Sveda Vidhim (pertaining to the group of herbs used in Panchakarma or purification treatments).

Types of swedana:
स्वेदस्तापोपनाहोष्मद्रवभेदाच्चतुर्विधः|
Kinds of sweating treatments – Swedana Prakara
1. Tapa- fomentation,
2. Upanaha- warm poultice,
3. Ushma- warm steam and
4. Drava – pouring of warm liquid

तापोऽग्नितप्तवसनफालहस्ततलादिभिः||१||

Tapa Sweda is done by touching the affected part of the body with heated cloth, metal plate, palm of the hand etc.

Upanaha dravyas:

उपनाहो वचाकिण्वशताह्वादेवदारुभिः|
धान्यैः समस्तैर्गन्धैश्च रास्नैरण्डजटामिषैः||२||
उद्रिक्तलवणैः स्नेहचुक्रतक्रपयःप्लुतैः|
केवले पवने, श्लेष्मसंसृष्टे सुरसादिभिः||३||

UpanahaSweda is application of poultice prepared from
Vacha (Acorus calamus), Kinva-yeast, Shatahva (Dill),
Devadaru – (Himalayan cedar (bark) – Cedrus deodara) etc. any kind of grains, all substances having pleasant smell, roots of Rasna (Pluchea lanceolata) and Castor (Eranda); or meat;
each one added with more salt, fats-oil ghee etc. Chukra- Vinegar, Takra- Buttermilk and milk.

It is preferred in people with only Vata imbalance. In cases of vata being associated with kapha (vata-kapha imbalance) poultice should be administered with the Surasadi Gana group of herbs. In cases of vata being associated with pitta (vata-pitta imbalance), poultice prepared with padmakadi gana group of herbs is used. The poultice prepared with these herbs is called Salvana Upanaha and can be applied often.

पित्तेन पद्मकाद्यैस्तु साल्वणाख्यैः पुनःपुनः|
स्निग्धोष्णवीर्यैर्मृदुभिश्चर्मपट्टैरपूतिभिः||४||
अलाभे वातजित्पत्रकौशेयाविकशाटकैः| बद्धं रात्रौ दिवा मुञ्चेन्मुञ्चेद्रात्रौ दिवाकृतम्||५||

After applying the poultice (Upanaha), the part of the body should be bandaged with soft piece of leather which does not have bad smell, which has been oiled; it should be slightly warmed and tied;
If leather is not available, leaves of plants which balance Vata, silk cloth, or woollen cloth may be used. Poultice tied during night should be removed during day and that tied during day should be removed during night.

ऊष्मा तूत्कारिकालोष्टकपालोपलपांसुभिः| पत्रभङ्गेन धान्येन करीषसिकतातुषैः||६||
अनेकोपायसन्तप्तैः प्रयोज्यो देशकालितः|

Ushma Sweda- Here the steam of the hot substance is directed towards the body part. Steam may be obtained by Utkarika- (boiling grains, pulses, seeds etc).

Stones, pebbles, mud, leaves pieces, grains, dried dung of animals like cow, Sheep, Goat etc, Sand, Husk etc are also used for this purpose.

शिग्रुवारणकैरण्डकरञ्जसुरसार्जकात्||७|| शिरीषवासावंशार्कमालतीदीर्घवृन्ततः|
पत्रभङ्गैर्वचाद्यैश्च मांसैश्चानूपवारिजैः||८|| दशमूलेन च पृथक् सहितैर्वा यथामलम्|
स्नेहवद्भिः   सुराशुक्तावारिक्षीरादिसाधितैः||९|| कुम्भीर्गलन्तीर्नाडीर्वा   पूरयित्वा
रुजार्दितम्|
वाससाऽऽच्छादितं गात्रं स्निग्धं सिञ्चेद्यथासुखम्||१०||

Drava Sweda - Warm liquid is prepared by boiling bits of leaves of drumstick, Varanaka , Eranda – (Castor), Karanja, Surasa, Arjaka, Shireesa, Vasa , Vamsha, Arka, Malati (Jasmine) or Dirghvrinta, with drugs of vachadi gana – vide chapter 15, meat of animals of Marshy land and of those living in water, drugs of Dashamula, each one separately or all together, mixed with fats – oil, ghee etc. appropriate to the Dosha; Sura- beer, Sukta- fermented gruel, water and milk.

This medicated liquid should be filled into pot, jug with spout, or a tube and poured slowly and steadily over the painful part covered with cloth.

तैरेव वा द्रवैः पूर्णं कुण्डं सर्वाङ्गगेऽनिले|
अवगाह्यातुरस्तिष्ठेदर्शःकृच्छ्रादिरुक्षु च||११||

In case of Vata affecting the entire body, the same- medicated water may be filled into the tub and the patient made to sit in it. This method can be adopted in piles, Dysuria etc.

Sweda vidhi – procedure of Sweating therapy:
निवातेऽन्तर्बहिःस्निग्धो जीर्णान्नः स्वेदमाचरेत्|

Sweating should be administered to him who has been given Snehana - both internally- by drinking fats and externally- anointing oil over the body, who is staying in a room devoid of breeze and after his meal has been completely digested.

व्याधिव्याधितदेशर्तुवशान्मध्यवरावरम्||१२||

Sweating may be mild, moderate or strong depending upon the condition of the disease, Patient, habitat and season.

कफार्ते रूक्षणं रूक्षो, रूक्षः स्निग्धं कफानिले|

Person suffering from diseases of Kapha should be given sweating treatment in dry condition- without the use of fat internally and externally and with dry liquid – without addition of fats;

In case of Kapha and Vata- increased together the patient should be given sweating in dry condition and liquid mixed fats – should be used for sweating.

आमाशयगते वायौ कफे पक्वाशयाश्रिते||१३||
रूक्षपूर्वं तथा स्नेहपूर्वं स्थानानुरोधतः|

When vata is localized in the Amashaya- stomach, dry sweating should be given.

When Kapha is localized in Pakvasaya- (intestines), oil-sweating should be given.

अल्पं वङ्क्षणयोः, स्वल्पं दृङ्मुष्कहृदये न वा||१४||

Sweating should be very mild / nil over the groins and also on the eye, scrotum and heart. 14b

Benefits of sweating treatment – care to be taken - Swedanaphala and Upacana:

शीतशूलक्षये स्विन्नो जातेऽङ्गानां च मार्दवे|
स्याच्छनैर्मृदितः स्नातस्ततः स्नेहविधिं भजेत्||१५||

Diminution of cold and pain and softness of the organ occur from Sweating. Afterwards the body should be massaged slowly, given bath –in warm water and allowed comforts as prescribed in lubrication therapy.

Ati Swedana phala – effects of excess Sweating:

पित्तास्रकोपतृण्मूर्च्छास्वराङ्गसदनभ्रमाः|
सन्धिपीडा ज्वरः श्यावरक्तमण्डलदर्शनम्||१६||
स्वेदातियोगाच्छर्दिश्च, तत्र स्तम्भनमौषधम्|
विषक्षाराग्न्यतीसारच्छर्दिमोहातुरेषु च||१७||

Aggravation of Pitta and vitiation of blood,

thirst, loss of consciousness, weakness of voice and body,

Bhrama – Delusion, Dizziness

Sandhipeeda– pain in the joints ,

Jvara – fever, appearance of black- blue, red patches on the skin, and vomiting are produced by excess of Sweating therapy;

For that , Stambhana treatment should be done. It is the same procedure, useful in diarrhoea and bleeding disorders.

Withholding, stopping, hindering of elimination is the treatment, so also for patients suffering from poison, caustic Alkali and Barding by fire; Diarrhoea, vomiting and unconsciousness.

Qualities of substances used for Swedana, Sthambhana:

स्वेदनं गुरु तीक्ष्णोष्णं प्रायः, स्तम्भनमन्यथा|

द्रवस्थिरसरस्निग्धरूक्षसूक्ष्मं च भेषजम्||१८||

स्वेदनं, स्तम्भनं श्लक्ष्णं रूक्षसूक्ष्मसरद्रवम्|

प्रायास्तिक्तं कषायं च मधुरं च समासतः||१९||

Generally substances which are heavy, penetrating and hot in potency are used in Swedana therapy.

Substances of opposite qualities are used in Sthambhana (withholding, hindrances to elimination)

Drugs which are liquid, sthira – static, mobile, unctuous, dry and penetrating bring about sweating.

Those which are smooth, dry, thin, mobile and liquid, bitter, Astringent and sweet in taste are generally Stambhana.

स्तम्भितः स्याद्बले लब्धे यथोक्तामयसङ्क्षयात्|

Stambhana is useful in diarrhoea and bleeding disorders,

With this treatment, the person gains Strength and gets relieved of symptoms of excess sweating.

Symptoms of excess Sthambana:

स्तम्भत्वक्स्नायुसङ्कोचकम्पहृद्वाग्धनुग्रहैः||२०||

पादौष्ठत्वक्करैः श्यावैरतिस्तम्भितमादिशेत्|

Contraction of skin and tendons, tremors, stiffness of region of heart, choking of voice, locked jaw, black discoloration of the feet, lips, skin and hands.

Persons unsuitable for Svedana:

न स्वेदयेदतिस्थूलरूक्षदुर्बलमूच्छिंतान्||२१|| स्तम्भनीयक्षतक्षीणक्षाममद्यविकारिणः|

तिमिरोदरवीसर्पकुष्ठशोषाढ्यरोगिणः||२२|| पीतदुग्धदधिस्नेहमधून् कृतविरेचनान्|

भ्रष्टदग्धगुदग्लानिक्रोधशोकभयादितान्||२३|| क्षुत्तृष्णाकामलापाण्डुमेहिनः पितपीडितान्|

गर्भिणीं पुष्पितां सूतां, मृदु चात्ययिके गदे||२४||

Aswedayah – persons Unsuitable for Sweating:-
Atishoola – excessively obese
Atirooksha – highly dry
Durbala – weak, debilitated
Murchita – fainted, unconscious
Those who are fit for Sthambhana treatment
Kshataksheena – wounded, injured
Patients with Ama condition
Madyavikari – chronic alcoholics
Night blindness
Visarpa – herpes
Kushta - skin diseases
Shosha – emaciated
who have recently consumed milk, curds, fat,
Who have just undergone Virechana treatment
Who are burnt,
Who are tired, suffering from anger, grief, fear, excess thirst, hunger,
Kamala – liver diseases
Pandu – anemia
Meha – urinary disorders
People with Pitta imbalance
women who are pregnant, menstruating – during periods and delivered –
recently. In case of emergency diseases, it should be done mildly – for the
above. 21-24

Persons suitable for Svedana:
श्वासकासप्रतिश्यायहिध्माध्मानविबन्धिषु|
स्वरभेदानिलव्याधिश्लेष्मामस्तम्भगौरवे||२५||
अङ्गमर्दकटीपार्श्वपृष्ठकुक्षिहनुग्रहे|
महत्वे मुष्कयोः खल्यामायामे वातकण्टके||२६||
मूत्रकृच्छ्रार्बुदग्रन्थिशुक्रघाताढ्यमारुते|
स्वेदं यथायथं कुर्यात्तदौषधविभागतः||२७||
Shwasa – dysnoea, COPD, Asthma
Kasa – cough,
Pratishyaya – running nose, allergic rhinitis
Hidhma – hiccup,
Adhmana – bloating

Vibandha – constipation
Svarabheda – altered voice, hoarseness
Vatavyadi – diseases of Vata imbalance
Angamarda – bodyache
stiffness in lower back, flanks, back, abdomen and jaws
enlargement of the scrotum, contractions of toes and fingers, tetanus sprains, dysuria, Malignant tumour- cancer, benign tumour, obstruction to the flow of semen and urine, and Adhyamaruta- Thigh stiffness.

Anagni Sweda – Sweating without fire source:
स्वेदो हितस्त्वनाग्नेयो वाते मेदःकफावृते| निवातं गृहमायासो गुरुप्रावरणं भयम्||२८||
उपनाहाहवक्रोधा भूरिपानं क्षुधाऽऽतपः|
Sweating without source of fire is suitable in diseases of vata enveloped by Medas and Kapha.
Nivatasadana – Staying in air tight room,
Ayasa – stressful physical activity,
Gurupravarana – covering oneself with thick blankets
Bhaya – fear,
Upanaha – bandaging wrapping with cloth etc.
Fighting, wrestling
Krodha – anger
Bhuripana – excess drinking of water
Kshudha – withholding hunger
Atapa – Sun exposure

Swedaphala – Effects of Sweating:
स्नेहक्लिन्नाः कोष्ठगा धातुगा वा स्रोतोलीना ये च शाखास्थिसंस्थाः|
दोषाः स्वेदैस्ते द्रवीकृत्य कोष्ठं नीताः सम्यक् शुद्धिभिर्निर्हियन्ते|
Doshas which have been lubricated by oleation therapy, residing either in the alimentary tract, tissues, or lurking in the channels of the extremities bones etc are liquefied by Sweating therapy, brought into the alimentary canal to be eliminated out of the body completely, by appropriate purification therapies.
So, sweating is done after oleation, but be fore elimination of Doshas by Panchakarma.

इति श्रीवैद्यपतिसिंहगुप्तसूनुश्रीमद्वाग्भटविरचितायामष्टाङ्गहृदयसंहितायां सूत्रस्थाने

स्वेदविधिर्नाम नाम सप्तदशोऽध्यायः||१५||

Thus ends the chapter Swedavidhi- the Seventeenth of Sutrasthana of Astangahrdaya Samhita.

18

वमनविरेचनविधिमध्यायम्‌
(vamana virechana vidhim adhyayam)

The 18th chapter of Sutrasthanam of Ashtanga Hridayam is named as Vamana Virechana Vidhim Adhyayam. This chapter explains in detail regarding Vamana and Virechana Panchakarma procedures. Who are best suited for these therapies, who are not, what are the signs to observe during the procedure, complications and treatments for such complications.

अथातो वमनविरेचनविधिमध्यायं व्याख्यास्याम:
इति ह स्माहुरात्रेयादयो महर्षय:॥

Atreya and other sages pledge that henceforth they will be explaining the chapter named VamanaVirechanaVidhim (pertaining to Emesis and Purgation therapies).

Conditions for administering emesis and purgation therapies

कफे विदध्याद्वमनं संयोगे वा कफोल्बणे| तद्वद्विरेचनं पित्ते

Vamana – Emesis should be administered for increase of Kapha either alone or in combination with other Doshas where Kapha is predominant.

Virechana – purgation should be administered to treat increase of Pitta – alone or in combination with other Doshas where Pitta is predominant.

Persons suitable for Vamana procedure – Vamana Arha:

विशेषेण तु वामयेत्॥१॥
नवज्वरातिसाराधःपित्तासृग्राजयक्ष्मिणः।
कुष्ठमेहापचीग्रन्थिश्लीपदोन्मादकासिनः॥२॥
श्वासहृल्लासवीसर्पस्तन्यदोषोर्ध्वरोगिणः।

Emesis should be administered to persons suffering from

Navajwara – fever of recent origin

Atisara – diarrhoea, dysentery

Adha:pitta – Pitta imbalance in lower part of abdomen

Pittasruk – Bleeding disorder due to Pitta imbalance

Rajayakshma – Chronic Respiratory disorder

Kushta – skin diseases

Meha – diabetes, urinary tract disorders

Apachi, Granthi – Goitre, tumour, fibroid

Shleepada – Elephantiasis, Filariasis

Unmada – Schizophrenia

Kasa – cough, cold

Shwasa – Chronic Respiratory tract disease, Asthma

Hrullasa – nausea

Visarpa – herpes

Stanyadosha – vitiated breast milk

Urdhvaroga – diseases affected neck and above region

Persons not suitable for Vamana – Vamana Anarha:

अवाम्या गर्भिणी रूक्षः क्षुधितो नित्यदुःखितः ॥ ३ ॥
बालवृद्धकृशस्थूलहृद्रोगिक्षतदुर्बलाः ।
प्रसक्तवमथुप्लीहतिमिरकृमिकोष्ठिनः ॥ ४ ॥
ऊर्ध्वप्रवृत्तवाय्वस्रदत्तवस्तिहतस्वराः ।
मूत्राघात्युदरी गुल्मी दुर्वमो ऽत्यग्निरर्शसः ॥ ५ ॥
उदावर्तभ्रमाष्ठीलापार्श्वरुग्वातरोगिणः ।
ऋते विषगराजीर्णविरुद्धाभ्यवहारतः ॥ ६ ॥
प्रसक्तवमथोः पूर्वं प्रायेणामज्वरो ऽपि च ।
धूमान्तैः कर्मभिर्वर्ज्याः सर्वैरेव त्वजीर्णिनः ॥ ७ ॥

Garbhini – The pregnant woman,

Rooskha – persons who are dry –not undergone oleation therapy,

Kshudhita – hungry,

Nitya Dukhita – constantly grief–stricken,

children, old persons,

Krusha – the emaciated,

Sthula – the obese,

Hrudrogi – patient of heart disease,

Kshata – the wounded,

Durbala – weak, debilitated,

who are having bouts of vomiting,

Pleeha – enlargement of spleen,

Timira – blindness,

Krimikoshta – intestinal parasites,

upward movement of vata and Asra– blood,

Soon after administration of Vamana,

who have loss of speech, dysuria,

Udara – ascites, intestinal obstruction, tumour of the abdomen,

who faced difficulties during Vamana therapy,

who have strong digestive activity,

Arsha – haemorrhoids

Urdhva Vata – upward movement of air – reverse peristalsis,

Giddiness / Dizziness – enlargement of the prostate,

Parshvavata – pain in the flanks and diseases caused by vata;

Person suffering from poisoning,

indigestion and who have consumed incompatible foods.

Persons not suitable for Virechana– Virechana Arha:

विरेकसाध्या गुल्मार्शोविस्फोटव्यङ्गकामलाः ।
जीर्णज्वरोदरगरच्छर्दिप्लीहहलीमकाः ॥ ८ ॥
विद्रधिस्तिमिरं काचः स्यन्दः पक्वाशयव्यथा ।
योनिशुक्राश्रया रोगाः कोष्ठगाः कृमयो व्रणाः ॥ ९ ॥
वातास्रमूर्ध्वगं रक्तं मूत्राघातः शकृद्ग्रहः ।
वाम्यश्च कुष्ठमेहाद्याः

persons suitable for purgation therapy:–

Diseases requiring purgation therapy are–

Gulma – Tumours of the abdomen,

Arsha – Piles,

Visphota– blisters,

Vyanga – discoloured patch on face,

Kamala – Jaundice, Liver disease

Jeernajwara – Chronic fever,
Udara – ascites, intestinal obstruction
Poisoning, Chronic poisoning
Chardi – Vomiting
Pleeha – Disease of the spleen, Splenomegaly,
Haleemaka – advanced jaundice,
Vidradhi – Abscess
Timira – blindness,
Kacha, Syanda – Cataract
pain in the large intestine,
Diseases of male and female uro–genital system
wounds/ Ulcers,
Vatasra – Gout,
Urdhwarakta – bleeding disorders of upper parts of the body (such as nasal bleeding)
Diseases of blood vitiation,
Mutraghata – Dysuria
Shakrut graham – constipation
Those persons who are Suitable for emesis therapy– enumerated in earlier verses commencing with " those suffering from Kustha" are curable– to be treated with purgation therapy. 8–10a
Those diseases are –
Kushta – skin diseases
Meha – diabetes, urinary tract disorders
Apachi, Granthi – Goitre, tumour, fibroid
Shleepada – Elephantiasis, Filariasis
Unmada – Schizophrenia
Kasa – cough, cold
Shwasa – Chronic respiratory tract disease, Asthma
Hrullasa – nausea
Visarpa – herpes
Stanyadosha – vitiated breast milk
Urdhvaroga – diseases affecting neck and above region

Persons not unsuitable for Virechana– Virechana Anarha:

न तु रेच्या नवज्वरी ॥ १० ॥
अल्पाग्न्यधोगपित्तास्रक्षतपाय्वतिसारिणः ।

सशल्यास्थापितक्रूरकोष्ठातिस्निग्धशोषिणः ॥ ११ ॥

Navajwara – fever of recent origin

Alpa Agni – poor digestive activity,

Adhoga Raktapitta – bleeding disease of lower part of the body (such as bleeding per rectum)

wounds, ulcers of the rectum

Atisara – diarrhoea, dysentery

Sashalya – foreign bodies;

Who have been administered decoction enema,

Krurakoshta – Persons who naturally have hard bowel movement,

Atisnigdha – who have undergone excess of Oleation treatment

Shosha – emaciated

Vamana Vidhi – Procedure of emesis therapy:

अथ साधारणे काले स्निग्धस्विन्नं यथाविधि ।

श्वोवम्यमुत्क्लिष्टकफं मत्स्यमाषतिलादिभिः ॥ १२ ॥

निशां सुप्तं सुजीर्णान्नं पूर्वाह्ने कृतमङ्गलम् ।

निरन्नमीषत्स्निग्धं वा पेयया पीतसर्पिषम् ॥ १३ ॥

वृद्धबालाबलक्लीबभीरून् रोगानुरोधतः ।

आकण्ठं पायितान् मद्यं क्षीरं इक्षुरसं रसम् ॥ १४ ॥

यथाविकारविहितां मधुसैन्धवसंयुताम् ।

कोष्ठं विभज्य भैषज्यमात्रां मन्त्राभिमन्त्रिताम् ॥ १५ ॥

ब्रह्मदक्षाश्विरुद्रेन्द्रभूचन्द्रार्कानिलानलाः ।

ऋषयः सौषधिग्रामा भूतसङ्घाश्च पान्तु वः ॥ १६ ॥

रसायनमिवर्षीणां अमराणां इवामृतम् ।

सुधेवोत्तमनागानां भैषज्यमिदमस्तु ते ॥ १७ ॥

नमो भगवते भैषज्यगुरवे वैडूर्यप्रभराजाय ॥ १७+१ ॥

तथागतायार्हते सम्यक्सम्बुद्धाय ॥ १७+२ ॥

तद्यथा ॥ १७+३ ॥

भैषज्ये भैषज्ये महाभैषज्ये समुद्गते स्वाहा ॥ १७+४ ॥

प्राङ्मुखं पाययेत्

Next, during temperate seasons, after administering oleation and sweating therapy properly,

on the day previous to the day of emesis,

The patient is made sure that he has slept well the previous night.

Patient is made sure that his previous food is well digested

In the morning of the previous day to Vamana, at first, Auspicious rituals are carried out.

Next, Kapha Dosha is excited in the patient by administering peya (drink) / thin gruel prepared from fish, Masha (black gram), Tila (Sesame) etc. added with little quantity of fats, in the morning.

On the day of Vamana, again, it is made sure that the patient's previous food has got digested and he has slept well.

He is either maintained on an empty stomach or a little quantity of ghee is given.

The Aged, children, the debilitated, VIPs and cowards, should be made to drink wine, milk, sugarcane juice or meat juice added with honey and Saindhava salt, appropriate to the disease, to their maximum capacity.

Afterwards, determining the nature of his bowels (Intestines – Koshta), the emetic drug is administered sanctifying it with the following hymn–

"let Brahma, Daksa, Ashvinis, Rudra, Indra, the Earth, Moon, Sun, Air, Fire, Sages, comity of herbs, and of living beings protect you; let this medicine be to you like Rasayana for the Sages, Nectar for gods and Sudha for the good serpents; Om, Salutations to the medicine." Uttering these hymns, he should drink the medicine, facing east. 12–18a

Note: The medicine given for Vamana depends on the disease. It usually contains Madanaphala (Randia spinosa), Licorice etc. Various combinations of Vamana drugs are discussed in a later chapter.

पीतो मुहूर्तम् अनुपालयेत् । तन्मना जातहल्लासप्रसेकश्छर्दयेत् ततः ॥ १८ ॥
अङ्गुलीभ्याम् अनायस्तो नालेन मृदुनाथवा ।
गलताल्वरुजन् वेगान् अप्रवृत्तान् प्रवर्तयन् ॥ १९ ॥
प्रवर्तयन् प्रवृत्तांश्च जानुतुल्यासने स्थितः ।
उभे पार्श्वे ललाटं च वमतश्चास्य धारयेत् ॥ २० ॥
प्रपीडयेत् तथा नाभिं पृष्ठं च प्रतिलोमतः ।

After consuming the medicine, he should wait for one Muhurta – 48 minutes for the commencement of vomiting, with keen intent.

With the appearance of oppression in the chest and salivation he should try to vomit

If the bouts are not coming up easily, he should tickle his throat either with his fingers or a soft tube without injuring the throat,

Sitting on a seat of the height of one's knee, the bouts of vomiting should be held supported by another person.

His umbilical region and back should be massaged in upward direction.

कफे तीक्ष्णोष्णकटुकैः पित्ते स्वादुहिमैरिति ॥ २१ ॥ वमेत् स्निग्धाम्ललवणैः संसृष्टे मरुता कफे ।

In case of increase of Kapha, vomiting should be induced with drugs having properties like penetrating, hot and Pungent (Teekshna, Ushna, Katu);
In case of Pitta – with drugs of sweet and cold properties and
In case of association of Vata with Kapha, with drugs of Unctuous, sour and salt properties. (Snigdha Amla Lavana).

पित्तस्य दर्शनं यावच्छेदो वा श्लेष्मणो भवेत् ॥ २२ ॥

Vomiting should be allowed till the appearance– coming out of Pitta or complete expulsion of Kapha.

हीनवेगः कणाधात्रीसिद्धार्थलवणोदकैः । वमेत् पुनः

If bouts are insufficient, they should be induced again and again by drinking water boiled with Kana, Dhatri, Siddhartha and salt (long pepper, Amla, White mustard and black salt).

Vishama yoga:
पुनः तत्र वेगानाम् अप्रवर्तनम् ॥ २३ ॥
प्रवृत्तिः सविबन्धा वा केवलस्यौषधस्य वा ।
अयोगस्तेन निष्ठीवकण्डूकोठज्वरादयः ॥ २४ ॥

Less bouts – Ayoga – Non – commencement of bouts, bouts coming on with hindrance or elimination of the medicine only– are the features of Ayoga– inadequate bouts. From it arise, excess of expectoration, itching, appearance of skin rashes, fever etc.

Samyak Yoga:
निर्विबन्धं प्रवर्तन्ते कफपित्तानिलाः क्रमात् ।
(मनःप्रसादः स्वास्थ्यं चावस्थानं च स्वयं भवेत् ।
वैपरीत्यमयोगानां न चातिमहती व्यथा ॥ २५+(१) ॥)
सम्यग्योगे

Kapha, Pitta and vata coming out in successive order, without any hindrance,
calmness of the mind and cessation of vomit bouts on its own,
absence of features of inadequate bouts and

feeling of not too much of discomfort are the features of samyagyoga-proper bout.

Ati yoga:

अतियोगे तु फेनचन्द्रकरक्तवत् ॥ २५ ॥

वमितं क्षामता दाहः कण्ठशोषस्तमो भ्रमः ।

घोरा वाय्वामया मृत्युर्जीवशोणितनिर्गमात् ॥ २६ ॥

In Atiyoga– excess bouts the vomited materials will be frothy, with glistering particles and blood;

The patient will experience weakness, burning sensation, dryness of the throat, giddiness, powerful disease of vata origin and even death due to discharge of life supporting blood.

Care after vomiting therapy – Vamanottara Upachara:

अतियोगे तु फेनचन्द्रकरक्तवत् ॥ २५ ॥

वमितं क्षामता दाहः कण्ठशोषस्तमो भ्रमः ।

घोरा वाय्वामया मृत्युर्जीवशोणितनिर्गमात् ॥ २६ ॥

After the patient had proper bouts of vomiting, he should be comforted with encouraging words, made to inhale anyone kinds of smoke (Dhuma)– mild, medium, or strong, and then allowed to follow the regimen of after–care of oleation therapy.

ततः सायं प्रभाते वा क्षुद्वान् स्नातः सुखाम्बुना ।

भुञ्जानो रक्तशाल्यन्नं भजेत् पेयादिकं क्रमम् ॥ २८ ॥

Then, either in the evening or next morning, after feeling hungry, after a bath with warm water, he can eat mass prepared with red rice or if he is not feeling hungry he should adhere to the following regimen of Peya (Thin gruel) etc. This regimen is called as Samsarjana Karma.

Samsarjana – PeyadiAhara Karma:

पेयां विलेपीमकृतं कृतं च यूषं रसं त्रीन् उभयं तथैकम् ।

क्रमेण सेवेत नरोऽन्नकालान् प्रधानमध्यावरशुद्धिशुद्धः ॥ २९ ॥

Regimen of liquid Diet –

Persons who have had the maximum, medium and minimum purificatory therapies, should consume Peya– thin Gruel,

Vilepi– thick Gruel,

AkrutaYusa– soup not processed with fat, salt, sours etc.

Krutayusa– Soup processed with fat, salt and Sours and

Rasa– meat juice– in Successive order, for three, two and one Annakala- time of meal respectively. 29

Note:

Eating periods = Anna Kala. Each day has two anna kala. – morning and evening.

If the maximum vomiting bouts were observed (Ati Yoga), then, the patient should take Peya, Vilepi, AkrutaYusha, KrutaYusha and Mamsarasa – for three eating periods (Annakala) each. The patient will not have any food except these. Likewise, for the medium vomiting bouts, the number of eating periods is two each and for lesser bouts (Heena Yoga), the number of eating periods (Anna kala) is one each.

Benefits of Samsarjana Karma:

यथाऽणुरग्निस्तृणगोमयाद्यैः सन्धुक्ष्यमाणो भवति क्रमेण ।
महान् स्थिरः सर्वपचस्तथैव शुद्धस्य पेयादिभिरन्तराग्निः ॥ ३० ॥

Just as a spark of fire after being fed by grass, powder of dry cow dung etc, gets augmented gradually and becomes great, steady, and capable of burning everything, similarly, the internal digestion fire, by the Samsarjana regimen, in the patient who has undergone Vamana karma, gains strength. 30

Vega Samkhya– Mana– Number of Bouts and quantity:

जघन्यमध्यप्रवरे तु वेगाश्चत्वार इष्टा वमने षडष्टौ ।
दशैव ते द्विवत्रिगुणा विरेके प्रस्थस्तथा स्यादि्द्विवचतुर्गुणश्च ॥ ३१ ॥

For Vamana,

Heenayoga – Minimum bouts – 4 bouts

Madhyamavega – Moderate – 6 bouts

Atiyoga – Maximum bouts – 8 bouts

For Virechana –

Heenayoga – 10 bouts of purgation or half prastha of purgated material (384 grams)

Madhyamayoga – 20 bouts – 1 prastha of material (768 grams)

Atiyoga – 30 bouts. – 2 prastha (1,536 grams).

Expulsion of Kapha and Pitta

पित्तावसानं वमनं विरेकादद्दर्ध कफान्तं च विरेकम् आहुः ।
द्विव्रान् सविट्कान् अपनीय वेगान् मेयं विरेके वमने तु पीतम् ॥ ३२ ॥

Vomiting therapy is allowed till the expulsions of pitta,
Purgation therapy is allowed till Kapha comes out;
Measurement to be done after rejecting 2 – 3 bouts, containing faeces in case of Virechana and after rejecting the medicine– emetic Drug in case of Vamana.

Virechana Vidhi– Purgation therapy procedure:
अथैनं वामितं भूयः स्नेहस्वेदोपपादितम् ।
श्लेष्मकाले गते ज्ञात्वा कोष्ठं सम्यग्विरेचयेत् ॥ ३३ ॥
After Vamana therapy, patient is given Samsarjana regimen. After that, he is again given Snehana and Swedana treatment.
After that, in the morning, after Kapha time has lapsed (after around 9 – 10 AM,) Virechana drug should be given (should be given the Purgation medicine). The kind and quantity of purgation medicine should be determining the nature of his Kostha (alimentary tract, bowels).

बहुपित्तो मृदुः कोष्ठः क्षीरेणापि विरिच्यते ।
प्रभूतमारुतः क्रूरः कृच्छ्राच्छ्यामादिकैरपि ॥ ३४ ॥
A person with predominant pitta is considered Mrudukoshta (soft intestines), In these people even milk will induce purgation.
A person with predominant vata is considered Krurakoshta, (hard bowels, intestines), In these people even Trivrit (a purgative herb) might cause purgation with great difficulty.

कषायमधुरैः पित्ते विरेकः कटुकैः कफे ।
स्निग्धोष्णलवणैर्वायौ
For Pitta disease, Kashaya – astringent and Madhura – sweet drugs should be used for purgation.
For Kapha disease, Katu (pungent) herbs should be given for purgation.
For Vata, drugs with Snigdha – unctuous, oily, Ushna (hot) and Lavana (salt) taste should be given to induce purgation.

अप्रवृत्तौ तु पाययेत् ॥ ३५ ॥
उष्णाम्बु स्वेदयेदस्य पाणितापेन चोदरम् ।
If bouts of purgation do not commence, he should drink hot water and his abdomen should be fomented with palms of the hand, made warm.

उत्थानेऽल्पे दिने
तस्मिन्भुक्त्वान्येद्युः पुनः पिबेत् ॥ ३६ ॥
अदृढस्नेहकोष्ठस्तु पिबेदूर्ध्वं दशाहतः ।
भूयोऽप्युपस्कृततनुः स्नेहस्वेदैर्विरेचनम् ॥ ३७ ॥
यौगिकं सम्यगालोच्य स्मरन् पूर्वमतिक्रमम् ।

If, on the day of consuming the purgative drug, the patient responds poorly, he should be allowed to take his food on that day and the purgative drugs administered again on the next day;

Persons who have unstable and un–lubricated alimentary tract, should consume the purgative drugs after ten days – during which Snehana and sweating therapies should be done because the body which has been well prepared with Snehana and sweating therapies, will be able to have purgation properly;

then the purgative drug should be administered after considering all aspects and remembering the procedures described earlier.

हृत्कुक्ष्यशुद्धिररुचिरुत्क्लेशः श्लेष्मपित्तयोः ॥ ३८ ॥
कण्डूविदाहः पिटिकाः पीनसो वातविड्ग्रहः ।
अयोगलक्षणं योगो वैपरीत्ये यथोदितात् ॥ ३९ ॥

Discomfort in the region of the heart and abdomen, anorexia, exacerbation / excitation of kapha and pitta in the intestines (since they are not expelled properly following purgation) or expulsion of doshas i.e. kapha and pitta from the mouth, itching, burning sensation, eruption on the skin, rhinitis, obstruction of flatus and feces (constipation) are the symptoms of deficit purgation in case of proper administration of purgation, the opposite symptoms of the above mentioned are found.

Symptoms of excessive purgation – Virechana Atiyoga:
विट्पित्तकफवातेषु निःसृतेषु क्रमात् स्रवेत् ।
निःश्लेष्मपित्तमुदकं श्वेतं कृष्णं सलोहितम् ॥ ४० ॥
मांसधावनतुल्यं वा मेदःखण्डाभमेव वा ।
गुदनिःसरणं तृष्णा भ्रमो नेत्रप्रवेशनम् ॥ ४१ ॥
भवन्त्यतिविरिक्तस्य तथातिवमनामयाः ।

After the elimination of feces, pitta, kapha and vata in successive order, there will be elimination of watery material devoid of kapha or pitta, which is white, black or slightly red in color, resembling the water in which meat has been washed or resembling a piece of fat prolapse of the rectum, thirst, giddiness, sunken eyes and diseases caused by excessive vomiting are the symptoms of excessive purgation.

After–care in purgation therapy – Virechana Paschat Karma:

सम्यग्विरिक्तमेनं च वमनोक्तेन योजयेत् ॥ ४२ ॥

धूमवर्ज्येन विधिना ततो वमितवानिव ।

क्रमेणान्नानि भुञ्जानो भजेत् प्रकृतिभोजनम् ॥ ४३ ॥

The person who has undergone proper purgation therapy should be administered with all other therapies described in emesis therapy, except inhalation of medicated smoke later, he should follow the same procedure of dietetic regimen in the same way as of emesis therapy and then resume his normal food.

Indications for fasting in the after–care of purgation therapy – virechana paschat kale langhana yogyah:

मन्दवह्निमसंशुद्धमक्षामं दोषदुर्बलम् ।

अदृष्टजीर्णलिङ्गं च लङ्घयेत् पीतभेषजम् ॥ ४४ ॥

स्नेहस्वेदौषधोत्क्लेशसङ्गैरिति न बाध्यते ।

On the day of consuming the purgation medicine, if the patient experiences (one or more of the) weak digestion,

coated feeling inside the gut due to deficit bouts, absence of emaciation caused by elimination therapy (purgation here), debility due to increase of doshas and

absence of symptoms of digestion of medicines, he should be put on fasting. Following fasting, he will not be harmed by the obstruction caused in the channels by the doshas which have been exacerbated due to oleation and sudation (but not been expelled).

Importance of graduated liquid diet - Peyadi Samsarjana:

संशोधनास्त्रविस्रावस्नेहयोजनलङ्घनैः ॥ ४५ ॥

यात्यग्निर्मन्दतां तस्मात् क्रमं पेयादिमाचरेत्।

The digestive activity becomes weak by administration of purification therapies bloodletting therapy, oleation therapies and fasting, Hence, the regimen of thin gruel etc. should be followed (to kindle the digestive activity).

Importance of nourishing therapy – Tarpanadi krama:

सुताल्प पित्तश्लेष्माणं मद्यपं वातपैत्तिकम्॥४६॥

पेयान्न पाययेतेषां तर्पणादिक्रमोहितः।

Thin gruel should not be given when (in those in whom) only small quantities of pitta and kapha are expelled out,

to alcohol addicts, and to those in whom vata and pitta are predominant for these people, nourishing therapy etc. are suitable (should be administered).

Status of expelled doshas in vomiting and purgation treatments:

अपक्वं वमनं दोषान् पच्यमानं विरेचनम् ॥ ४७ ॥

निर्हरेद्वमनस्यातः पाकं न प्रतिपालयेत् ।

Emesis treatment brings out the doshas in an unprocessed form whereas purgation therapy brings out the doshas which are in the process of being processed. Therefore, in case of emesis therapy, the physician should not wait for doshas to get processed.

Need of purgative foods – Bhedaniya bhojya:

दुर्बलो बहुदोषश्च दोषपाकेन यः स्वयम् ॥ ४८ ॥

विरिच्यते भेदनीयैर्भोज्यैस्तम् उपपादयेत् ।

The person who is weak, who has a great amount of increased doshas in the body, would develop purgation on his own (even without consuming purgation medicine) as an effect of maturity of doshas (which happens spontaneously in these people). These people should be treated with foods which are purgative in nature.

Indications for administration of mild, strong and repeatedly small dose of purgatives:

दुर्बलः शोधितः पूर्वमल्पदोषः कृशो नरः ॥ ४९ ॥

अपरिज्ञातकोष्ठश्च पिबेन् मृद्वल्पम् औषधम् ।

वरं तदसकृत्पीतम् अन्यथा संशयावहम् ॥ ५० ॥

हरेद्बहुंश्चलान् दोषान् अल्पान् अल्पान् पुनः पुनः ।

दुर्बलस्य मृदुद्रव्यैरल्पान् संशमयेतु तान् ॥ ५१ ॥

Durbala - People who are weak,

Shodhita - who have undergone cleansing therapy,

Alpadosha - who have small amount of imbalanced doshas,

Krusha - who are emaciated

Aparijnata Koshta - whose bowel nature is not known should be given mild purgative, in a small dose, it is ideal to give the medicine in small doses often, or else i.e. if large dose of medicine is given in these conditions, it creates a doubt of death the purgation drug given in (small and) repeated doses will eliminate the circulating abundant doshas little by little in a weak person, small quantity of doshas should only be mitigated by medicines which are mild acting and liquid.

Effects of doshas which are stagnated – Anirhrta Dosha:

क्लेशयन्ति चिरं ते हि हन्युर्वैनमनिर्हृताः ।

The same doshas which are excessive in quantity trouble the person greatly and even cause death if (they are) not expelled out by purification treatments.

Preparation of patient having weak digestion and hard bowels for purgation therapy:

मन्दाग्निं क्रूरकोष्ठं च सक्षारलवणैर्घृतैः ॥ ५२ ॥

सन्धुक्षिताग्निं विजितकफवातं च शोधयेत् ।

Mandagni - Person having weak digestion,

Krurakoshta - hard bowels,

Sa kshara Lavana - should be administered ghee processed with alkali and salt, (with this) when his digestive capacity gets increased and morbid kapha and vata get destroyed, he should be given purification therapies.

Indications for enema and suppository before purgation therapy:

रूक्षबहुवनिलक्रूरकोष्ठव्यायामशीलिनाम् ॥ ५३ ॥

दीप्ताग्नीनां च भैषज्यम् अविरेच्यैव जीर्यति ।

तेभ्यो वस्तिं पुरा दद्यात्ततः स्निग्धं विरेचनम् ॥ ५४ ॥

शकृन्निर्हृत्य वा किञ्चित् तीक्ष्णाभिः फलवर्तिभिः ।

प्रवृत्तं हि मलं स्निग्धो विरेको निर्हरेत् सुखम् ॥ ५५ ॥

Rooksha - In persons who are dry,

Bahu Anila - who have great increase of vata,

Krura koshta - who has hard bowel,

Vyayama sheelina - who are indulged in exercise regularly and

Deeptagni - who have strong digestion strength, the purgation medicine gets digested without producing purgation, for these people, an enema should be given first and then purgative medicine which is unctuous should be given or the feces should be removed first by using a strong rectal suppository. The unctuous purgation easily expels the doshas thus initiated in their movement

Indications for administering mild oleation before purgation therapy:
विषाभिघातपिटिकाकुष्ठशोफविसर्पिणः ।
कामलापाण्डुमेहार्तान्नातिस्निग्धान् विशोधयेत् ॥ ५६ ॥
सर्वान् स्नेहविरेकैश्च रूक्षैस्तु स्नेहभावितान् ।
Visha, Abhighata, Persons who are suffering from poisoning, trauma,
Pitika - skin eruptions,
Kushta - skin diseases,
Shopha - inflammation / swelling,
Visarpa - herpes,
Kamala - jaundice,
Pandu - anemia and
Meha - diabetes / urinary disorders
should be given purgation therapy without administering too much oleation (small quantity of mild oleation is sufficient for these people). All of them should be given fatty / unctuous purgation; those who have had oleation earlier should be administered dry (non–unctuous) purgatives.

Use of oleation and sudation in between the cleansing measures:
कर्मणां वमनादीनां पुनरप्यन्तरेऽन्तरे ॥ ५७ ॥
स्नेहस्वेदौ प्रयुञ्जीत स्नेहमन्ते बलाय च ।
In between (each) emesis etc cleansing therapies, oleation and sudation therapies should be used once again at the end of each therapy, oleation should be done to restore strength in the body

Note – this means to tell that oleation and sudation should be interspersed in between each cleansing therapy, like oleation and sudation should be done before emesis, in between emesis and purgation, in between purgation and enema therapy etc.

Similey for understanding cleansing treatments:
मलो हि देहादुत्क्लेश्य ह्रियते वाससो यथा ॥ ५८ ॥
स्नेहस्वेदैस्तथोत्क्लिष्टः शोध्यते शोधनैर्मलः ।
Just like the dirt from the cloth gets cleansed by washing the cloth, similarly

the doshas get loosened from the body getting excited by the administration of oleation and sudation therapies get expelled by administration of purification therapies.

Effects of purification therapies done without oleation and purgation therapies:

स्नेहस्वेदावनभ्यस्य कुर्यात् संशोधनं तु यः ॥ ५९ ॥
दारु शुष्कमिवानामे शरीरं तस्य दीर्यते ॥ ५९ab ॥

When the person undertakes cleansing / purification therapies (emesis and purgation) without undergoing oleation and sweating therapies. His body gets broken just like a dried log of wood (gets broken) when it is bent.

Benefits of purification therapies – Shodhana Phala:

बुद्धिप्रसादं बलमिन्द्रियाणां धातुस्थिरत्वं ज्वलनस्य दीप्तिम् ।
चिराच्च पाकं वयसः करोति संशोधनं सम्यगुपास्यमानम् ॥ ६०a ॥

Clarity of mind, strength of the sense organs, stability of the tissues, kindled digestive power and slow ageing occur (as benefits) when purification therapies are properly undertaken.

इति श्रीवैद्यपतिसिंहगुप्तसूनुश्रीमद्वाग्भटविरचितायामष्टाङ्गहृदयसंहितायां सूत्रस्थाने वमनविरेचनविधिर्नामाष्टादशोऽध्यायः ॥ १८ ॥

Thus ends the 18th chapter of Ashtangahridaya Samhita Sutrasthana, named Vamana Virechana Vidhi Adhyayam, written by Shrimad Vagbhata, son of Shri Vaidyapati Simhagupta.

19

बस्तिविधिमध्यायम् (basti vidhim adhyayam)

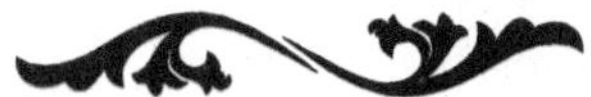

The 19th chapter of Sutrasthanam of Ashtanga Hridayam is named as Basti Vidhi Adhyayam. This chapter explains in detail about types, methods, indications and contra indications of nasal instillation of medicine – Nasya therapy.

अथातो बस्तिविधिमध्यायं व्याख्यास्याम: इति ह स्माहुरात्रेयादयो महर्षय:॥
Atreya and other sages pledge that henceforth they will be explaining the chapter named Basti vidhimadhyaya (pertaining to therapeutic enema therapy).

Basti – best remedy for vitiated vata, types of enema therapies
वातोल्बणेषु दोषेषु वाते वा वस्तिरिष्यते ।
उपक्रमाणां सर्वेषां सोऽग्रणीस्त्रिविधस्तु सः ॥ १ ॥
निरूहोऽन्वासनं वस्तिरुत्तरः
Basti is described for
diseases with imbalanced Doshas having predominance of Vata
or for diseases with Vata imbalance alone.
It is the best among all treatments.
It is of three kinds– viz
Niruha is also called Asthapana Basti or Decoction enema in which decoction mixed with salt, herbal paste, honey, fat is administered.
Anuvasana, also known as snehabasti or fat enema. Here, ghee, oil, fat etc are administered. Herbal oils such as Narayana Taila, Herbal ghritas are

more commonly used for this purpose. (If needed, Saindhava lavana (rock salt) is added).

Uttarabasti administered through the urethral route.

Notes– Basti means urinary bladder. In ancient times the urinary bladder of animals like buffalo etc were used as a bag to hold the enema material like decoctions, oil etc.

Persons suitable for decoction enema:

तेन साधयेत् ।

गुल्मानाहखुडप्लीहशुद्धातीसारशूलिनः ॥ २ ॥

जीर्णज्वरप्रतिश्यायशुक्रानिलमलग्रहान् ।

वर्ध्माश्मरीरजोनाशान् दारुणांश्चानिलामयान् ॥ ३ ॥

Patients suffering from

Gulma – Tumours of the abdomen

Anaha – bloating, fullness

Khuda – gout,

Pleeha – Disease of the spleen, Splenomegaly

Shuddha atisara – Diarrhoea un–associated with other diseases

Shula – abdominal pain

Jeerna jwara – Chronic fever

Pratishyaya – rhinitis

Shukra, Anila, Mala Graha – obstruction of semen, flatus and constipation,

Vardhma – enlargement of the scrotum / hernia

Ashmari – Urinary calculi,

Rajonasha – Amenorrhoea, female infertility and grievous diseases of vata origin.

Unsuitable for Niruha

Asthapana Anarha – Anasthapya

अनास्थाप्यास्त्वतिस्निग्धः क्षतोरस्को भृशं कृशः ।

आमातीसारी वमिमान् संशुद्धो दत्तनावनः ॥ ४ ॥

श्वासकासप्रसेकार्शोहिध्माध्मानाल्पवह्नयः ।

शूनपायुः कृताहारो बद्धच्छिद्रोदकोदरी ॥ ५ ॥

कुष्ठी च मधुमेही च मासान् सप्त च गर्भिणी ।

Atisnigdha – Who have had excess oleation therapy;

Urakshata – chest injury

Krusha – highly emaciated,

Ama Atisara – diarrhoea, dysentery due to Ama or diarrhoea of recent onset,

Vami – vomiting,

Samshuddha – who have undergone purification therapies (Panchakarma),

Datta Navana – who have been administered nasal medication

Shvasa – Asthma, Dyspnoea

Kasa – cough, cold

Praseka – excessive salivation

Arsha – haemorrhoids

Hidhma – hiccups

Adhmana – Abdominal bloating

Alpavahni– low digestion strength

Shunapayu – Swelling in the rectum

Kruta Ahara – Who have just taken food

Badhodara – intestinal obstruction

Chidra Udara – Intestinal rupture

Udakodara – Ascites

Kushta – skin diseases

Madhumeha – diabetes

Pregnant woman in the seventh month.

Patients suitable for Anuvasana Basti

Anuvasana Arha – Anuvasya

आस्थाप्या एव चान्वास्या विशेषादतिवहनयः ॥ ६ ॥

रूक्षाः केवलवातार्ता

Person suitable for Asthapana are suitable for Anuvasana (fat enema). Especially those who have strong digestion power, who are dry, not undergone Snehana therapy and those suffering from diseases of vata.

Patients not suitable for Anuvasana:

नानुवास्यास्त एव च ।

येऽनास्थाप्यास्तथा पाण्डुकामलामेहपीनसाः ॥ ७ ॥

निरन्नप्लीहविड्भेदिगुरुकोष्ठकफोदराः ।

अभिष्यन्दिभृशस्थूलकृमिकोष्ठाढ्यमारुताः ॥ ८ ॥

पीते विषे गरेऽपच्यां श्लीपदी गलगण्डवान् ।

Persons unsuitable for Anuvasana (fat enema) are all those unsuitable for Niruha basti, those suffering from

Pandu – anaemia,
Kamala – Jaundice,
Meha – diabetes, urinary tract disorders
Peenasa – rhinitis
Niranna on empty stomach
Pleeha - disease of the spleen, Splenomegaly
Vid bhedi – diarrhoea,
Guru koshta – hard bowels – constipated,
Kaphodara – Kapha type of Ascites
Abhishyandi – a type of eye disorder (conjunctivitis)
Bhrusha Sthula – profound obesity,
KrumiKoshta – Intestinal worm infestation
Adhyamaruta – gout;
Who have consumed poison, those suffering from artificial poison, goitre, filariasis and scrofula.

Bastinetra – enema nozzle:
तयोस्तु नेत्रं हेमादिधातुदार्वस्थिवेणुजम् ॥ ९ ॥
गोपुच्छाकारमच्छिद्रं श्लक्ष्णर्जु गुलिकामुखम् ।
Enema nozzle should be made from metals like gold, silver, wood, bone or bamboo;
Gopuchhakara – resembling the tail of the cow in shape,
Achidra – without holes (except at the ends), smooth, straight and with
Gulikamukha – tip shaped like a pill.

Measurements for children:
ऊनेऽब्दे पञ्च पूर्णऽस्मिन्न् आसप्तभ्योऽङ्गुलानि षट् ॥ १० ॥
सप्तमे सप्त तान्यष्टौ द्वादशे षोडशे नव ।
द्वादशैव परं विंशाद्वीक्ष्य वर्षान्तरेषु च ॥ ११ ॥
वयोबलशरीराणि प्रमाणमभिवर्धयेत् ।
For children less than 1year of age, nozzle should be five angula– fingers breadth of patient's own finger in length;
1 – 7 years of age, it should be 6 angula;
7 year it should be 7 Angula,
12 years – 8 Angula
16 years – 9 Angula
20 years and onwards it should be 12 Angulas only.

These measurements may be slightly increased for those of other age groups based on age, strength and body build.

Diameter of the orifice (Basti netra):

स्वाङ्गुष्ठेन समं मूले स्थौल्येनाग्रे कनिष्ठया ॥ १२ ॥

पूर्णेऽब्देऽङ्गुलमादाय तदद्धर्धाद्धर्धप्रवर्धितम् ।

त्र्यङ्गुलं परमं छिद्रं मूलेऽग्रे वहते तु यत् ॥ १३ ॥

मुद्गं माषं कलायं च क्लिन्नं कर्कन्धुकं क्रमात् ।

Its orifice at its root should be 1 Angula in diameter for children of one year of age.

Diameter of the orifice should be increased by ½ angula for different age groups and its maximum is 3 Angula diameters.

At its tip, the orifice should allow free movement of soaked Mudga (green gram), Masha (black gram), Kalaya (round pea) and seed of Karkandhu (Jujube) respectively.

Karnika – Ridges:

मूलच्छिद्रप्रमाणेन प्रान्ते घटितकर्णिकम् ॥ १४ ॥ वर्त्याग्रे पिहितं मूले यथास्वं द्व्यङ्गुलान्तरम् ।

कर्णिकादि्वतयं नेत्रे कुर्यात्

Near the orifice at its root, a Karnika– ear–like ridge of the same size of the orifice should be constructed – at the time of preparing the nozzle, another Karnika– ridge should be made at a distance of two Angula– towards its tip. The orifice at the tip should be kept closed with a plug of cloth.

Basti Putaka– Enema bag:

तत्र च योजयेत् ॥ १५ ॥

अजाविमहिषादीनां वस्तिं सुमृदितं दृढम् ।

कषायरक्तं निश्छिद्रग्रन्थिगन्धशिरं तनुम् ॥ १६ ॥

ग्रथितं साधु सूत्रेण सुखसंस्थाप्यभेषजम् ।

वस्त्यभावेऽङ्कपादं वा न्यसेद्वासोऽथवा घनम् ॥ १७ ॥

Urinary bladder of goats, sheep, buffalo or other animals was used as enema bag. The bladder should be sturdy, well beaten, made red by tanning with astringent substances.

The bladder should be devoid of holes, hard spots.

It should not be torn.

To such a bladder, the big end of the nozzle is adjusted and tied with threads.

If the bladder is not available, skin of thigh and legs of animals or thick cloth may be utilized for making the bag.

Niruha Matra (quantity of medicine for decoction enema):

निरूहमात्रा प्रथमे प्रकुञ्चो वत्सरे परम् ।

प्रकुञ्चवृद्धिः प्रत्यब्दं यावत् षट् प्रसृतास्ततः ॥ १८ ॥

प्रसृतं वर्द्धयेदूर्ध्वं द्वादशाष्टादशस्य तु । आसप्ततेरिदं मानं दशैव प्रसृताः परम् ॥ १९ ॥

For a child up to 1 year age, the quantity of Niruha basti is 1 prakuncha = 1 Pala = 48 g.

For each succeeding year it should be increased by 1 pala (48 g) till it becomes six Prasruta– 12 pala = 576 g;

So for a 12 year old, the quantity is 12 Pala = 576 g.

Further on, it should be increased by one Prasruta (2 Palas= 96 g). Each year till it becomes twelve Prasta– 24 Palas = 1,152 g.

At 18 years, it is 24 Pala.

18 – 70 years – 24 Pala.

After 70 years, 10 Prasruta = 20 Pala = 960 grams / ml

Anuvasana Matra– quantity for oil enema:

यथायथं निरूहस्य पादो मात्राऽनुवासने ।

The quantity for oil enema should be one fourth of the quantity of that of decoction enema, as prescribed for each age group.

Anuvasana Vidhi procedure of fat Enema –
preparation and position of patient:

आस्थाप्यं स्नेहितं स्विन्नं शुद्धं लब्धबलं पुनः ॥ २० ॥

अन्वासनार्हं विज्ञाय पूर्वमेवानुवासयेत् ।

शीते वसन्ते च दिवा रात्रौ केचित्ततोऽन्यदा ॥ २१ ॥

अभ्यक्तस्नातमुचितात् पादहीनं हितं लघु ।

अस्निग्धरूक्षमशितं सानुपानं द्रवादि च ॥ २२ ॥

कृतचङ्क्रमणं मुक्तविण्मूत्रं शयने सुखे ।

नात्युच्छ्रिते न चोच्छीर्षं संविष्टं वामपार्श्वतः ॥ २३ ॥

The person suitable for Niruha (Asthapana) Basti should be administered Snehana (oleation) and Swedana (sweating therapy) followed by Vamana and Virechana.

After he regains strength, determining that he is fit, he is given Sneha Basti.

Then, the following procedure is adopted.

During cold seasons (Hemanta and Shishira Rutus) and Vasanta (spring) it should be given during day time, in other seasons during night.

He should be given Abhyanga and bath, then accustomed food, less by one fourth of the usual quantity; satiable, light, easily digestible, neither with too oily nor very dry, followed by an after–drink of appropriate liquid.

Next he should walk for some time, eliminate faeces and urine and lie on a comfortable cot, neither too high nor too low, on his left side, folding his right thigh, and extending the left thigh.

Administration of Sneha basti:

सङ्कोच्य दक्षिणं सक्थि प्रसार्य च ततोऽपरम् ।
अथास्य नेत्रं प्रणयेत् स्निग्धे स्निग्धमुखं गुदे ॥ २४ ॥
उच्छ्वास्य वस्तेर्वदने बद्धे हस्तमकम्पयन् ।
पृष्ठवंशं प्रति ततो नातिद्रुतविलम्बितम् ॥ २५ ॥
नातिवेगं न वा मन्दं सकृदेव प्रपीडयेत् । सावशेषं च कुर्वीत वायुः शेषे हि तिष्ठति ॥ २६ ॥

Next, the enema nozzle is lubricated. The air inside the bag is expelled out and well fastening of the nozzle is confirmed.

It should be pressed without shaking the hands, in the direction of the vertebral column, neither too fast nor too slow, neither with great force nor with low pressure but in one attempt, a little quantity of liquid material be allowed to remain in the bag.

Regimen after administration of Sneha Basti:

दत्ते तूत्तानदेहस्य पाणिना ताडयेत् स्फिजौ ।
तत्पार्ष्णिभ्यां तथा शय्यां पादतश्च त्रिरुत्क्षिपेत् ॥ २७ ॥
ततः प्रसारिताङ्गस्य सोपधानस्य पार्ष्णिके ।
आहन्यान्मुष्टिनाङ्गं च स्नेहेनाभ्यज्य मर्दयेत् ॥ २८ ॥
वेदनार्तमिति स्नेहो न हि शीघ्रं निवर्तते ।
योज्यः शीघ्रं निवृत्तेऽन्यः स्नेहोऽतिष्ठन्नकार्यकृत् ॥ २९ ॥
दीप्ताग्निं त्वागतस्नेहं सायाह्ने भोजयेल्लघु ।

After the administration and removing the nozzle, the person should be placed with his face upwards, his buttocks beaten gently by the hands of the physician, then by patients own heels;

the foot of the cot should be lifted up thrice;

Next he must lie extending the entire body, with a pillow under his heels, oil should be smeared all over the body and all the parts of it beaten with fist or massaged, concentrating on the painful areas of the body, so that the fat enema liquid inside the rectum does not come out soon.

If it comes out soon, another oil enema should be administered immediately because Sneha which does not remain inside does not serve the purpose. If the person has good digestion strength and if the fat comes out after the stipulated time, he can be given light food in the evening.

Time for retaining of Sneha within colon:

निवृत्तिकालः परमस्त्रयो यामास्ततः परम् ॥ ३० ॥ अहोरात्रमुपेक्षेत परतः फलवर्तिभिः ।
तीक्ष्णैर्वा वस्तिभिः कुर्याद्यत्नं स्नेहनिवृत्तये ॥ ३१ ॥

The maximum time for the fat to come out is 3 Yama– nine hours; after that, it can be awaited for one day and night; later on, after 24 hours after administration, attempt should be made to remove it by force, with the help of Phalavarti (rectal suppositories) made from fruits or with the help of Teekshna Basti (strong decoction enema).

Severe dryness

अतिरौक्ष्यादनागच्छन्नचेज्जाड्यादिदोषकृत् ।
उपेक्षेतैव हि ततोऽध्युषितश्च निशां पिबेत् ॥ ३२ ॥

If it does not come out due to severe dryness inside and does not produce any troubles like lassitude etc., it should be neglected and allowed to remain inside for the night;

Drink for next morning:

प्रातर्नागरधान्याम्भः कोष्णं केवलमेव वा । अन्वासयेत्तृतीयेऽह्नि पञ्चमे वा पुनश्च तम् ॥ ३३ ॥
यथा वा स्नेहपक्तिः:

Next morning he is made to drink warm water either processed with ginger and coriander or plain.

Again he should be given fat enema on the third or fifth day, or till the fat gets well–digested.

People eligible to take unctuous enema daily – Nitya Sneha basti Sevaneeya

स्यादतोऽत्युल्बणमारुतान् । व्यायामनित्यान् दीप्ताग्नीन् रूक्षांश्च प्रतिवासरम् ॥ ३४ ॥
For people having an intense increase of vata, who do exercise every day, who have good digestive power and those who are very dry can be given

sneha basti daily.

Sneha basti as preparation for decoction enemas:

इति स्नेहैस्त्रिचतुरैः स्निग्धे स्रोतोविशुद्धये । निरूहं शोधनं युञ्ज्यादस्निग्धे स्नेहनं तनोः ॥ ३५ ॥

After administering 3–4 such sneha bastis, if the body is found to be well lubricated, Shodhana Niruha basti should be administered next, to clear the channels, if the body is not well lubricated, the fat enemas only should be continued.

Procedure of decoction enema – Niruha basti Vidhi:

पञ्चमेऽथ तृतीये वा दिवसे साधके शुभे ।
मध्याह्ने किञ्चिदावृत्ते प्रयुक्ते बलिमङ्गले ॥ ३६ ॥
अभ्यक्तस्वेदितोत्सृष्टमलं नातिबुभुक्षितम् ।
अवेक्ष्य पुरुषं दोषभेषजादीनि चादरात् ॥ ३७ ॥
वस्तिं प्रकल्पयेद्वैद्यस्तद्विद्यैर्बहुभिः सह ।

On the 3rd or 5th day after completion of Sneha basti, at an auspicious day decided as per astrology, sometime after the passage of mid–day, after performing auspicious rites and rituals, after Abhyanga and Swedana, after the elimination of urine and faeces, after making sure that the patient has not taken a heavy meal, after carefully considering the person, dosha status, drugs and dose etc.; the physician, accompanied by many experts of enema therapy, should administer Asthapana Basti to the patient.

Preparation of decoction for enema – Niruha dravya kalpana:

क्वाथयेद्द्विंशतिपलं द्रव्यस्याष्टौ फलानि च ॥ ३८ ॥
ततः क्वाथाच्चतुर्थांशं स्नेहं वाते प्रकल्पयेत् ।
पित्ते स्वस्थे च षष्ठांशमष्टमांशं कफेऽधिके ॥ ३९ ॥
सर्वत्र चाष्टमं भागं कल्काद्भवति वा यथा ।
नात्यच्छसान्द्रता वस्तेः पलमात्रं गुडस्य च ॥ ४० ॥ मधुपट्वादिशेषं च युक्त्या

The drugs / herbs (mentioned in the prescription for preparation of Kashaya) should be taken in 20 pala (960 grams) quantity and madana phala i.e. fruits of Randia dumetorum should be taken in 8 numbers the above mentioned ingredients should be made into a Kashaya .

(Note – the decoction is prepared with 16 parts water i.e. 15.360 litres and the contents boiled until ¼ quantity remains. Thus, 3.840 litres of decoction will remain roughly)

To this Kashaya, sneha dravya i.e. oil, ghee etc are added in ¼ quantity as that of kashaya for treatment of vata conditions / disorders (i.e. 960 grams), in 1/6 quantity as that of kashaya for treatment of pitta conditions / disorders and in healthy persons (i.e. 640 grams) and 1/8 quantity as that of kashaya for treatment of kapha disorders, the quantity of kalka of some drugs / herbs to be added to the kashaya for all the doshas and for healthy persons shall be 1/8 part of the decoction (i.e. 480 grams). The decoction should neither be too thin nor too thick after mixing all the above said ingredients.

Next, 1 pala (48 grams) of jaggery / molasses and appropriate quantity of honey and salt are also added.

Administration of decoction enema – Kashaya basti pranidhana:

सर्वं तद् एकतः । उष्णाम्बुकुम्भीबाष्पेण तप्तं खजसमाहतम् ॥ ४१ ॥

प्रक्षिप्य वस्तौ प्रणयेत् पायौ नात्युष्णशीतलम् । नातिस्निग्धं न वा रूक्षं नातितीक्ष्णं न वा मृदु ॥ ४२ ॥

नात्यच्छसान्द्रं नोनातिमात्रं नापटु नाति च । लवणं तद्वद् अम्लं च

All these are then mixed together, churned well with a churner and made warm by keeping its vessel either in hot water or by steam from a pot, it should then be filled into the basti putaka (enema bag). The medicine or basti dravya should neither be too hot or too cold, neither too fatty nor too dry, neither too strong nor mild, neither too thick nor too thin, neither too much nor too less in quantity, neither with too much salt nor without it, similarly the sour substances too (neither too much nor without their inclusion) is then pushed into the rectum.

Difference of opinion on quantity of fats, honey, salt, paste and liquids to be added to the enema liquid:

पठन्त्यन्ये तु तद्विदः ॥ ४३ ॥

मात्रां त्रिपलिकां कुर्यात् स्नेहमाक्षिकयोः पृथक् ।

कर्षार्धं माणिमन्थस्य स्वस्थे कल्कपलद्वयम् ॥ ४४ ॥

सर्वद्रवाणां शेषाणां पलानि दश कल्पयेत् ।

Some others, who are well versed in basti or enema therapy opine that the quantity of sneha dravya or fats i.e., oil, ghee and honey should be 3 pala (144 grams) individually, quantity of rock salt for healthy will be ardha karsha (6 grams), the paste of the drugs should be 2 pala (96 grams) and of all the other liquids put together should be 10 pala (480 grams).

Order of mixing enema substances basti dravya mishrana krama:

माक्षिकं लवणं स्नेहं कल्कं क्वाथमिति क्रमात् ॥ ४५ ॥

आवपेत निरूहाणां एष संयोजने विधिः ।

Honey, salt, fat (oil, ghee etc), paste of drugs / herbs and decoction are to be grinded and mixed in successive order this shall be the method of mixing the materials for Niruha basti.

After–care following the completion of decoction enema:

उत्तानो दत्तमात्रे तु निरूहे तन्मना भवेत् ॥ ४६ ॥

कृतोपधानः सञ्जातवेगश्चोत्कटकः सृजेत् ।

After receiving the enema, the patient should lie with his face upwards with a pillow under his head, focussing on (mentally intent) on the enema, after getting the urge (to evacuate), he should eliminate the faeces sitting on his heels.

Maximum time required for exit of decoction enema and measures to be taken when the decoction enema doesn't come out on its own:

आगतौ परमः कालो मुहूर्तो मृत्यवे परम् ॥ ४७ ॥ तत्रानुलोमिकं स्नेहक्षारमूत्राम्लकल्पितम् ।

त्वरितं स्निग्धतीक्ष्णोष्णं वस्तिमन्यं प्रपीडयेत् ॥ ४८ ॥ विदद्यात् फलवर्तिं वा स्वेदनोत्त्रासनादि च

स्वयमेव निवृत्ते तु द्विवतीयो वस्तिरिष्यते ॥ ४९ ॥ तृतीयोऽपि चतुर्थोऽपि यावद्वा सुनिरूढता ।

The maximum time for return of administered basti dravya is one muhurta (48 minutes). If it doesn't return by itself after the mentioned time period, it is said to be fatal. Hence, another Anulomana basti (purging enema) prepared with fats, alkalis, urine of animals like cow and sour substances, which possess unctuous, penetrating and hot properties should be administered immediately or a phala varti (rectal suppository) should be introduced. Swedana karma and frightening should also be resorted to, if the enema liquid comes out on its own accord, then second, third or fourth enemas can be given or as many enemas as required until he develops symptoms of proper enema therapy.

Measures to be done after proper elimination of enema liquid:

विरिक्तवच्च योगादीन् विद्यात् योगे तु भोजयेत् ॥ ५० ॥ कोष्णेन वारिणा स्नातं

तनुधन्वरसौदनम् ।

विकारा ये निरूढस्य भवन्ति प्रचलैर्मलैः ॥ ५१ ॥ ते सुखोष्णाम्बुसिक्तस्य यान्ति भुक्तवतः शमम् ।

The symptoms of bouts of kashaya basti i.e., signs of proper and improper elimination are similar to those of virechana after the appearance of the symptoms of proper elimination (proper administration of kashaya basti), the patient should take a warm water bath and eat rice mass along with the juice of meat of animals living in deserts. The complications of kashaya basti caused by the circulating doshas will subside by warm water bath and prescribed food.

Measures to be taken in those troubled by increased vata:

अथ वातार्दितं भूयः सद्य एवानुवासयेत् ॥ ५२ ॥

If the patient becomes troubled by increased vata, he should be given Anuvasana basti immediately once again on the same day itself.

Signs of proper, less and excessive administration of decoction enema:

सम्यग्धीनातियोगाश्च तस्य स्युः स्नेहपीतवत्|

The symptoms of samyak (proper), heena (inadequate) and ati (excessive) administration of decoction enema therapy are the same as those of snehana (drinking of fat) therapy.

Signs of properly done unctuous (oil, lubricating) enema therapy:

किञ्चित्कालं स्थितो यश्च सपुरीषो निवर्तते ॥ ५३ ॥

सानुलोमानिलः स्नेहस्तत् सिद्धमनुवासनम् ।

The sneha (oil, ghee etc.) given through enema coming out along with faeces after staying inside for a short time, followed by flatus moving down are the symptoms of properly given anuvasana basti.

Number of unctuous enemas in relation to the doshas:

एकं त्रीन् वा बलासे तु स्नेहवस्तीन् प्रकल्पयेत् ॥ ५४ ॥

पञ्च वा सप्त वा पित्ते नवैकादश वाऽनिले ।

पुनस्ततोऽप्ययुग्मांस्तु पुनरास्थापनं ततः ॥ ५५ ॥

1–3 anuvasana bastis should be administered for the treatment of kapha predominant diseases, anuvasana bastis for pitta predominant diseases and 9–11 anuvasana bastis for vata predominant diseases again on uneven alternative days, i.e., 3rd, 5th, 7th etc days, kashaya bastis should be administered.

Diet arrangement for different doshas in enema after-care:

कफपितानिलेष्वन्नं यूषक्षीररसैः क्रमात् ।

In kapha, pitta and vata disorders, food should be given along with soup prepared with rice, grains etc., milk and meat soup respectively (with soup in kapha, with milk in pitta and with meat soup in vata).

Enema for increased vata:

वातघ्नौषधनिःक्वाथत्रिवृतासैन्धवैर्युतः ॥ ५६ ॥ वस्तिरेकोऽनिले स्निग्धः स्वाद्वम्लोष्णो रसान्वितः ।

In case of vata vruddhi, one enema consisting of decoction of herbs which pacify vata, trivrit (Operculina turpethum), rock salt, mixed with fats, liquids of sweet and sour taste, made warm and administered will be ideal.

Enema for increased pitta:

न्यग्रोधादिगणक्वाथपद्मकादिसितायुतौ ॥ ५७ ॥ पित्ते स्वादुहिमौ साज्यक्षीरेक्षुरसमाक्षिकौ ।

In case of pitta vruddhi, two enemas consisting of decoction of herbs of Nyagrodhadi gana and Padmakadi gana of herbs made sweet by adding sugar and cold and mixed with ghee, milk, sugarcane juice and honey will be ideal.

Enema for increased kapha:

आरग्वधादिनिःक्वाथवत्सकादियुतास्त्रयः ॥ ५८ ॥ रूक्षाः सक्षौद्रगोमूत्रास्तीक्ष्णोष्णकटुकाः कफे ।

In case of kapha vruddhi, three enemas consisting of decoction of herbs of Aragwadhadi gana and Vatsakadi gana of herbs, dry in nature, mixed with honey, urine of cow, possessing penetrating, hot and pungent properties is ideal.

Enema for increased kapha:

त्रयस्ते सन्निपातेऽपि दोषान् घ्नन्ति यतः क्रमात् ॥ ५९ ॥

In case of tridosha vruddhi (increase of all the three doshas together), these three kinds of enemas (mentioned above for vata, pitta and kapha) will bring down the doshas when given in that order.

Superiority of the above mentioned three dosha mitigating enemas:

त्रिभ्यः परं वस्तिमतो नेच्छन्त्यन्ये चिकित्सकाः । न हि दोषश्चतुर्थोऽस्ति पुनर्दीयेत यं प्रति ॥ ६० ॥

Other physicians do not desire any enema other than these three enemas because there is no fourth dosha for which another enema needs to be given.

Three other kinds of enema:

उत्क्लेशनं शुद्धिकरं दोषाणां शमनं क्रमात् ।
त्रिधैव कल्पयेद्वस्तिमित्यन्येऽपि प्रचक्षते ॥ ६१ ॥
दोषौषधादिबलतः सर्वमेतत् प्रमाणयेत् ।

Yet others say that only three kinds of enema are to be prepared, (they are) utkleshana basti – that which causes exacerbation of doshas, shodhana basti – that which causes purification, by expelling the doshas and shamana basti – that which causes mitigation of doshas by subsiding them inside the body, without expelling them. In that order all these are to be justified on the basis of strength of the doshas, drugs, etc.

Limits of doing basti therapy:

सम्यङ्निरूढलिङ्गं तु नासम्भाव्य निवर्तयेत् ॥ ६२ ॥

The administration of kashaya basti should not be stopped until the symptoms of proper enema are not obtained.

Karma Basti – treatment with 30 enemas:

प्राक् स्नेह एकः पञ्चान्ते द्वादशास्थापनानि च ।
सान्वासनानि कर्मैवं वस्तयस्त्रिंशदीरिताः ॥ ६३ ॥

A course of 30 enemas in which one Anuvasana basti is given at the beginning and five Anuvasana bastis at the end (of the course), with twelve kashaya bastis and twelve anuvasana bastis alternatively in the middle (in between the above said unctuous enemas at the beginning and end) is called karma basti.

Pattern of Karma basti –

Anuvasana basti days –

1st day, 2nd, 4th, 6th, 8th, 10th, 12th, 14th, 16th, 18th, 20th, 22nd and 24th days

Kashaya basti days –

3rd, 5th, 7th, 9th, 11th, 13th, 15th, 17th, 19th, 21st, 23rd, 25th days

26th, 27th, 28th, 29th, 30th days – anuvasana basti

Kala Basti – treatment with 15 enemas:

कालः पञ्चदशैकोऽत्र प्राक् स्नेहोऽन्ते त्रयस्तथा ।

षट् पञ्चवस्त्यन्तरिताः

A course of 15 enemas in which 1 anuvasana basti is given at the beginning and three anuvasana bastis at the end (of the course), with 6 kashaya bastis and 5 anuvasana bastis alternatively in the middle (in between the first and last anuvasana bastis) is known as kala basti.

Pattern of Kala basti –

1st day – anuvasana basti

2nd, 4th, 6th, 8th, 10th and 12th days – Niruha basti

3rd, 5th, 7th, 9th and 11th days – anuvasana basti

13th, 14th, 15th days – anuvasana basti

Yoga Basti – treatment with 8 enemas:

योगोऽष्टौ वस्तयोऽत्र तु ॥ ६४ ॥

त्रयो निरूहाः स्नेहाश्च स्नेहावाद्यन्तयोरुभौ ।

A course of 8 enemas in which 1 anuvasana basti is given at the beginning and 1 anuvasana basti at the end (of the course), with 3 kashaya bastis and 3 anuvasana bastis alternatively in the middle (in between the first and last anuvasana bastis) is known as yoga basti.

Pattern of Yoga basti –

Anuvasana basti – 1st day, 3rd, 5th & 7th days and on 8th day

Niruha basti – 2nd, 4th & 6th days

Unctuous or decoction enemas should not be administered alone, in excess:

स्नेहवस्तिं निरूहं वा नैकमेवातिशीलयेत् ॥ ६५ ॥

उत्क्लेशाग्निवधौ स्नेहान्निरूहान्मरुतो भयम् ॥

तस्मान्निरूढः स्नेह्यः स्यान्निरूह्यश्चानुवासितः ॥ ६६ ॥

स्नेहशोधनयुक्त्यैवं वस्तिकर्म त्रिदोषजित् ।

Either anuvasana basti or kashaya basti alone should not be administered (in excess and continuously) more of anuvasana basti – unctuous (oil, lubricating, fat) enema may cause nausea and loss of digestion strength, more of kashaya basti may cause fear of increase of vata hence those who are given kashaya basti should also be given with anuvasana basti and those who are given anuvasana basti should also be given with kashaya basti will balance the three doshas only when it is both lubricating and purifying /

cleansing (as caused by anuvasana basti and kashaya basti respectively).

Matra Basti – Low dose fat enema:

ह्रस्वया स्नेहपानस्य मात्रया योजितः समः ॥ ६७ ॥ मात्रावस्तिः स्मृतः स्नेहः

The anuvasana basti consisting of fat/oil quantity equivalent to the minimum quantity of fats used for oral consumption (sneha pana) is known as matra basti.

Indications and benefits of Matra Basti:

शीलनीयः सदा च सः । बालवृद्धाध्वभारस्त्रीव्यायामासक्तचिन्तकैः ॥ ६८ ॥

वातभग्नाबलाल्पाग्निनृपेश्वरसुखात्मभिः । दोषघ्नो निष्परीहारो बल्यः सृष्टमलः सुखः ॥ ६९ ॥

It (matra basti) should always be administered in children, the aged, who are habituated to long walking, carrying heavy weights, excessive sexual activity, excessive exercise, who think too much, who are suffering from diseases of vata, fractures, debility, those having poor digestive activity, for kings, wealthy persons and persons who live happily. Matra Basti conquers the doshas, does not need strict regimen, gives strength, eliminates the wastes (urine, faeces etc.), easily and is comfortable (to undergo).

Uttara basti – urethral and vaginal enema (douche):

वस्तौ रोगेषु नारीणां योनिगर्भाशयेषु च ।

द्वित्रास्थापनशुद्धेभ्यो विदध्याद्वस्तिमुत्तरम् ॥ ७० ॥

In diseases of urinary bladder and diseases of vagina and uterus in women, Uttara basti (enema administered through urethral route for both men and women or vaginal route for women) should be administered, to those who have purified by two or three kashaya bastis given through the rectal route.

Enema nozzle for Uttara basti:

आतुराङ्गुलमानेन तन्नेत्रं द्वादशाङ्गुलम् ।

वृत्तं गोपुच्छवन्मूलमध्ययोः कृतकर्णिकम् ॥ ७१ ॥

सिद्धार्थकप्रवेशाग्रं श्लक्ष्णं हेमादिसम्भवम् ।

कुन्दाश्वमारसुमनःपुष्पवृन्तोपमं दृढम् ॥ ७२ ॥

The basti netra or nozzle for administering uttara basti should be of 12 angula in length, in terms of patients own fingers, rounded (tubular), which looks like a cow's tail at its end, should have ridges at the root and middle should have an orifice of mustard seed size, it should be smooth and made up of gold, silver etc. metals, resembling the stalk of flowers such as kunda, ashwamara and sumanas, it should be strong in consistency.

Enema liquid for Uttara basti:

तस्य वस्तिर्मृदुलघुर्मात्रा शुक्तिर्विकल्प्य वा ।

The enema liquid meant for uttara basti should be mild in strength light (easily acting) its quantity should be one sukti i.e. 24 grams .

Procedute of urethral / vaginal enema – Uttara basti Vidhi:

अथ स्नाताशितस्यास्य स्नेहवस्तिविधानतः ॥ ७३ ॥

ऋजोः सुखोपविष्टस्य पीठे जानुसमे मृदौ ।

हृष्टे मेढ्रे स्थिते चर्जौ शनैः स्रोतोविशुद्धये ॥ ७४ ॥

सूक्ष्मां शलाकां प्रणयेत्तया शुद्धेऽनुसेवनि ।

आमेहनान्तं नेत्रं च निष्कम्पं गुदवत्ततः ॥ ७५ ॥

पीडितेऽन्तर्गते स्नेहे स्नेहवस्तिक्रमो हितः ।

वस्तीननेन विधिना दद्यात् त्रींश्चतुरोऽपि वा ॥ ७६ ॥

अनुवासनवच्छेषं सर्वमेवास्य चिन्तयेत् ।

Next, the patient who has been given bath and food according to the regimen prescribed for anuvasana basti, the person should be stable and steadily placed, should be seated comfortably on soft seat of one's knee height, the erect penis should be held straight by the physician and a thin probe should be inserted gently (by the physician) to clear the channel (urinary or vaginal tract), after thus cleansing the passage, the enema nozzle should be inserted along the line of the suture, to the entire length of the urethral passage, till the cavity of the urinary bladder is reached, without shaking and the enema bag should be pressed gently as explained in rectal enema, pushing the fat (oil, ghee etc.) into the urinary bladder, this is the ideal method for administering urethral enema in this manner, three or four enemas should be given, all other procedures including after–care, diet etc. are planned (and implemented) similar to that of fat enema therapy.

When to administer Uttara Basti in women, during or after menstrual period in women?

स्त्रीणामार्तवकाले तु योनिर्गृह्णात्यपावृतेः ॥ ७७ ॥

विदधीत तदा तस्मादनृतावपि चात्यये ।

योनिविभ्रंशशूलेषु योनिव्यापद्यसृग्दरे ॥ ७८ ॥

In women, the uterus (uterine passage) will be open only during the menstrual period, therefore, vaginal / uterine enema should be administered during the menstrual period only. It can be given even apart from the menstrual period in case of emergency, in diseases such as prolapsed and pain of uterus / vagina, in other diseases of uterus and vagina and in menorrhagia

Nozzle for vaginal / uterine enema & urethral enema in women:

नेत्रं दशाङ्गुलं मुद्गप्रवेशं चतुरङ्गुलम् ।

अपत्यमार्गे योज्यं स्याद् द्व्यङ्गुलं मूत्रवर्त्मनि ॥ ७९ ॥

मूत्रकृच्छ्रविकारेषु बालानां त्वेकमङ्गुलम् ।

The length of basti netra or nozzle for administering vaginal / uterine enema should be 10 angulas, permitting the entry of a grain of green gram, it should be inserted to a length of four angula in case of vaginal passage and to a length of 2 angulas in case of urethral passage in diseases like dysuria etc. and in case of children, it shall be one angula.

Dosage of enema liquid for vaginal / uterine enema in women:

प्रकुञ्चो मध्यमा मात्रा बालानां शुक्तिरेव तु ॥ ८० ॥

The medium quantity of enema is one prakuncha (48 grams) and for children the dose is 1 shukti (i.e., 24 grams).

Administering uttara basti in women:

उत्तानायाः शयानायाः सम्यक् सङ्कोच्य सक्थिनी ।

ऊर्ध्वजान्वास्त्रिचतुरानहोरात्रेण योजयेत् ॥ ८१ ॥

वस्तींस्त्रिरात्रमेवं च स्नेहमात्रां विवर्धयन् ।

त्र्यहमेव च विश्रम्य प्रणिदध्यात् पुनस्त्र्यहम् ॥ ८२ ॥

The woman, who is lying on a cot with her face upwards, flexing the thighs and legs folded at the knees, should be administered with vaginal / urethral enema, 3–4 times in a day and night, it should be continued for 3 days only, increasing the quantity of unctuous enema liquid daily, after a gap of 3 days, it should be administered again for another 3 days.

General period of administration of enema and relation to other purification treatments in terms of time–gap:

पक्षादिवरेको वमिते ततः पक्षान्निरूहणम् ।

सद्यो निरूढश्चान्वास्यः सप्तरात्रादिवरेचितः ॥ ८३ ॥

Virechana should be administered after a fortnight after vamana and kashaya basti should be administered a fortnight after purgation therapy. Anuvasana basti should be administered immediately after kashaya basti but 7 days after virechana.

Similey to explain the mode of action of enema liquid:

यथा कुसुम्भादियुत्तात्तोयाद्रागं हरेत्पटः ।
तथा द्रवीकृताद्देहाद्वस्तिर्निहरते मलान् ॥ ८४ ॥

Just as the cloth absorbs the color from the water boiled with kusumbha etc. coloring materials, the enema absorbs the doshas from the moistened body

Importance of enema therapy – Basti Chikitsa Shreshtata

शाखागताः कोष्ठगताश्च रोगा मर्मोर्ध्वसर्वावयवाङ्गजाश्च ।
ये सन्ति तेषां न तु कश्चिदन्यो वायोः परं जन्मनि हेतुरस्ति ॥ ८५ ॥
विट्श्लेष्मपित्तादिमलोच्चयानां विक्षेपसंहारकरः स यस्मात् ।
तस्यातिवृद्धस्य शमाय नान्यद्वस्तेर्विना भेषजमस्ति किञ्चित् ॥ ८६ ॥
तस्माच्चिकित्सार्ध इति प्रदिष्टः कृत्स्ना चिकित्साऽपि च वस्तिरेकैः ।

For all the ailments located in the shakha (extremities, tissues), koshta (alimentary tract, visceral organs) and marma (vital organs), all the organs above the shoulders, there is no other cause more important than vata dosha. Vata is the one responsible for transportation and destruction of the increased faeces, kapha, pitta and other wastes (excreta) of the body.

To balance this intensely increased vata, there is no treatment more efficient other than the enema treatment. Hence it is described as half of the treatment (of all other treatments in the world put together) of all diseases, while some others opine that it is full treatment by itself.

Importance of venesection – Siravyadha pradhanyata:

तथा निजागन्तुविकारकारि रक्तौषधत्वेन सिराव्यधोऽपि ॥८९॥

Similarly, Sira Vyadha – venesection treatment is considered to be effective in vitiated blood conditions.

इति श्रीवैद्यपतिसिंहगुप्तप्रसूनुश्रीमद्वाग्भटविरचितायामष्टाङ्गहृदयसंहितायां सूत्रस्थाने बस्तिविधिर्नामैकोनविंशतितमोऽध्यायः॥१९॥

Thus ends the 19th chapter of Ashtangahridaya Samhita Sutrasthana, named Basti Vidhi Adhyayam, written by Shrimad Vagbhata, son of Shri Vaidyapati Simhagupta.

20

नस्यविधिमध्यायम् (nasya vidhim adhyayam)

The 20th chapter of Sutrasthanam of Ashtanga Hridayam is named as Nasya Vidhi Adhyayam. This chapter explains in detail about types, methods, indications and contra indications of nasal instillation of medicine – Nasya therapy.

अथातो नस्यविधिमध्यायं व्याख्यास्यामः इति ह स्माहुरात्रेयादयो महर्षयः॥

Atreya and other sages pledge that henceforth they will be explaining the chapter named Nasyavidhimadhyaya (pertaining to nasal administration of medicines).

Meaning and intention of Nasya:

ऊर्ध्वजत्रुविकारेषु विशेषान्नस्यम् इष्यते । नासा हि शिरसो द्वारं तेन तद् व्याप्य हन्ति तान् ॥ १ ॥

Nasya is especially useful in the treatment of diseases of the parts of the body above shoulder level. Nose is considered as the gateway of head. The nasal medication spreads through the nose and reaches all parts of head and neck and cures the diseases of head and neck.

Three kinds of Nasal medication:

विरेचनं बृंहणं च शमनं च त्रिधापि तत् ।

Nasya is of three kinds, they are –

Virechana nasya (purgatory errhines)
Brumhana nasya (nourishing errhines)
Shamana nasya (palliative errhines)

Virechana Nasya:
विरेचनं शिरःशूलजाड्यस्यन्दगलामये ॥ २ ॥
शोफगण्डकृमिग्रन्थिकुष्ठापस्मारपीनसे ।
Virechana nasya is beneficial in –
Shirashoola - headache,
Shira Jadya Syanda - loss of movement of the head/heaviness/stiffness in the head and neck,
Galamaya - neck disorders
eye diseases/conjunctivitis, diseases of the throat,
Shopha - swelling,
Ganda - enlargement of glands around the throat/goiter,
Krumi - worm infestation,
Granthi - cystic swelling/small tumors/fibroids,
Kushta - skin diseases,
Apasmara - memory related disorders/epilepsy,
Peenasa - rhinitis

Brimhana Nasya:
बृंहणं वातजे शूले सूर्यावर्ते स्वरक्षये ॥ ३ ॥ नासास्यशोषे वाक्सङ्गे कृच्छ्रबोधेऽवबाहुके ।
Brimhana Nasya is beneficial in – headache of vata origin, headache that increases by the day, loss of voice, dryness of nose and mouth, difficulty/ obstruction of speech, difficulty in opening the eyes, difficulty in speaking and stiffness of arms/difficulty of movement of arm along with pain.

Palliative errhines – Shamana Nasya:
शमनं नीलिकाव्यङ्गकेशदोषाक्षिराजिषु ॥ ४ ॥
Shamana Nasya is beneficial in –
Nilika - blue spots/patches on the skin,
Vyanga - discolored patches/spots on the face,
Kesha Dosha - diseases of the hairs/hair fall,
Akshi Raji streaks of engorged blood vessels formed in the eyes

Materials used in the three types of Nasya:

यथास्वं यौगिकैः स्नेहैर्यथास्वं च प्रसाधितैः । कल्कक्वाथादिभिश्चाद्यं मधुपट्वासवैरपि ॥ ५ ॥

बृंहणं धन्वमांसोत्थरसासृक्खपुरैरपि । शमनं योजयेत् पूर्वैः क्षीरेण सलिलेन वा ॥ ६ ॥

The Virechana nasya is administered by the use of fatty substances like oil etc. suitable in destroying the related diseases or with the fats processed with appropriate herbs or with fats processed with paste of medicinal herbs, decoction etc. or processed and added with honey, salt, and fermented infusions.

Brimhana nasya is done using juice of meat or blood of animals living in desert-like lands, mixed with plant extracts, resin, gums etc.

Shamana nasya is done using the juice of meat, blood etc., as used in nourishing nasal medications, milk or water.

Other kinds of Nasya:

मर्शश्च प्रतिमर्शश्च द्विधा स्नेहोऽत्र मात्रया । कल्कादयैरवपीडस्तु स तीक्ष्णैर्मूर्धरेचनः ॥ ७ ॥

ध्मानं विरेचनश्चूर्णो

Marsha and pratimarsha are two subtypes of sneha nasya (unctuous nasal medication) and are based on the quantity of fats used.

Avapeeda Nasya is used in the form of paste, fresh decoction, fresh juice etc. (not in the form of fats) and it is strong purgation to the head (purges off the doshas accumulated in the head and neck)

Dhmana is a type of nasal medication used in the form of powder and is virechaka (purging) in nature.

Method of using Dhmana nasya (churna nasya) prayoga vidhi:

युञ्ज्यात् तं मुखवायुना ।

षडङ्गुलद्विमुखया नाड्या भेषजगर्भया ॥ ८ ॥ स हि भूरितरं दोषं चूर्णत्वादपकर्षति ।

The Dhmana Nasya is administered by blowing the powder inside the nose with the help of air from the mouth.

The powder is filled in a tube of 6 angula length, open at both ends (and blown into the nose by blowing air at one opening while the powder enters the nostril of the patient through the other end of the tube)

It pulls out the greatly imbalanced doshas (from head and neck) because it is in the form of powder.

Quantity of nasal drops administered in nasal medication – Nasya Matra:

प्रदेशिन्यङ्गुलीपर्वद्वयान् मग्नसमुद्धृतात् ॥ ९ ॥ यावत् पतत्यसौ बिन्दुर्देशाष्टौ षट्
क्रमेण ते ।

मर्शस्योत्कृष्टमध्योना मात्रास्ता एव च क्रमात् ॥ १० ॥ बिन्दुद्वयोनाः कल्कादेर्

The quantity of liquid that drops after immersing two digits of the index
finger in any liquid and taking the finger out, that quantity of liquid forms
one bindu i.e., 1 drop

10, 8 and 6 drops are the maximum, moderate and minimum doses
respectively of marsha nasal medication (oil/fat nasya).

When the nasal drops are administered in the form of paste, juice, decoction
etc., i.e., avapidaka nasya, the doses are less by two drops (in comparison to
that of fat nasal drops), i.e., the maximum, medium and minimum doses are
8, 6 and 4 drops respectively.

Persons unsuitable to undergo nasal medication – Nasya Anarhah:

योजयेन् न तु नावनम् ।

तोयमद्यगरस्नेहपीतानां   पातुमिच्छताम्   ॥   ११   ॥

भुक्तभक्तशिरःस्नातस्नातुकामसुतासृजाम् ।

नवपीनसवेगार्तसूतिकाश्वासकासिनाम् ॥ १२ ॥ शुद्धानां दत्तवस्तीनां तथानार्तवदुर्दिने ।

अन्यत्रात्ययिकाद् व्याधेर्

Nasya should not be administered to the persons (in below said conditions)
–

Toya, Madya Gara, Sneha Peeta - who have just consumed water, wine,
artificial poisons and fats (as part of snehana therapy) or

Patum Iccatam - those who wish to consume the above said materials very
soon,

for those who have taken food just now, who have taken head bath, who
desires to take bath soon, who have undergone blood-letting therapy/or
who have had severe bleeding due to other causes,

Nava Peenasa - who are having acute rhinitis,

Vegarta - those who are getting natural urges of the body,

the woman who has recently delivered,

Kasa, Shwasa - those suffereing from dyspnea and cough,

Shuddha - those who have undergone purification therapies (panchakarma
therapies), who have just been given enema treatment, at unsuitable seasons
and on sunless cloudy days (cloudy climate)

except in emergency diseases (wherein nasal medication needs to be given)

Regulations for administration of Nasya:

अथ नस्यं प्रयोजयेत् ॥ १३ ॥

प्रातः श्लेष्मणि मध्याह्ने पित्ते सायन्निशोश्चले । स्वस्थवृत्ते तु पूर्वाह्णे शरत्कालवसन्तयोः ॥ १४ ॥

शीते मध्यन्दिने ग्रीष्मे सायं वर्षासु सातपे । वाताभिभूते शिरसि हिध्मायामपतानके ॥ १५ ॥

मन्यास्तम्भे स्वरभ्रंशे सायं प्रातर्दिने दिने । एकाहान्तरमन्यत्र

Therefore, the nasya should be administered in (the below mentioned conditions) in the morning time for increased Kapha conditions)

in the midday/noon for pitta (in pita increase)

in the evenings or night for vata (in vata increase).

For healthy people (to maintain health), in autumn and spring seasons, nasal medication shall be administered in the mid-day.

In cold/winter season, it should be given in the midday,

In summer it should be administered in the evening,

In the rainy season/monsoon, it need to be done when there is sunlight/ heat of sun,

It should be done both in the evening and morning, daily in – diseases of head caused by vitiated vata, hiccough, tetanus, convulsive disorders, stiffness of the neck, cervical spondylosis, hoarseness of voice, in other diseases it should be done with a gap of one day.

Number of days the nasal medication need to be done at a stretch:

सप्ताहं च तदाचरेत्॥ १६ ॥

The nasya therapy shall be done for a period of 7 days at a stretch (and not for more than 7 days), 7 days shall be a course

Procedure of nasal medication – Nasya Vidhi:

स्निग्धस्विन्नोत्तमाङ्गस्य प्राक्कृतावश्यकस्य च । निवातशयनस्थस्य जत्रूर्ध्वं स्वेदयेत् पुनः ॥ १७ ॥

अथोतानर्जुदेहस्य पाणिपादे प्रसारिते । किञ्चिदुन्नतपादस्य किञ्चिन् मूर्धनि नामिते ॥ १८ ॥

नासापुटं पिधायैकं पर्यायेण निषेचयेत् । उष्णाम्बुतप्तं भैषज्यं प्रणाड्या पिचुनाथवा ॥ १९ ॥

दत्ते पादतलस्कन्धहस्तकर्णादि मर्दयेत् । शनैरुच्छिद्य निष्ठीवेत् पार्श्वयोरुभयोस्ततः ॥ २० ॥

आभेषजक्षयाद् एवं द्विस्त्रिर्वा नस्यमाचरेत् । मूर्छायां शीततोयेन सिञ्चेत् परिहरन् शिरः ॥ २१ ॥

The person who has undergone the rituals of morning routine, should undergo head massage followed by mild sudation. He should then be made to sleep on a cot, in a room devoid of breeze.

The parts of the body above his shoulders should be given mild sweating once again, he is made to lie down straight, facing upwards (towards the ceiling), extending his arms and lower limbs. The medicine slightly warmed up with the help of hot water (the medicine is passively heated by keeping the nasya medicine bowl in a vessel containing hot water until lukewarm) should be taken either in a tube or soaked in a piece of cloth. And the medicine which is made warm is instilled into each nostril alternately, keeping the other nostril closed (while the medicine is instilled in one nostril, the other nostril is closed by pressing it with fingers). The person should sleep with a little elevation of his feet and with little bending backwards of his head (so as to enable easy instilling of drops). After instilling the medicine into the nostrils, his soles, neck, palms, ears etc. should be massaged mildly.

The person should then turn to his sides and spit out (the medicine coming into his mouth from the nose) till the entire medicine comes out. In this manner, two or three nasal medications should be administered. If the person goes unconscious (after the nasya therapy), cold water should be sprinkled over his face while avoiding the head.

Time of administration of unctuous/fat errhines:

स्नेहं विरेचनस्यान्ते दद्याद् दोषाद्यपेक्षया । नस्यान्ते वाक्शतं तिष्ठेद् उत्तानो

Nasya with sneha (fat materials) should be given at the end of Virechana Nasya after duly considering the involved doshas. After the nasal medication procedure is completed, he should lie supine i.e. facing upwards for a period of uttering one hundred syllables (approximately 100 seconds)

Post care after administering fat errhines – Sneha Nasya:

धारयेत् ततः ॥ २२ ॥ धूमं पीत्वा कवोष्णाम्बुकवडान् कण्ठशुद्धये ।

After nasya, one should inhale smoke of medicated herbs (Dhumapana), he should hold lukewarm water as gargle (in his mouth and throat), many times, in order to cleanse his throat.

Symptoms of properly administered Sneha nasya - (with oil or ghee):

सम्यक्स्निग्धे सुखोच्छ्वासस्वप्नबोधाक्षपाटवम् ॥ २३ ॥

In case of properly administered sneha nasya, the below mentioned symptoms can be observed – expiration (breathing out of air) without difficulty,

easy and good sleep, easy awakening from sleep and keenness of sense organs.

Symptoms of inadequately administered Sneha Nasya:

रूक्षेऽक्षिस्तब्धता शोषो नासास्ये मूर्धशून्यता ।

In case of dryness or inadequate lubrication following sneha nasya, the below mentioned symptoms are seen – stiffness/lack of movements of the eyes, emaciation/dryness of the nose and mouth and feeling of emptiness inside the head

Symptoms of excessively administered Sneha nasya:

स्निग्धेऽति कण्डूगुरुताप्रसेकारुचिपीनसाः ॥ २४ ॥

In case of excessive lubrication following excessive administration of sneha nasya, the below mentioned symptoms can be observed – itching, feeling of heaviness of the head, excessive salivation, anorexia and rhinitis.

Symptoms of properly, inadequately and excessively administered Virechana nasya:

सुविरिक्तेऽक्षिलघुतावक्त्रस्वरविशुद्धयः । दुर्विरिक्ते गदोद्रेकः क्षामतातिविरेचिते ॥ २५ ॥

When the virechana nasya is administered properly, it causes lightness of the eyes, clarity of mouth and voice, inadequate virechana nasya causes exacerbation of the diseases and excessive administration of virechana nasya leads to emaciation.

Indications of pratimarsha nasal medication:

प्रतिमर्शः क्षतक्षामबालवृद्धसुखात्मसु । प्रयोज्योऽकालवर्षेऽपि

Pratimarsha type of nasya shall be administered to – wounded, emaciated, children, aged people and those who lead a happy and conservative life.
It can even be administered during unsuitable time, season and day and also during the rainy season.

Note: Pratimarsha nasya is a type of sneha nasya. The drops in this are used in lower doses. Therefore, it can be used in many diseases as a cure.

Contraindications of pratimarsha nasya:

न त्विष्टो दुष्टपीनसे ॥ २६ ॥

मद्यपीतेऽबलश्रोत्रे कृमिदूषितमूर्धनि । उत्कृष्टोत्क्लिष्टदोषे च हीनमात्रतया हि सः ॥ २७ ॥

Pratimarsha nasya is not suitable in (the below mentioned conditions) –

Dushta Peenasa - Infective/allergic rhinitis,

Madya Peeta - those who have drunk wine/alcohol,

Abala Shrotre - people with low perception of sound, low hearing capacity,

Krimi Dushita Murdha - head infested with worms,

severe dosha imbalance and move from one place to the other in the body

(It is not suitable in the above-mentioned conditions because) it is of less quantity.

Proper time to administer Pratimarsha nasya:

निशाहर्भुक्तवान्ताहःस्वप्नाध्वश्रमरेतसाम् । शिरोऽभ्यञ्जनगण्डूषप्रस्रावाञ्जनवर्चसाम् ॥ २८ ॥

दन्तकाष्ठस्य हासस्य योज्योऽन्तेऽसौ द्विबिन्दुकः । पञ्चसु स्रोतसां शुद्धिः क्लमनाशस्त्रिषु क्रमात् ॥ २९ ॥

दृग्बलं पञ्चसु ततो दन्तदाढर्यं मरुच्छमः ।

Pratimarsha nasya shall be administered in the below mentioned 15 time periods –

Nisha - at night,

Aha - during day time,

Bhukta - after intake of food,

Vanta - after an episode of vomiting,

Aha Svapna - after day sleeping,

Adhva - after walking,

Shrama - after exertion,

Retas - after coitus,

Shiro Abhyanga - after head massage,

Gandusha - after gargling,

Prasrava - after urination,

Anjana - after administration of collyrium,

Varcasa - after defecation,

Dantakashta - after brushing teeth,

Hasya - at the end of laughing.

Its dose is 2 drops.

Among these, the first five helps in cleansing the body channels (at night, at morning, after food, after vomiting and after day sleep),

the next three (6-8) will relieve exhaustion (after walking, after exhaustion and after intercourse),

the next five (9-13) will strengthen the eyes (after head massage, after gargles, after urination, after collyrium and after defecation),

the last two (14 & 15) will strengthen the teeth and pacify the vitiated vata respectively (after brushing teeth and at the end of laughing).

Unsuitable age for different therapies – Kriya Nishiddha Vaya:

न नस्यम् ऊनसप्ताब्दे नातीताशीतिवत्सरे ॥ ३० ॥ न चोनाष्टादशे धूमः कवडो नोनपञ्चमे ।

न शुद्धिरूनदशमे न चातिक्रान्तसप्ततौ ॥ ३१ ॥

Nasya should not be administered to those who are less than 7 years of age and also for those who are above 80 years of age,

Dhuma Nasya - inhalation of medicated smoke should not be administered for children/youth below 18 years of age,

mouth gargling should not be administered for children below five years of age, purification therapies (panchakarma) should not be administered for children below 10 years of age and above 70 years of age.

Evaluation of Pratimarsha nasya:

आजन्ममरणं शस्तः प्रतिमर्शस्तु वस्तिवत् । मर्शवच्च गुणान् कुर्यात् स हि नित्योपसेवनात् ॥ ३२ ॥

न चात्र यन्त्रणा नापि व्यापद्भ्यो मर्शवद् भयम् ।

Just like the basti treatment, pratimarsha nasya is also admired to be good from birth to death (can be administered from birth until death, at all ages).

Pratimarsha nasya, when done daily, bestows benefits just like marsha type of nasya.

Either it does not require following any restrictions during the treatment, nor it carries any risks like marsha nasya.

Only oil should be used for nasal medication:

तैलमेव च नस्यार्थे नित्याभ्यासेन शस्यते ॥ ३३ ॥ शिरसः श्लेष्मधामत्वात् स्नेहाः स्वस्थस्य नेतरे ।

Only medicated oil is ideal for daily use of nasya (pratimarsha nasya to be specific), because the head is the chief site of kapha and no fat other than oil can keep it healthy.

Differences between Marsha Nasya and Pratimarsha Nasya:
आशुकृच्चिरकारित्वं गुणोत्कर्षापकृष्टता ॥ ३४ ॥ मर्शे च प्रतिमर्शे च विशेषो न भवेद्यदि ।
को मर्शं सपरीहारं सापदं च भजेत् ततः ॥ ३५ ॥ अच्छपानविचाराख्यौ कुटीवातातपस्थिती ।
अन्वासमात्रावस्ती च तद्वदेव विनिर्दिशेत् ॥ ३६ ॥

Immediate and delayed action, more and less benefits are the results (specific differences) of marsha and pratimarsha nasal medications respectively.

If there is no difference between them, who will resort to marsha type of nasya which are associated with restrictions related to food and activities and also with some risks and complications.

In the same way, are advocated the below mentioned treatment duals (following the same differences)

acchapana i.e., drinking of pure fat alone and vicharana sneha i.e., intake of fat mixed with foods etc.

kuti pravesha rasayana (i.e., kind of rejuvenation therapy wherein the person needs to stay in a specially constructed cottage for many weeks and consume rejuvenating and anti-ageing medicines) and vata atapika rasayana (i.e., wherein the patient can take the rejuvenation therapy without being confined to living in the cottage, while attending his daily routine works),

anuvasana vasti i.e., fat enema in large quantity and matra vasti i.e., fat enema in small quantity.

Preparation and use of Anu Taila oil for nasal medication:
जीवन्तीजलदेवदारुजलदत्वक्सेव्यगोपीहिमं ॥ ३७a ॥
दार्वीत्वङ्मधुकप्लवागुरुवरीपुण्ड्राह्वबिल्वोत्पलम् ॥ ३७b ॥
धाव्न्यौ सुरभिं स्थिरे कृमिहरं पत्रं त्रुटीं रेणुकां ॥ ३७चc ॥
किञ्जल्कं कमलाद् बलां शतगुणे दिव्येऽम्भसि क्वाथयेत् ॥ ३७d ॥
तैलाद् रसं दशगुणं परिशेष्य तेन तैलं पचेत सलिलेन दशैव वारान् ।
पाके क्षिपेच्च दशमे सममाजदुग्धं नस्यं महागुणमुशन्त्यणुतैलमेतत् ॥ ३८ ॥

Jivanti - Leptadenia reticulata,

Jala – Valerian,

Devadaru - Cedrus deodara,

Jalada - Cyperus rotundus,

Tvak – cinnamon,

Sevya - Vetiveria zizanioides,

Gopi - Hemidesmus indicus,

Hima – camphor,

Darvi tvak – bark of Berberis aristata,

Madhuka – Glycyrrhiza glabra,

Plava – smaller variety of Cyperus rotundus,

Aguru – Aquilaria agallocha,

Vari – Asparagus racemosus,

Pundrahva – Nymphaea lotus,

Bilva – Bael,

Utpala – Nymphaea stellata,

Dhavanyau – Solanum indicum and Solanum xanthocarpum,

Surabhi – Boswellia serrata/Pluchea lanceolata,

Sthire – Desmodium gangeticum and Uraria picta,

Krimihara – Eembelia ribes,

Patra – Cinnamomum tamala,

Truti – cardamom,

Renuka - Vitex negundo,

Kinjalaka - stamens of lotus,

Kamala – lotus,

Bala - Sida cordifolia, all these herbs should be boiled and processed in one hundred parts of rain water and the decoction should be reduced to one tenth part. To this decoction, equal quantity of sesame oil is added and cooked for ten times. During the tenth cooking/processing, an equal quantity of goat milk (equal to that of the oil) is added and cooked (until cooking is completed). This oil is known as anutaila, when used as nasal drops, bestows great benefits.

Benefits of nasal medication – Nasya Phala:

घनोन्नतप्रसन्नत्वक्स्कन्धग्रीवास्यवक्षसः । दृढेन्द्रियास्तपलिता भवेयुर्नस्यशीलिनः ॥ ३९ ॥

In persons who are accustomed to nasya, the skin, shoulders, neck, face and chest becomes thick, well developed and bright/attractive, the sense organs become strong and the grey hairs would disappear.

इति श्रीवैद्यपति सिंहगुप्त सूनु श्रीमत् वाग्भट विरचितायाम् अष्टाङ्गहृदयसंहिताया सूत्रस्थाने नस्य विधिः नाम विंशो अध्यायः ॥२०॥

Thus ends the 20th chapter of Ashtangahridaya Samhita Sutrasthana, named Nasya Vidhim Adhyayam, written by Shrimad Vagbhata, son of Shri Vaidyapati Simhagupta.

21

धूमपानविधिमध्यायम्‌ (dhumapana vidhim adhyayam)

The 21st chapter of Sutrasthanam of Ashtanga Hridayam is named as Dhumapana Vidhi Adhyayam. In this chapter, we are learning in detail about herbal smoking, its benefits, indications, timing, contraindication etc.

अथातो धूमपानविधिमध्यायं व्याख्यास्यामः इति ह स्माहुरात्रेयादयो महर्षयः॥

Atreya and other sages pledge that henceforth they will be explaining the chapter named Dhumapana vidhimadhyaya (pertaining to inhalation of herbal therapeutic smoke).

Purpose of administering medicated smoking:

जत्रूर्ध्वकफवातोत्थविकाराणामजन्मने । उच्छेदाय च जातानां पिबेद् धूमं सदात्मवान् ॥ १ ॥

The person who takes care of his health by following disciplinary measures related to food and life activities should inhale herbal smoke daily to prevent the non-manifested diseases and to root out (treat, destroy) the manifested diseases occurring above the shoulders, arising from vitiated kapha and vata.

Types of dhumapana according to dosha balancing actions:

स्निग्धो मध्यः स तीक्ष्णश्च वाते वातकफे कफे । योज्यो

a. snigdha / mrdu / prayogika i.e. unctuous / lubricating,

b. madhya i.e. medium and

c. teekshna i.e. strong

(are the three types of medicated smoking)

These should be administered to balance vata, vata-kapha and kapha respectively

Types of medicated smoking in relation to their Dosha balancing actions:

न रक्तपित्तार्तिविरिक्तोदरमेहिषु ॥ २ ॥ तिमिरोर्ध्वानिलाध्मानरोहिणीदत्तवस्तिषु ।

मत्स्यमद्यदधिक्षीरक्षौद्रस्नेहविषाशिषु ॥ ३ ॥ शिरस्यभिहते पाण्डुरोगे जागरिते निशि ।

Dhumapana should not be advised in the below mentioned conditions –

Raktapitti - those suffering from bleeding disorders,

virikta - person who has just undergone purgation therapy,

udara - abdominal / intestinal disorders or obstruction, ascites,

mehi - those suffering from diabetes, urinary disorders,

timira - cataract,

urdhwa anila - pathological upward movement of vata,|

adhmana - flatulence / bloating,

rohini - a serious disease of throat, diphtheria,

dattavasti - for those who have been administered with enema,

matsya madya dadhi ksheera kshaudra sneha visha - those who have just eaten fish, wine, curds, milk, honey, fats and poison,

shirasyabhiahata - those who have injured their head,

panduroga - those suffering from anemia,

nishi jagarita - those who have kept awake at night.

Effects of medicated smoking done at improper time or in excess:

रक्तपित्तान्ध्यबाधिर्यतृण्मूर्छामदमोहकृत् ॥ ४ ॥ धूमोऽकालेऽतिपीतो वा

If the dhumapana procedure is done at improper time or when done in excess, it leads to (the manifestation of below mentioned conditions) –

raktapitta – bleeding disorders,

andhya – blindness,

badhirya – deafness,

trit moorcha – excessive thirst and loss of consciousness

mada – intoxication

moha kṛt – hallucination / bewilderment / delusion / idiocy

Treatment for ill-effects caused by taking medicated smoking at

improper time or in excess:

तत्र शीतो विधिर्हितः ।

To treat ill-effects caused by medicated smoking done at improper time or in excess, cold regimen is the ideal treatment

Proper time of administration and indications of different types of dhumapana:

क्षुतजृम्भितविण्मूत्रस्त्रीसेवाशस्त्रकर्मणाम् ॥ ५ ॥ हासस्य दन्तकाष्ठस्य धूममन्ते पिबेन् मृदुम् ।

कालेष्वेषु निशाहारनावनान्ते च मध्यमम् ॥ ६ ॥ निद्रानस्याञ्जनस्नानच्छर्दितान्ते विरेचनम् ।

Mild, lubricating smoke should be inhaled after (at the end of) –

- kshut - at the end of sneezing

- jrumbhita - after yawning

- vit - after defecation

- mootra - after urination

- stree seva - after copulation

- shastra karma - after surgical operation

- hasya – after bouts of laughing

- use of dantakashtha – at the end of brushing the teeth

Medium strength dhuma should be inhaled in the below mentioned time periods –

- nisha ante – at the end of the night

- ahara ante – at the end of the meals

- navana ante – at the end of nasal medication / errhine therapy

Strong type of virecanam or purgative smoke should be inhaled (in the below mentioned conditions)

- nidra ante – at the end of sleep

- nasya ante – at the end of errhine therapies

- anjana ante – at the end of / after applying collyrium

- snana ante – after having taken bath

- chardita ante – after vomiting

Smoking apparatus – Dhuma yantra:

वस्तिनेत्रसमद्रव्यं त्रिकोशं कारयेद् ऋजु ॥ ७ ॥ मूलाग्रेऽङ्गुष्ठकोलास्थिप्रवेशं धूमनेत्रकम् ।

Dhuma netra or smoking nozzle / apparatus should be prepared from the same materials as those used to prepare the enema nozzle (from metals like gold, silver, iron etc.). It should have three chambers, should be straight and should permit the entry of the thumb and seed of jujube through the orifices at the root and tip respectively.

Measurements of dhumanetra in different types of dhumapana:

तीक्ष्णस्नेहनमध्येषु त्रीणि चत्वारि पञ्च च ॥ ८ ॥ अङ्गुलानां क्रमात् पातुः प्रमाणेनाष्टकानि तत् ।

त्रीणि अष्टकानि चत्वारि अष्टकानि पञ्च अष्टकानि च

For teekshna (strong), snehana (lubricating) and madhya (medium) medicated smoking, the length of the nozzle should be of the dimensions - 3x8=24 angulas,

4x8=32 angulas and

5x8=40 angulas respectively.

Procedure - Dhumapana Vidhi:

ऋजूपविष्टस्तच्चेता विवृतास्यस् त्रिपर्ययम् ॥ ९ ॥ पिधायैच्छिद्रमेकैकं धूमं नासिकया पिबेत् ।

The patient should sit straight being attentive with his mouth open three (times) smokes should be inhaled through the nose, through each nostril alternatively,

while closing one nostril, he should inhale the medicated smoke through the other nostril (alternatively)

Note: the inhalation of medicated smoke is said to be done thrice, inhaling the smoke and letting it out forms one bout, three such bouts should be done at a time

Application of dhumapana according to the localization of doshas:

प्राक् पिबेन् नासयोत्क्लिष्टे दोषे घ्राणशिरोगते ॥ १० ॥

उत्क्लेशनार्थं वक्त्रेण विपरीतं तु कण्ठगे ।

If the aggravated doshas are located in the nose and head, smoke should be first inhaled through the nose to provoke and mobilize the doshas,

The inhalation of smoke should be first done through the mouth (and next through the nose) when the doshas are located in the throat.

The method of inhalation of smoke is opposite (reverse order) to that which is done when the doshas are localized in the nose and head, i.e. the smoke should first be inhaled through the nose and later by the mouth. Here, when doshas are already provoked, the inhalation should be first done through the mouth and later through the nose. To provoke the doshas, the inhalation should be done first through the nose and then through the mouth.

मुखेनैवोद्वमेद् धूमं
The smoke (inhaled either from mouth or nose) should be let out only through the mouth.

Effect of letting out smoke through the nose:
नासया दृग्विघातकृत् ॥ ११ ॥
Exhaling smoke through the nose leads to loss of vision.

How many times to inhale smoke:
आक्षेपमोक्षैः पातव्यो धूमस् तु त्रिस् त्रिभिस् त्रिभिः ।
Smoke should be inhaled thrice with three times inhaling and three times exhaling alternatively.

Number of times of taking smoke in different types of dhumapana:
अह्नः पिबेत् सकृत् स्निग्धं द्विर्मध्यं शोधनं परम् ॥ १२ ॥ त्रिश् चतुर्वा
The snigdha dhuma should be taken only once (one set of three inhalations and three exhalations) during the day time.
The madhya type of dhuma inhalation should be done twice (in two sets of 3 inhalations and 3 exhalations).
The virechana dhumapana should be done thrice or four times (3-4 sets of 3 inhalations and 3 exhalations).

Herbs for Mrudu Dhuma:
मृदौ तत्र द्रव्याण्यगुरु गुग्गुलु । मुस्तस्थौणेयशैलेयनलदोशीरवालकम् ॥ १३ ॥
वराङ्गकौन्तीमधुकबिल्वमज्जैलवालुकम् । श्रीवेष्टकं सर्जरसो ध्यामकं मदनं प्लवम् ॥ १४ ॥
शल्लकी कुङ्कुमं माषा यवाः कुन्दुरुकस्तिलाः । स्नेहः फलानां साराणां मेदो मज्जा वसा घृतम् ॥ १५ ॥
In mridu dhumapana, following are the most useful herbs –
Aguru – Aquilaria agollocha
Guggulu – Commiphora mukul
Musta – Cyperus rotundus
Sthauneya – Taxus baccata
Shaileya – Parmelia perlata

Nalada – Nardostachys jatamansi
Usheera – Vetiver
Valaka – Gisekia pharnaceoides
Varanga – Cinnamon
Kaunti - Vitex agnus
Madhuka – Licorice
Bilva majja – fruit pulp of bael fruit
Elavaluka – Prunus cerasus
Shriveshtaka - Pinus roxburghii
Sarjarasa – exudates / resin of Shorea robusta
Dhyamaka - Cymbopogon martini
Madana - Randia dumetorum
Plava - smaller variety of Cyperus rotundus
Shallaki – Boswellia serrata
Kumkuma - Crocus sativus
Masha – Black gram
Yava - Barley
Kunduruka - exudates / resin of Boswellia serrata
Tila - Sesame
oil obtained from fruits and pith of the trees
Meda – fat
Majja – bone marrow
Vasa – muscle fat
Ghrita - ghee.

Herbs for Shamana Dhuma:
शमने शल्लकी लाक्षा पृथ्वीका कमलोत्पलम् । न्यग्रोधोदुम्बराश्वत्थप्लक्षलोध्रत्वचः सिता
॥ १६ ॥
यष्टीमधु सुवर्णत्वक् पद्मकं रक्तयष्टिका । गन्धाश्चाकुष्ठतगरास्
For shamana dhuma, which does pacification of doshas, the below
mentioned herbs are useful –
Shallaki – Boswellia serrata
Laksha – lac
Prithvika – greater cardamom
Kamala – lotus
Utpala – water lily
Tvacha - barks of –

- nyagrodha – Ficus benghalensis
- udumbara – Ficus glomerata
- ashvattha – Ficus religiosa
- plaksha – Ficus lacor
- rodhra – Symplocos racemosa
sita - sugar
yashtimadhu – licorice
suvarna tvak – Cassia fistula
padmaka - Prunus cerasoides
raktayashtika – Rubia cordifolia
fragrant herbs like Saussurea lappa, Valeriana wallichii etc.

Herbs for Teekshna Dhuma:

तीक्ष्णे ज्योतिष्मती निशा ॥ १७ ॥ दशमूलमनोह्वालं लाक्षा श्वेता फलत्रयम् ।
गन्धद्रव्याणि तीक्ष्णानि गणो मूर्धविरेचनः ॥ १८ ॥

For teekshna dhuma, which does evacuation of doshas, the below mentioned herbs are useful –
jyotishmati, nisha – turmeric, dashamoola – 10 roots
manohvala - realgar and orpiment
laksha – lac, shveta – Bauhinia variegata / Clitorea ternatea
Triphala
teekshna gandha dravya – herbs and substances having strong fragrance and
murdha virechana gana - herbs comprising of head cleansing group of herbs

Preparation of Dhumavarti (smoke wick):

जले स्थितामहोरात्रमिषीकां द्वादशाङ्गुलाम् । पिष्टैर् धूमौषधैरेवं पञ्चकृत्वः प्रलेपयेत् ॥ १९ ॥

वर्तिरङ्गुष्ठकस्थूला यवमध्या यथा भवेत् । छायाशुष्कां विगर्भां तां स्नेहाभ्यक्तां यथायथम् ॥ २० ॥

धूमनेत्रार्पितां पातुमग्निप्लुष्टां प्रयोजयेत् ।

A reed (tall, grass like plant) of 12 angula in length should be soaked in water for a day and night and smeared with the paste of the medicines useful for medicated smoking for five times (five layers, after every layer gets dried, another layer of paste is applied, this is done for five times). Thus, a wick which has the thickness of the middle of the thumb and that of barley in the middle should be prepared. It should then be dried in the shade. Removed of its reed (the reed should be gradually removed from the wick, this leaves the wick to have hollowness in its entire length), smeared with any suitable fat material (oil, ghee). The wick should be inserted into the smoking nozzle, lit with fire and the smoke should be inhaled.

Kasaghna Dhuma (Antitussive type of smoke for cough):
शरावसम्पुटच्छिद्रे नाडीं न्यस्य दशाङ्गुलाम् ॥ २१ ॥
अष्टाङ्गुलां वा वक्त्रेण कासवान् धूमम् आपिबेत् ॥ २१ऊअब् ॥
A tube either of 10 or 8 angulas in length should be fixed to a hole made in the capsule prepared by placing two earthen saucers one over the other and binding their ends and the person suffering from cough is made to inhale the smoke through the mouth.

Benefits of dhumapana:
कासः श्वासः पीनसो विस्वरत्वं पूतिर्गन्धः पाण्डुता केशदोषः ।
कर्णास्याक्षिस्रावकण्डुवर्तिजाड्यं तन्द्रा हिध्मा धूमपं न स्पृशन्ति ॥ २२ऊ ॥
kasa - cough

shvasa - dyspnea, shortness of breath, asthma

peenasa – rhinitis

visvaratva - disorders of voice, hoarseness of voice

pooti gandha – pūtiḥ gandhaḥ - bad odor in the nose and smell

panduta – pallor (of face)

keshadosha - disorders of hairs

karnasrava akshisrava – discharges from ears, mouth and eyes

kandu – itching

arti – pain

jadya – stiffness / inactivity of ears, mouth and eyes

tandra – tandrā – stupor

hidhma – hidhmā – hiccough

These diseases do not affect the person who is habituated to dhumapana therapy regularly.

इति श्रीवैद्यपति सिंहगुप्तसूनु श्रीमत् वाग्भट विरचित अष्टाङ्गहृदयसंहितायां सूत्रस्थाने धूमपानविधिः नाम एकविंशतितमो अध्यायः ॥२१॥
Thus ends the 21st chapter of Ashtangahridaya Samhita Sutrasthana, named Dhumapana Vidhim Adhyayam, written by Shrimad Vagbhata, son of Shri Vaidyapati Simhagupta.

22

गण्डूषविधिमध्यायम्
(gandusha vidhim adhyayam)

The 22nd chapter of Sutrasthanam of Ashtanga Hridayam is named as Gandusha Vidhi Adhyayam. In this chapter, we learn about a few oral, ear and head therapy, their benefits, procedures etc. The chapter is called Gandushadi Vidhi Adhyaya, because it starts with an explanation of Gandusha – mouth gargling.

अथातो गण्डूषविधिमध्यायं व्याख्यास्याम: इति ह स्माहुरात्रेयादयो महर्षय:॥

Atreya and other sages pledge that henceforth they will be explaining the chapter named Gandusha vidhimadhyaya (pertaining to inhalation of herbal therapeutic smoke).

Types of Gandusha (liquid medicine held in the mouth to its full):

चतु: प्रकारो गण्डूष: स्निग्ध: शमनशोधनौ ।

रोपणश्च

Full mouth gargle is of four types –

Snigdha - lubricating

Shamana – palliative

Shodhana – purifying

Ropana – healing

Usage of four types of gandusha:

त्रयस्तत्र त्रिषु योज्याश्चलादिषु ॥ १ ॥

अन्त्यो व्रणघ्नः

Among the four types of gandusha, the first three should be used for balancing the three vata etc. doshas (vata, pitta and kapha) and the last one should be used for healing the wounds.

Note:

- The lubricating gargle, wherein oils and fats are used, is administered to balance vata disorders
- The palliative gargle should be used for balance pitta disorders and
- The purifying gargles shall be used for balancing kapha disorders
- The healing gargles are used for healing the wounds and ulcers

Snigdha gandusha:

स्निग्धोऽत्र स्वाद्वम्लपटुसाधितैः ।

स्नेहैः

Among these, the Snigdha gandusha is done by using the oil processed with herbs of sweet, sour and salt tastes.

Shamana Gandusha:

संशमनस्तिक्त-कषाय-मधुरौषधैः ॥ २ ॥

The shamana gandusha is done with herbs having bitter, astringent and sweet tastes.

Shodhana gandusha:

शोधनस्तिक्तकट्वम्लपटूष्णै

The shodhana gandusha is made with herbs having bitter, pungent, sour and salty tastes and hot properties.

Ropana gandusha:

रोपणः पुनः ।

कषाय-तिक्तकैः

The ropana gandusha is done with herbs having astringent and bitter tastes.

Gandusha Dravya (medicines used):

तत्र स्नेहः क्षीरं मधूदकम् ॥ ३ ॥

शुक्तं मद्यं रसो मूत्रं धान्याम्लं च यथायथम् ।

कल्कैर्युक्तं विपक्वं वा यथास्पर्शं प्रयोजयेत् ॥ ४ ॥

Below mentioned medicines are commonly used for gandusha procedure –
sneha - fats, oil, ghee, etc
ksheera – milk
madhoodaka – honey mixed water
shukta- fermented liquid, fermented gruel
madya - wine
rasa – meat juice
mootra - urine of animals
dhanyamla - wash of grains fermented by keeping overnight for several days
The gargle liquids may be mixed with herbal pastes, the liquids may be cooked or raw, the liquids shall be used such that it is comfortable to touch and hold in the mouth.

Benefits of gandusha with Tila kalka udaka (sesame seed paste mixed in water):
दन्तहर्षे दन्तचाले मुखरोगे च वातिके ।
सुखोष्णमथवा शीतं तिलकल्कोदकं हितम् ॥ ५ ॥
गण्डूष धारणे
Water mixed with sesame seed paste, either in lukewarm or cold form, is useful for gandusha in conditions mentioned below –
dantaharsha – tingling sensation in the teeth
dantachala – loose / shaking teeth
Vatika mukharoga – diseases of the mouth caused by vitiated vata

Liquids beneficial for daily gandusha:
नित्यं तैलं मांसरसोऽथवा ।
For daily use (for full mouth gargle), sesame oil or meat soup shall be used (they are the best for daily use)

Benefits of holding ghee and milk full mouth gargles:
ऊषादाहान्विते पाके क्षते चागन्तुसम्भवे ॥ ६ ॥
विषे क्षाराग्निदग्धे च सर्पिर्धार्यं पयोऽथवा ।
Doing gandusha with ghee or milk is beneficial in the below mentioned conditions –
Oosha dahanvite - local or general burning sensation
paka – ulcerations of the mouth
kshate agantu sambhave – injuries and wounds caused by foreign materials

visha kshara agni dagdha – wounds caused by contact with poisons, alkalis and burns caused by fire

Benefits of Madhu Gandusha (full mouth gargles with honey):
वैशद्यं जनयत्याशु सन्दधाति मुखे व्रणान् ॥ ७ ॥
दाहतृष्णाप्रशमनं मधुगण्डूषधारणम् ।
Madhu gandusha brings about cleanliness of the mouth and removes sliminess, quickly heals mouth ulcers and pacifies burning sensation and relieves thirst.
Benefits of Dhanyamla gandusha (full mouth gargle with fermented grain water)

धान्याम्लमास्यवैरस्य मलदौर्गन्ध्यनाशनम् ॥ ८ ॥
तदेवालवणं शीतं मुखशोषहरं परम् ।
Dhanyamla gandusha removes distaste, dirt accumulated in the mouth, teeth and tongue and foul smell from the mouth. The same fermented grain wash, if used without addition of salt and in cold form, is best to remove the dryness of the mouth.

Benefits of ksharambu gandusha (full mouth gargles with alkaline water):
आशु क्षाराम्बुगण्डूषो भिनत्ति श्लेष्मणश्चयम् ॥ ९ ॥
Ksharambu gandusha quickly destroys / breaks the accumulated kapha.

Benefits of sukha ushna udaka gandusha (full mouth gargles with warm water):
सुखोष्णोदकगण्डूषैर्जायते वक्त्रलाघवम् ।
Sukha ushna udaka gandusha brings about lightness and cleansing of the mouth (causes freshness of mouth).

Procedure of gandusha:
निवाते सातपे स्विन्नमृदितस्कन्धकन्धरः ॥ १० ॥
गण्डूषमपिबन् किञ्चिदुन्नतास्यो विधारयेत् ।
The person who wishes to do gandusha should be seated in a place devoid of breeze but should be seated where there is sunlight. And his shoulders and neck should be massaged and fomented (provided with heat through steam or hot compresses). He should hold the gandusha dravya (gargle medicament) by keeping his face slightly lifted up.

Time duration of gandusha:

कफपूर्णास्यता यावत् स्रवद्घ्राणाक्षताथवा ॥ ११ ॥

Liquid should be held until the mouth gets filled with kapha or until there are secretions from nose and eyes.

Difference between Kavala (partial mouth gargle) and Gandusha (full mouth gargle):

असञ्चार्यो मुखे पूर्णे गण्डूषः कवलोऽन्यथा ॥ ११-a ॥

Filling the mouth with fluids upto full capacity, not permitting any movement of the fluid inside the mouth is called gandusha. Whereas kavala is opposite to gandusha, taking the liquid into the mouth and moving it all around by gargling for specific duration.

Benefits of Kavala (partial mouth gargle):

मन्याशिरःकर्णमुखाक्षिरोगाः प्रसेककण्ठामयवक्त्रशोषाः ।

हल्लासतन्द्रारुचिपीनसाश्च साध्या विशेषात् कवडग्रहेण ॥ १२ ॥

By doing kavala, the below mentioned conditions will be cured diseases of the neck, head, ears, mouth and eyes, excessive salivation, diseases of the throat, dryness of the throat, nausea, stupor, drowsiness, anorexia, tastelessness and rhinitis.

Pratisarana and its benefits (Coating the mouth with medicaments):

कल्को रसक्रिया चूर्णस्त्रिविधं प्रतिसारणम् ॥ १३अब् ॥

युञ्ज्यात् तत् कफरोगेषु गण्डूषविहितौषधैः ।

Pratisarana or coating the mouth with herbs is of three kinds, they are –

kalka – in the form of medicinal pastes

rasakriya – in the form of solidified decoction and

choorna - in the form of powder

It should be administered in diseases of kapha origin, with the same herbs as suggested in full mouth gargle.

Mukhalepa (Application of paste of herbs over the face):

मुखालेपस्त्रिधा दोषविषहा वर्णकृच्च सः ॥ १४ ॥

Mukhalepa is of three kinds, they are –

doshaha – that which removes the doshas

vishaha – that which removes the poisons / toxins and

varnakrit – and that which improves color and complexion.

Mukhalepa for balancing the doshas

उष्णो वातकफे शस्तः शेषेष्वत्यर्थशीतलः ।

Mukhalepa is beneficial when applied warm for balancing vata and kapha doshas and in others (to balance other dosha i.e. pitta) it should be applied in excessively cold form.

Thickness of mukhalepa:

त्रिप्रमाणश्चतुर्भागत्रिभागार्धाङ्गुलोन्नतिः ॥ १५ ॥

The thickness to which the facial herbal pastes are applied are of three forms –

Chaturbhaga angula – ¼ angula thickness

Tribhaga angula – 1/3 angula thickness

Ardha angula – ½ angula thickness

Rules for removal of mukhalepa

अशुष्कस्य स्थितिस्तस्य शुष्को दूषयति च्छविम् ।

तम् आर्द्रयित्वापनयेत्तदन्तेऽभ्यङ्गमाचरेत् ॥ १६ ॥

Mukhalepa shall be left in place until it becomes dry. When it gets dry, it vitiates the skin complexion and color (therefore it should be removed soon after it becomes dry). It should be moistened and then removed (when moistened, it can be easily removed, or else it will hurt the face). At the end i.e., after removal of the paste, a gentle oil massage should be given to the face.

Things not to do while applying mukhalepas:

विवर्जयेद्दिवास्वप्न-भाष्याग्न्यातप-शुक्क्रुधः ।

Following should be avoided one who wishes to apply mukhalepa -

divasvapna – day sleeping

bhashya – excessive speaking

agni – exposure to fire

atapa – exposure to the sunlight / heat of the sun

shukkrudha - grief and anger.

Contraindications for mukhalepa:

न योज्यः पीनसेऽजीर्णे दत्तनस्ये हनुग्रहे ॥ १७ ॥

अरोचके जागरिते

Mukhalepa should not be administered to persons suffering from –

peenasa – rhinitis

ajeerna – indigestion

datta nasya – to those who have been administered with nasal medication / errhines

hanugragha – lockjaw

arochaka – anorexia, tastelessness

jaagarita – those who have awakened the whole night, those suffering from insufficiency of sleep.

Benefits of mukhalepa:

स तु हन्ति सुयोजितः ।

अकालपलितव्यङ्गवलीतिमिरनीलिकाः ॥ १८ ॥

The same (herbal facial packs) when done properly cures / destroys –

Akala palita – premature graying of hairs

vyanga – discolored patches on the face / freckles

valee – wrinkles on the face

timira –blindness, darkness in front of the eyes

neelika - blue spots on face bluish vision (a type of blindness).

Mukhalepa in different seasons:

कोलमज्जा वृषान् मूलं शाबरं गौरसर्षपाः ।

सिंहीमूलं तिलाः कृष्णा दार्वीत्वङ् निस्तुषा यवाः ॥ १९ ॥

दर्भमूलहिमोशीरशिरीषमिशितण्डुलाः ।

कुमुदोत्पलकल्हारदूर्वामधुकचन्दनम् ॥ २० ॥

कालीयकतिलोशीरमांसीतगरपद्मकम् ।

तालीशगुन्द्रापुण्ड्राह्वयष्टीकाशनतागुरु ॥ २१ ॥

इत्य् अर्धार्धोदिता लेपा हेमन्तादिषु षट् स्मृताः ।

The following six facial applications mentioned in each half line of the above said verses are said to be ideal for six seasons commencing with Hemanta i.e. early winter season respectively –

Paste of the pulp of jujube fruit, root of Adhatoda vasica, Symplocos racemosa and white mustard seeds are ideal for Hemanta Rtu i.e., early winter.

Roots of Adhatoda vasica, black sesame, bark of Berberis aristata and dehusked barley is ideal for Shishira Rtu i.e,. late winter season.

Paste of roots of Desmostachya bipinnata, camphor, Vetiveria zizanioides, Albizia lebbeck, fennel seeds and rice are ideal for Vasanta Rtu i.e., spring season.

Paste of water lily, blue variety of water lily, water plant, Cynodon dactylon, Licorice and sandalwood is ideal for Greeshma Rtu i.e., summer season

Paste of dried rood and stem of Coscinium fenestratum, sesame, Vetiver, Nardostachys jatamansi, Valeriana wallichii and Prunus cerasoides is ideal in Varsha Rtu, i.e., Rainy season.

Paste of Abies webbiana, Typha elephantiana, Saccharum officinarum, licorice, Saccharum spontaneum, Arundo donax / Cyperus rotundus and Aquilaria agallocha is ideal in Sharad Rtu, i.e., Autumn season.

Benefits of mukhalepa:

मुखालेपनशीलानां दृढं भवति दर्शनम् ॥ २२ ॥
वदनं चापरिम्लानं श्लक्ष्णं तामरसोपमम् ।

For those who are habituated (regularly apply) to application of herbal pastes on the face, the vision (perception of eye) becomes strong and keen, face never loses its luster, never becomes dull. The face becomes smooth and brilliant resembling a lotus flower in appearance

Murdhna Taila (Oil treatments related to head):

अभ्यङ्गसेकपिचवो वस्तिश्चेति चतुर्विधम् ॥ २३ ॥
मूर्धतैलं बहुगुणं तद्विद्यादुत्तरोत्तरम् ।

Oil treatments done over the head are of four types, they are –

abhyanga – head massage with herbal oils

seka – pouring of oil over the head in continuous stream

pichu – keeping cloth soaked in oil over the entire area of the scalp for a predetermined time period

basti - making the oil stand on the head with the help of a cabin constructed over the head to hold the oil / oil pooling over the head

Each successive one among these four are said to be more effective (than their previous ones) i.e. Shiro Vasti is the best and most effective one among the four treatments done on the head.

Shiro Abhyanga (Head massage):

तत्राभ्यङ्गः प्रयोक्तव्यो रौक्ष्यकण्डूमलादिषु ॥ २४ ॥

Among these treatments, head massage (applying oil over the head and giving a gentle massage) should be done in cases of (to cure) dryness, itching and dirtiness.

Shiro Seka / Shiro Parisheka (Pouring of oil over the head in stream):

अरूंषिकाशिरस्तोददाहपाकव्रणेषु तु ।
परिषेक:

Pouring oil in thin stream over the head is useful in (treating) –

arumshika – ulcerations in the scalp

shiratoda – headache, pricking pain in the scalp / head

daha – burning sensation

paka – suppuration

vrana – and in wounds

Shiro Pichu (Oil swabs used over the head)

पिचु: केशशातस्फुटनधूपने ॥ २५ ॥
नेत्रस्तम्भे च

Oil-soaked cloth / cotton swabs, applied over the scalp is useful in (treating) –

keshashata– hair fall

sphutana – cracking of the skin of scalp

dhoopana – feeling of burning sensation, feeling as if smoke is being eliminated from the scalp

netrastambha – stiffness / loss of movements of the eye.

Shiro Basti (Oil pooling over the head):

वस्तिस्तु प्रसुप्त्यर्दितजागरे ।
नासास्यशोषे तिमिरे शिरोरोगे च दारुणे ॥ २६ ॥

Oil pooling over the head is useful in (treating) the below mentioned conditions –

prasupti – loss of sensation of the scalp

ardita – facial palsy / facial paralysis

jagara – loss of sleep

nasa asya shosha – dryness of the nose and mouth

timira – blindness

daruna shiroroga – dreadful diseases of the head

Procedure of Shiro Vasti:

विधिस्तस्य निषण्णस्य पीठे जानुसमे मृदौ ।
शुद्धाक्तस्विन्नदेहस्य दिनान्ते गव्यमाहिषम् ॥ २७ ॥
द्वादशाङ्गुलविस्तीर्णं चर्मपट्टं शिरःसमम् ।
आकर्णबन्धनस्थानं ललाटे वस्त्रवेष्टिते ॥ २८ ॥
चैलवेणिकया बद्ध्वा माषकल्केन लेपयेत् ।
ततो यथाव्याधि शृतं स्नेहं कोष्णं निषेचयेत् ॥ २९ ॥
ऊर्ध्वं केशभुवो यावदङ्गुलं

The patient who has been subjected to cleansing (after administration of vamana and virechana) should be given oil massage and steaming treatments. And should be made to sit on a soft and comfortable seat / chair of the height of one's knee (knee height) at the end of the day. A strap of leather made from the skin of either cow or buffalo, 12 angulas in width (8-9 inches approximately), and equal to that of the head in circumference (such that it fits exactly over the head just like a cap), should be wrapped around the head, just above the ears, covered by a piece / strap of cloth over the forehead and should be fastened tight with the help of a thread. Then paste of black gram should be applied (to the joints and intervening spaces, at the junction of the leather cap and scalp, in order to prevent leakage of oil during the process of the treatment). After that, lukewarm medicated oil prescribed as per the disease, should be poured over the scalp (into the leather cap, and is made to stand in the cap) to a height of 1 angula over the skin of the roots of the hairs (over the scalp).

Time duration for Shiro Vasti:

धारयेच्च तम् ।
आवक्त्रनासिकोत्क्लेदाद् दशाष्टौ षट् चलादिषु ॥ ३० ॥
मात्रासहस्राण्यरुजे त्वेकं

The medicine (oil) should be held on the head until the secretions start coming from the mouth and nose. Or for a period of 10,000 matra kala, 8,000 matra kala and 6,000 matra kala for vata, pitta and kapha respectively. For those who are healthy, it should be held for 1,000 matra kala.

Note – 1 matra kala is the time required to blink the eye once

Shiro Vasti pashchat karma (Post treatment procedures):

स्कन्धादि मर्दयेत् । मुक्तस्नेहस्य

After the scheduled time period, the oil on the head should be removed and the shoulders etc. should be massaged.

Maximum number of days Shiro Vasti should be done:

परमं सप्ताहं तस्य सेवनम् ॥ ३१ ॥

Seven days shall be the maximum number of days for undergoing this therapy.

Karna Purana (Filling the ears with oil):

धारयेत् पूरणं कर्णे कर्णमूलं विमर्दयन् ।
रुजः स्यान् मार्दवं यावन् मात्राशतम् अवेदने ॥ ३२ ॥

The medicated oil / fat should be filled and held in the ears. The roots of the ears should be massaged, till the pain or disease subsides and for a time period of 1000 matra kala in case of healthy people.

Definition of Matra Kala:

यावत् पर्येति हस्ताग्रं दक्षिणं जानुमण्डलम् ।
निमेषोन्मेषकालेन समं मात्रा तु सा स्मृता ॥ ३३ ॥

The time period required for the finger of the right hand to move around the right knee joint once or the time equivalent to that required for closing and opening the eyelids once is defined as a Matra Kala.

Murdha Taila Phala (Benefits of oiling the head):

कचसदनसितत्वपिञ्जरत्वं परिफुटनं शिरसः समीररोगान् ।
जयति जनयतीन्द्रियप्रसादं स्वरहनुमूर्धबलं च मूर्धतैलम् ॥ ३४ ॥

Oiling of the head prevents / cures (the below mentioned conditions) - hair fall, graying of hairs, tawny-brown / reddish yellow color of hairs, cracking of the skin of the scalp, diseases of the head caused due to the imbalance of vata, causes clarity / pleasantness of the senses, imparts strength to voice, jaw and head.

इति श्री वैद्यपति सिंहगुप्त प्रसूनु श्रीमत् वाग्भट विरचितायाम् अष्टाङ्गहृदय संहितायां सूत्रस्थाने गण्डूषादिविधिः नाम द्वाविंशो अध्यायः ॥२२॥

Thus ends the 22nd chapter of Ashtangahridaya Samhita Sutrasthana, named Gandushadi Vidhim Adhyayam, written by Shrimad Vagbhata, son of Shri Vaidyapati Simhagupta.

23

आश्चोतनाञ्जनविधिमध्यायम् (ashchotana anjana vidhim adhyayam)

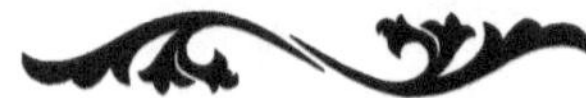

The 23rd chapter of Sutrasthanam of Ashtanga Hridayam is named as Ashchotana anjana Vidhi Adhyayam. This chapter deals with the detailed procedure of administration of Aschotana (eye drops) and Anjana therapies (eye salve/collyrium therapies).

अथातो आश्चोतनाञ्जनविधिमध्यायं व्याख्यास्याम: इति ह स्माहुरात्रेयादयो महर्षय:॥

Atreya and other sages pledge that henceforth they will be explaining the chapter named Ashchotana anjana vidhim adhyaya (pertaining to inhalation of herbal therapeutic smoke).

Benefits of Aschotana:

सर्वेषामक्षिरोगाणामादावाश्च्योतनं हितम् ।
रुक्तोदकण्डुघर्षाश्रुदाहरागनिबर्हणम् ॥ १ ॥

In all the eye disorders, eye drops are highly beneficial at the beginning,
eye drops helps to destroy –
ruk – eye pain,
toda – throbbing pain/pricking pain,
kandu – itching of the eyes,
gharsha – feeling of friction/as if something is being rubbed in the eyes,
arshu – excessive lacrimation/tears,
daha – burning sensation in the eyes and
raga – redness of the eyes.

Nature of eye drops for different doshas:

उष्णं वाते कफे कोष्णं तच्छीतं रक्तपित्तयोः ।

It should be –

warm in case of Vata imbalance,

lukewarm in case of Kapha imbalance and

cold in case of imbalance of blood and Pitta.

Method of administration of eye drops:

निवातस्थस्य वामेन पाणिनोन्मील्य लोचनम् ॥ २ ॥ शुक्तौ प्रलम्बयान्येन पिचुवर्त्या कनीनिके ।

दश द्वादश वा बिन्दून्द्व्यङ्गुलादवसेचयेत् ॥ ३ ॥ ततः प्रमृज्य मृदुना चैलेन कफवातयोः ।

अन्येन कोष्णपानीयप्लुतेन स्वेदयेन्मृदु ॥ ४ ॥

The eyes of the patient, who is lying on a cot, in a place devoid of breeze, should be opened with the left hand of the physician. Using the dropper, either made of a seashell or a wick is held in the right hand of the physician, just two angulas above the inner angle of the eye. 10 - 12 drops of the medicated liquid are put into the eye into the inner angle (inner canthus) of the eye, from a height of 2 angulas. Later, after the eyes are cleansed with the help of a soft cloth. Mild fomentation is given with a piece of cloth rinsed in warm water in case of disorders of Kapha and Vata.

Effects of very hot, very cold, excessively used, inadequately used eye drops:

अत्युष्णतीक्ष्णं रुग्रागदृङ्नाशायाक्षिसेचनम् । अतिशीतं तु कुरुते निस्तोदस्तम्भवेदनाः ॥ ५ ॥

कषायवर्त्मतां घर्षं कृच्छ्रादुन्मेषणं बहु । विकारवृद्धिधमत्यल्पं संरम्भमपरिस्रुतम् ॥ ६ ॥

Very hot and strong medicinal eye drops lead to manifestation of pain, redness and loss of vision.

Too cold eye drops cause pricking pain, loss of movements/stiffness of the eyes and pain.

Excessive use of eye drops produces roughness of the lids, friction and difficulty in opening the eyelids.

Inadequate/less use of eye drops causes worsening of the diseases, increase of redness of the eyes and absence of lacrimation.

Mode of action of eye drops:

गत्वा सन्धिशिरोघ्राणमुखस्रोतांसि भेषजम् । ऊर्ध्वगान् नयने न्यस्तं अपवर्तयते मलान् ॥ ७ ॥

The medicines instilled into the eye, entering into the channels of the joints, head, nose and face, eliminates the imbalanced doshas which have been accumulated and localized in the upper portion of the body.

Indications for Anjana (collyrium/eye salve):

अथाञ्जनं शुद्धतनोर्नेत्रमात्राश्रये मले । पक्वलिङ्गेऽल्पशोफातिकण्डूपैच्छिल्यलक्षिते ॥ ८ ॥

मन्दघर्षाश्रुरागेऽक्ष्णि प्रयोज्यं घनदूषिके । आर्ते पित्तकफासृग्भिर्मारुतेन विशेषतः ॥ ९ ॥

Application of anjana is beneficial in the below mentioned conditions –

the person who has undergone purification of his body by undergoing cleansing treatments like vamana, virechana etc.,

in whom the doshas are localized only in the eyes,

when the signs of fully ripened state of doshas like, presence of slight edema, severe itching and sliminess are found,

in presence of mild friction, excess lacrimation and redness in the eyes,

when the excretions of the eye are thick

and in persons who are troubled by vitiated Pitta, Kapha, blood and especially by Vata imbalance.

Types of Anjana:

लेखनं रोपणं दृष्टिप्रसादनमिति त्रिधा । अञ्जनं

Anjana is of three types, they are –

lekhana - scraping/scarifying,

ropana - healing

drishti prasadana – soothing to the eyes (that which makes the vision clear).

Lekhana Anjana (Scraping type of collyrium):

लेखनं तत्र कषायाम्लपटूष्णैः ॥ १० ॥

Among these, the lekhana anjana is prepared from herbs having astringent, sour and salt tastes and hot potency.

Ropana Anjana (Healing type of collyrium):

रोपणं तिक्तकैर्द्रव्यैः

The ropana anjana are prepared from bitter herbs.

Prasadana Anjana (Soothing/vision clearing type of collyrium):

स्वादुशीतैः प्रसादनम् ।

The prasadana Anjana is prepared from herbs having sweet taste and cold potency.

Pratyanjana (Counter-acting collyrium):

तीक्ष्णाञ्जनाभिसन्तप्ते नयने तत् प्रसादनम् ॥ ११ ॥ प्रयुज्यमानं लभते प्रत्यञ्जनसमाह्वयम् ।

For the eyes afflicted by side effects of teekshna Anjana (strong collyrium) the soothing collyrium are used. Such collyriums administered in the eyes to counteract the effects of the other collyriums are called Pratyanjana i.e., counter-acting collyrium/eye salve.

Anjana Shalaka (Collyrium apparatus):

दशाङ्गुला तनुर्मध्ये शलाका मुकुलानना ॥ १२ ॥ प्रशस्ता लेखने ताम्री रोपणे काललोहजा ।
अङ्गुली च सुवर्णोत्था रूप्यजा च प्रसादने ॥ १३ ॥

A shalaka or metal rod, 10 angulas (finger width) in length, thin in the middle, with its tip resembling a flower is best suited to be used as a collyrium applicator. For application of scraping collyrium, the applicator made of copper should be used. For application of healing collyrium, the applicator made up of iron or finger itself shall be used. For applying a soothing/vision clearing type of collyrium, the applicator made of gold or silver should be used.

Types of Anjana based on materials used:

पिण्डो रसक्रिया चूर्णस्त्रिधैवाञ्जनकल्पना । गुरौ मध्ये लघौ दोषे तां क्रमेण प्रयोजयेत् ॥ १४ ॥

The Anjana preparations are only of three types
pinda – used in pill form,
rasakriya – used in form of gel, confection (semisolid obtained after boiling the decoction until most of its liquid has been evaporated)
choorna - used in the form of powder
They should be used in
profound imbalance of doshas (pill form),
moderate imbalance of doshas (confection form) and
mild imbalance of doshas (powder form) respectively.

Dose of pinda and rasakriya types of Anjana (pill and confection type of collyriums):

हरेणुमात्रा पिण्डस्य वेल्लमात्रा रसक्रिया । तीक्ष्णस्य द्विगुणं तस्य मृदुनः

The quantity of pinda anjana prepared from strong herbs is one harenu. The quantity of pinda anjana prepared from mild herbs is twice that of the pill form, i.e., 2 harenu. The quantity of rasakriya anjana is equal to that of vella (Embelia ribes).

Dose of churna Anjana (powder form of collyriums):

चूर्णितस्य च ॥ १५ ॥ द्वे शलाके तु तीक्ष्णस्य तिस्रस्तदितरस्य च ।

The quantity of anjana used in the form of powder shall be two rods full when strong acting herbs are used and three rods full in case when mild herbs are used.

Wrong and right time for application of Anjana:

निशि स्वप्ने न मध्याह्ने म्लाने नोष्णगभस्तिभिः ॥ १६ ॥

अक्षिरोगाय दोषाः स्युर्वर्धितोत्पीडितद्रुताः ।

प्रातः सायं च तच्छान्त्यै व्यभ्रेऽर्केऽस्तोऽञ्जयेत् सदा ॥ १७ ॥

Application of Anjana should not be done at nights, during sleep, during afternoon and when the eyes are fatigued by strong rays of the sun. If collyrium is done during these times, the doshas get increased, spread to the other sites and get liquefied, leading to manifestation of diseases of the eyes. So, in order to mitigate the doshas, collyrium should be applied always either in the morning time or in the evening time when the sun is not present.

Contraindication of teekshna anjana application during day time:

वदन्त्यन्ये तु न दिवा प्रयोज्यं तीक्ष्णमञ्जनम् । विरेकदुर्बलं चक्षुरादित्यं प्राप्य सीदति ॥ १८ ॥

Some experts say that strong collyriums should not be applied during day time, because the eyes which have become weak following the purgation treatment given using strong herbs, will be further debilitated by the presence of the sun during day time.

Benefits of sleep on eye health:

स्वप्नेन रात्रौ कालस्य सौम्यत्वेन च तर्पिता । शीतसात्म्या दृगाग्नेयी स्थिरतां लभते पुनः ॥ १९ ॥

The eye being naturally predominant in the fire element and habituated to cold comforts, will regain its strength/stability yet again, after good sleep and being nourished by the coolant nature of the night.

Conditions for usage of lekhaneeya and teekshna Anjanas:

अत्युद्रिक्ते बलासे तु लेखनीयेऽथवा गदे । काममहन्यपि नात्युष्णे तीक्ष्णमक्ष्णि प्रयोजयेत् ॥ २० ॥

The lekhaneeya Anjana shall be used in conditions of extreme increase of Kapha or in diseases requiring scraping treatments and teekshna anjana can be applied to the eyes even during day time, if desired, only if the day is not hot.

Predominance of fire element in eyes:

अश्मनो जन्म लोहस्य तत एव च तीक्ष्णता । उपघातोऽपि तेनैव तथा नेत्रस्य तेजसः ॥ २१ ॥

The metals take their origin from their ores, similarly from the ores itself (the metals derive) their sharpness, bluntness etc. features. In the same way, the power and features and destruction of eyes are derived from the fire element itself.

Effect of Anjana in cold conditions:

न रात्रावपि शीतेऽति नेत्रे तीक्ष्णाञ्जनं हितम् । दोषमस्रावयेत् स्तब्धं कण्डूजाड्यादिकारि तत् ॥ २२ ॥

When there is severe cold, application of strong collyrium into the eye is not good even during night, because it does not cause elimination of the doshas from the eyes. Instead, it produces stiffness, itching, inactivity etc.

Anjana anarha (contraindications for collyrium/eye salve):

नाञ्जयेत् भीतवमितविरिक्ताशितवेगिते । क्रुद्धज्वरिततान्ताक्षिशिरोरुक्शोकजागरे ॥ २३ ॥

अदृष्टेऽर्के शिरःस्नाते पीतयोर्धूममद्ययोः । अजीर्णेऽग्न्यर्कसन्तप्ते दिवासुप्ते पिपासिते ॥ २४ ॥

Anjana should not be applied to the persons who are –

bheeta – in a state of fear,

vamita – those who have undergone emesis therapy,

virikta – those who have undergone purgation therapy,

ashita – those who have just consumed food,

vegita – during natural body urges like that of urine, feces, hunger etc,

kruddha – anger,

jvarita – those who are having fever,

tanta akshi – eye fatigue,

shiro ruk – headache,

shoka – grief, depressed,

jagara – loss of sleep,

adrishta arka – when the sun is not seen (totally covered with clouds),

shira snata – after head bath,

peeta dhooma – after inhalation of smoke,

madya - after drinking wine,

ajeerna – in presence of indigestion,

agni arka santapta – fatigued from exposure to fire and sun,

divasupta – after day sleeping,

pipasita – pipāsite – when thirsty.

Unsuitable Anjana:

अतितीक्ष्णमृदुस्तोकबहुवच्छघनकर्कशम् । अत्यर्थशीतलं तप्तमञ्जनं नावचारयेत् ॥ २५ ॥

The Anjana which is very strong or very mild, which is very little in quantity or very large, which is too thin or very thick in consistency, or is very rough/coarse, which is too cold or too hot should not be used.

Procedures that need to be done after applying Anjana:

अथानुमीलयन् दृष्टिं अन्तः सञ्चारयेच्छनैः ।

अञ्जिते वर्त्मनी किञ्चिच्चालयेच्चैवमञ्जनम् ॥ २६ ॥

तीक्ष्णं व्याप्नोति सहसा न चोन्मेषनिमेषणम् ।

निष्पीडनं च वर्त्मभ्यां क्षालनं वा समाचरेत् ॥ २७ ॥

After the administration of collyrium, the eyeball should not be moved up, it should be rotated slowly within the socket. The eyelids should be moved slightly. By all these acts, the strong collyrium quickly spreads to all places in the eye. Opening and closing of eyelids, squeezing or washing of the eyelids should not be done.

Proper time to wash the eyes after applying Anjana:

अपेतौषधसंरम्भं निर्वृतं नयनं यदा ।

व्याधिदोषर्तुयोग्याभिरदिभः प्रक्षालयेत् तदा ॥ २८ ॥

After the cessation of the activity of the collyrium medicine, when the eyes have regained strength, the eyes should be washed with water, as suitable with respect to the diseases, doshas and seasons.

Method of washing the eyes after Anjana:

दक्षिणाङ्गुष्ठकेनाक्षि ततो वामं सवाससा ।
ऊर्ध्ववर्त्मनि सङ्गृह्य शोध्यं वामेन चेतरत् ॥ २९ ॥

The physician should lift and hold the upper eyelid of the left eye of the patient with a piece of cloth, hold it with the help of his right thumb and fingers and wash the left eye of the patient with the help of his left hand he should wash the right eye of the patient.

Effects of not washing the eyes after the application of Anjana:

वर्त्मप्राप्तोऽञ्जनात् दोषो रोगान् कुर्यादतोऽन्यथा ।

If not washed, the Anjana remaining in the eyelids, excites the doshas which in turn give rise to eye diseases.

Indications of teekshna Anjana or Teekshna Dhuma:

कण्डूजाड्येऽञ्जनं तीक्ष्णं धूमं वा योजयेत् पुनः ॥ ३० ॥

When itching and inactivity are present following collyrium application, either a strong collyrium should be applied again or an inhalation of strong smoke of herbs should be done.

Remedy for eye fatigue caused by application of strong collyriums:

तीक्ष्ण अञ्जन अभितप्ते तु चूर्णं प्रत्यञ्जनं हिमम् ॥३० १/२॥

When the eyes get fatigued due to application of strong collyrium, a counter-eye salve which is in the form of powder and cold in effect should be applied.

इति श्री वैद्यपति सिंहगुप्त सूनु श्रीमत् वाग्भट विरचितायां अष्टाङ्गहृदय संहितायां सूत्रस्थान आश्चोतनाञ्जनविधिः नाम त्रयोविंशो अध्यायः॥२३॥

Thus ends the 23rd chapter of Ashtangahridaya Samhita Sutrasthana, named Aschotana Anjana Vidhim Adhyayam, written by Shrimad Vagbhata, son of Shri Vaidyapati Simhagupta.

24

तर्पणपुटपाकविधिमध्यायम्
(tarpana putapaka vidhim adhyayam)

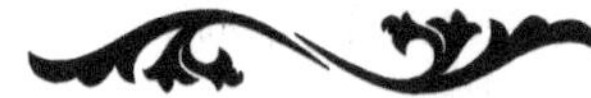

The 24th chapter of Sutrasthanam of Ashtanga Hridayam is named as Tarpana Putapaka Vidhi Adhyayam. This chapter deals with the detailed procedure of administration of Tarpana and Putapaka wherein medicinal liquids including oil / ghee / fat or juices are pooled around the eyes.

अथातो तर्पणपुटपाकविधिमध्यायं व्याख्यास्यामः इति ह स्माहुरात्रेयादयो महर्षयः॥

Atreya and other sages pledge that henceforth they will be explaining the chapter named Tarpana Putapaka vidhim adhyaya.

Indications for Tarpana treatment:

नयने ताम्यति स्तब्धे शुष्के रूक्षेऽभिघातिते । वातपित्तातुरे जिह्मे शीर्णपक्ष्माविलेक्षणे ॥ १ ॥

कृच्छ्रोन्मीलसिराहर्षसिरोत्पाततमोऽर्जुनैः । स्यन्दमन्थान्यतोवातवातपर्यायशुक्रकैः ॥ २ ॥

आतुरे शान्तरागाश्रुशूलसंरम्भदूषिके । निवाते तर्पणं योज्यं शुद्धयोर्मूर्धकाययोः ॥ ३ ॥

काले साधारणे प्रातः सायं वोत्तानशायिनः ।

Tarpana should be done in the following conditions –

when the eyes are fatigued, stiffness of the eye / loss of movements of the eye, roughness of the eyes, dryness of the eyes, injury of eye, in those patients suffering from Vata and Pitta disorders of the eye, irregularity / asymmetry of eye lashes or falling of eye lashes, clouded / unclear vision, difficulty in opening the eyes, feeling of darkness in front of his eyes, eye disorders like Siraharsha, Sirotpata, Arjuna, Anyatovata and Vataparyaya, conjunctivitis, glaucoma,

after the pacification of redness, lacrimation, pain, swelling and excreta of the eye.

Conditions where tarpana is advised

Tarpana should be conducted to a person who –

has purified both his head (by undergoing nasal treatment / errhines) and body (by cleansing treatments like emesis and purgation),

in a place devoid of breeze, in moderate / temperate season, at morning and evening, to a person who is lying with his face upwards (supine).

Procedure of Tarpana:

यवमाषमयीं पालीं नेत्रकोशाद्बहिः समाम् ॥ ४ ॥ द्व्यङ्गुलोच्चां दृढां कृत्वा यथास्वं सिद्धं आवपेत् ।

सर्पिर्निमीलिते नेत्रे तप्ताम्बुप्रविलायितम् ॥ ५ ॥ नक्तान्ध्यवाततिमिरकृच्छ्रबोधादिके वसाम् ।

आपक्ष्माग्रात्

Round walls, resembling a well, of uniform dimensions are constructed with the paste prepared from barley and black gram around both eye sockets, to a height of 2 angulas (finger width).

After confirming the steadiness of the wall, the medicated ghee prepared as per disease and liquefied by heating indirectly with hot water, should be poured gently into the well, over the closed eyelids after checking the temperature. The medications are poured up to the level of the eye lashes.

In diseases like night blindness, blindness caused by vata vitiation and difficulty to open the eyes etc., muscle fat (vasa) should be used instead of ghee.

Procedures after pouring the medicines, time of retention of medicines:

अथोन्मेषं शनकैस्तस्य कुर्वतः ॥ ६ ॥ मात्रा विगणयेत् तत्र वर्त्मसन्धिसितासिते ।

दृष्टौ च क्रमशो व्याधौ शतं त्रीणि च पञ्च च ॥ ७ ॥ शतानि सप्त च अष्टौ च, दश मन्थे, दशानिले।

पित्ते षट्, स्वस्थवृत्ते च बलासे पञ्च धारयेत् ॥ ८ ॥

After pouring the medicines, the patient is advised to open his eyes gradually (and keep blinking the eyes so as to expose his eyes to the medicines). While he does the blinking and holds the medicine, the time in terms of matra kala (1 matrakala is the time required to utter a soft syllable) should be counted to 100, 300, 500, 700 and 800 counts,

for diseases of eyelids, fornices, sclera, cornea, pupil and retina respectively; 1000 counts for glaucoma, 10 hundred counts i.e., 1000 counts for the diseases caused by Vata imbalance, 600 counts for diseases caused by Pitta imbalance, 500 counts for healthy persons and for diseases caused by Kapha imbalance.

These are the time limitations for retaining the medicines in various conditions while doing Tarpana.

Note –

Maximum retention time of medicines in various conditions of the eye while doing Tarpana treatment –

100 matrakala – for diseases of eyelids

300 matrakala – for diseases of fornices of the eyes

500 matrakala – for diseases of sclera

700 matrakala – for diseases of cornea

800 matrakala – for diseases of vision, pupil, retina

1000 matrakala – for glaucoma

1000 matrakala – for diseases caused by Vata imbalance

600 matrakala – for diseases caused by Pitta imbalance

500 matrakala – for diseases caused by Kapha imbalance and also for healthy persons.

Removal of medicines and the latter procedures:

कृत्वापाङ्गे ततो द्वारं स्नेहं पात्रे निगालयेत् ।

पिबेत् च धूमं नेक्षेत व्योम रूपं च भास्वरम् ॥ ९ ॥

After the specified time, the ghee should be removed and collected in a vessel through a hole made in the wall of the constructed chamber / socket near the outer angle of the eye. Then the person should be given herbal smoking. And he is also advised not to look at the bright sky or bright objects.

Number of days for doing Tarpana treatment:

इत्थं प्रतिदिनं वायौ पित्ते त्वेकान्तरं कफे ।

स्वस्थे तु द्व्यन्तरं दद्यात् आतृप्तेरिति योजयेत् ॥ १० ॥

Following the mentioned order of matra kala explained above, Tarpana treatment should be done daily in diseases of Vata, on alternative days in Pitta disorders, in diseases of Kapha and for healthy persons, it should be done with an interval of two days. It should be done until the eyes are properly nourished (until signs of proper Tarpana are observed).

Symptoms of samyak yoga, atiyoga and ayoga of Tarpana therapy (proper, excessive and inadequate):

प्रकाशक्षमता स्वास्थ्यं विशदं लघु लोचनम् ।
तृप्ते विपर्ययोऽतृप्तेऽतितृप्ते श्लेष्मजा रुजः ॥ ११ ॥

Tarpana done properly leads to – ability to tolerate bright light, good eye health, clarity of vision and lightness in the eyes.

Opposite to these are the symptoms of inadequately done Tarpana.

And when the tarpana is done in excess, the symptoms and disorders of Kapha imbalance will be observed.

Purpose of doing Putapaka eye treatment:

स्नेहपीता तनुरिव क्लान्ता दृष्टिर्हि सीदति ।
तर्पणानन्तरं तस्माद्दृग्बलाधानकारिणम् ॥ १२ ॥
पुटपाकं प्रयुञ्जीत पूर्वोक्तेष्वेव यक्ष्मसु ।

Just as the body becomes fatigued after the Snehana procedure, the eyes too become fatigued after the Tarpana treatment. Therefore, in order to restore the strength to the eyes, Putapaka therapy should be conducted in the diseases which have been mentioned earlier.

Types and indications of Putapaka:

स वाते स्नेहनः श्लेष्मसहिते लेखनो हितः ॥ १३ ॥
दृग्दौर्बल्येऽनिले पित्ते रक्ते स्वस्थे प्रसादनः ।

Snehana type of Putapaka (done using fats) should be done in disorders of Vata imbalance, lekhana type of Putapaka is beneficial in disorders of Kapha imbalance associated with Vata and prasadana type of putapaka is beneficial in weakness of the eyes and vision, in disorders caused by Vata, Pitta and blood and also in healthy persons.

Materials used in Snehana Putapaka:

भूशयप्रसहानूपमेदोमज्जवसामिषैः ॥ १४ ॥
स्नेहनं पयसा पिष्टैर्जीवनीयैश्च कल्पयेत् ।

The snehana putapaka therapy is done by making use of the below mentioned materials –

fat, bone marrow, muscle fat and juice of the meat of animals living in burrows, which bite and cut their foods and those which live in marshy lands or herbs of Jivaneeya group of herbs macerated with milk.

Materials used in Lekhana Putapaka:

मृगपक्षियकृन्मांसमुक्तायस्ताम्रसैन्धवैः ॥ १५ ॥
स्रोतोजशङ्खफेनालैर्लेखनं मस्तुकल्कितैः ।

Lekhana Putapaka is done by making use of –

Water of curds macerated with paste of – liver and meat of animals and birds, pearls and ash of iron and copper, rock salt, antimony sulfide, ash of conch shell and sea foam and orpiment.

Materials used in Prasadana Putapaka:

मृगपक्षियकृन्मज्जवसान्त्रहृदयामिषैः ॥ १६ ॥
मधुरैः सघृतैः स्तन्यक्षीरपिष्टैः प्रसादनम् ।

Prasadana Putapaka is done by using –

Breast milk or milk of cow macerated with liver, marrow, muscle fat, intestines, heart and meat of animals and birds, herbs having sweet taste and mixed with ghee.

Putapaka Kalpana (Recipe for Putapaka):

बिल्वमात्रं पृथक् पिण्डं मांसभेषजकल्कयोः ॥ १७ ॥ उरुबूकवटाम्भोजपत्रैः स्नेहादिषु क्रमात् ।

वेष्टयित्वा मृदा लिप्तं धवधन्वनगोमयैः ॥ १८ ॥ पचेत् प्रदीप्तैरग्न्याभं पक्वं निष्पीड्य तद्रसम् ।

नेत्रे तर्पणवद्युञ्ज्यात्

The meat of animals and paste of medicinal herbs should be separately made into balls of the size equal to that of a bael fruit each (48 grams). These balls should be wrapped in leaves of castor plant, banyan and amboja (lotus species) and smeared with fats in that order and given a coating of mud, (when the coating gets dried), the balls should be cooked in the intense fire of wood of Dhava (Anogeissus latifolia) or Dhanvana (Grewia tiliaefolia) or dried cow dung cakes (until the balls become red hot).

When the herbs (balls in the bolus) are cooked, they are taken out and their juice extracted from them. This juice should be used for treating the eyes just as explained in Tarpana procedure.

Time duration for Putapaka – Matra Kala:

शतं द्वे त्रीणि धारयेत्॥१९॥

लेखन स्नेहन अन्त्येषु

For lekhana and snehana Putapaka, the medicine should be retained for a time period of 200-300 matra kala.

In case of the last one i.e., prasadana putapaka, it should be retained for a time period of 300 matra kala.

Temperature of the medicines used in Putapaka:

कोष्णौ पूर्वौ हिमोऽपरः ।

The juice used in Putapaka should be lukewarm in case of lekhana and snehana Putapakas, whereas it should be used cold in prasadana Putapaka.

Use of Dhumapana in Putapaka:

धूमपोऽन्ते तयोरेव

Dhumapana is indicated in the same two forms i.e., snehana and lekhana types of Putapaka, at the end of the treatment.

Signs of samyak yoga, ati yoga and ayoga of putapaka (properly, excessively and inadequately done Putapaka):

योगास्तत्र च तृप्तिवत् ॥ २० ॥

The signs of properly, excessively and inadequately done putapaka are similar to those of Tarpana.

Contraindication of Tarpana and Putapaka:

तर्पणं पुटपाकं च नस्यानर्हे न योजयेत् ।

Both Tarpana and Putapaka should not be administered to those who are unfit for undergoing nasya (nasal medication therapy).

Pathya during Tarpana and Putapaka (Healthy foods and activities):

यावन्त्यहानि युञ्जीत दिवस्ततो हितभाग्भवेत् ॥ २१ ॥

मालतीमल्लिकापुष्पैर्बद्धाक्षो निवसेन्निशाम् ॥ २१ab॥

The healthy foods and activities should be followed for twice the number of days as those needed to conduct Tarpana or Putapaka treatment during nights, he should bind the eyes with a pad of flowers of malati and mallika (jasmine varieties).

Need for protecting and strengthening the eyes:

सर्वात्मना नेत्रबलाय यत्नं कुर्वीत नस्याञ्जनतर्पणाद्यैः ।
दृष्टिश्च नष्टा विविधं जगच्च तमोमयं जायत एकरूपम् ॥ २२a ॥

All our efforts should be done with heart to strengthen the eyes by following nasal medications (errhines), collyrium (eye salve), Tarpana and Putapaka eye therapies etc. Once the vision is lost, different things of the world will become alike since everything will appear dark.

इति श्री वैद्यपति सिंहगुप्त सूनु श्रीमद्वाग्भट विरचित अष्टाङ्गहृदयसंहिताया सूत्रस्थाने तर्पणपुटपाकविधिर्नाम चतुर्विंशो अध्यायः ॥२४॥

Thus ends the 24th chapter of Ashtangahridaya Samhita Sutrasthana, named Tarpana Putapaka Vidhim Adhyayam, written by Shrimad Vagbhata, son of Shri Vaidyapati Simhagupta.

25

यन्त्रविधिमध्यायम् (yantravidhim adhyayam)

The 25th chapter of Sutrasthanam of Ashtanga Hridayam is named as Yantra Vidhi Adhyayam. This chapter deals with the detailed procedure of administration of usage of blunt instruments in different conditions.

अथातो यन्त्रविधिमध्यायं व्याख्यास्याम: इति ह स्माहुरात्रेयादयो महर्षय:॥

Atreya and other sages pledge that henceforth they will be explaining the chapter named Yantra vidhim adhyaya.

Definition of Yantra (the blunt instruments):

नानाविधानां शल्यानां नानादेशप्रबोधिनाम् । आहर्तुमभ्युपायो यस्तद्यन्त्रं यच्च दर्शने ॥ १ ॥

अर्शोभिगन्दरादीनां शस्त्रक्षाराग्निनियोजने । शेषाङ्गपरिरक्षायां तथा वस्त्यादिकर्मणि ॥ २ ॥

घटिकालाबुशृङ्गं च जाम्बवौष्ठादिकानि च ।

The equipments used to extract different types of foreign bodies causing pain or discomfort in different parts of the body,

to look into pile masses (hemorrhoids), anal and rectal fistulae etc.

to apply sharp instruments, alkalis (cauterization by applying alkalis), and fire (cauterization by applying heat of fire),

to protect the remaining parts of the body other than the diseased parts in therapies / treatments like medicated enema etc.

and the pot (used as instrument), ground horn of animals (used as instruments), cylindrical smooth stones etc. – All these are known as yantra i.e., blunt surgical instruments.

Need for designing instruments:

अनेकरूपकार्याणि यन्त्राणि विविधान्यतः ॥ ३ ॥ विकल्प्य कल्पयेत् बुद्ध्या

The instruments are of different shapes, utilized in different functions, and of several kinds, hence they are to be designed and to be prepared with utmost intelligence.

Note - Instruments having different shapes and types are to be designed as per need so that they would be utilized in many functions.

Explanation of various instruments:

यथास्थूलं तु वक्ष्यते ।

तुल्यानि कङ्कसिंहर्क्षकाकादिमृगपक्षिणाम् ॥ ४ ॥

मुखैर्मुखानि यन्त्राणां कुर्यात् तत्सञ्ज्ञकानि च ।

The instruments shall be described grossly.

Those instruments which have their mouths resembling the mouths of heron, lion, bear, crow and other animals and birds shall be designed and prepared bearing the respective names of those animals and birds.

Swastika Yantra (Cruciform instruments):

अष्टादशाङ्गुलायामान्यायसानि च भूरिशः ॥ ५ ॥ मसूराकारपर्यन्तैः कण्ठे बद्धानि कीलकैः
।

विद्यात् स्वस्तिकयन्त्राणि मूलेऽङ्कुशनतानि च ॥ ६ ॥ तैर्दृढैरस्थिसंलग्नशल्याहरणमिष्यते ।

Swastika Yantras generally should be of 18 angulas (1 angula = 1 finger breadth) in length, made of iron, have shape resembling that of a lentil cotyledon at its edges, held together by a rivet bolt at their neck, slightly bent like an elephant goad at its handle. They are utilized in pulling out the foreign bodies stuck hard in the bones.

Samdamsha / Sandamsha Yantra (Forceps instruments):

कीलबद्धविमुक्ताग्रौ सन्दंशौ षोडशाङ्गुलौ ॥ ७ ॥

त्वक्सिरास्नायुपिशितलग्नशल्यापकर्षणौ ।

षडङ्गुलोऽन्यो हरणे सूक्ष्मशल्योपपक्ष्मणाम् ॥ ८ ॥

Sandamsha yantra, which is of two types, one type of forceps is with a catch at its tip and the other type is without a catch at its tip. The forceps with a catch is 16 angulas (finger breadth) in length, it is used for extracting foreign bodies which are stuck in the skin, veins, tendons and muscles.

The forceps without a catch is 6 angulas in length and it is useful for extracting small foreign bodies and eyelashes.

Muchundi (Forceps with teeth):

मुचुण्डी सूक्ष्मदन्तर्जुर्मूले रुचकभूषणा । गम्भीरव्रणमांसानामर्मणः शेषितस्य च ॥ ९ ॥

Forceps with teeth i.e., Muchundi yantra has small teeth,

straight, with tooth catch, hook at its root. Useful for extracting the fleshy parts from the deep-rooted wounds and remnants from the pterygium (disease of the eye), which has been cut.

Tala Yantra (Instruments with flat arms):

द्वे द्वादशाङ्गुले मत्स्यतालवत् द्व्येकतालके । तालयन्त्रे स्मृते कर्णनाडीशल्यापहारिणी ॥ १० ॥

The instrument which is of 12 angulas and is of two types (of same dimension),

One with 2 flat discs at its mouth and the other with 1 flat disc at its mouth, which resembles the palate of a fish is called Tala yantra i.e., instruments with flat arms, both types are useful for removing foreign bodies from the orifice of the ear.

Nadi Yantra (Tubular instruments - probes):

नाडीयन्त्राणि सुषिराणि एकानेकमुखानि च । स्रोतोगतानां शल्यानां आमयानां च दर्शने ॥ ११ ॥

क्रियाणां सुकरत्वाय कुर्यादाचूषणाय च । तद्विस्तारपरीणाहदैर्घ्यं स्रोतोऽनुरोधतः ॥ १२ ॥

Nadi yantras, i.e., the tubular instruments are hollow with one or more openings, for looking, recognizing and diagnosing the foreign bodies and diseases located in the channels of the body, for carrying out the treatment procedures in a comfortable way, for sucking out the unwanted things and fluids from the channels. The width, circumference (perimeter) etc. vary according to the size and shape etc. of the channels (into which they are inserted).

Nadi Yantra (Tubular instruments) measurement:

दशाङ्गुलार्धनाहान्तःकण्ठशल्यावलोकिनी । नाडी

The tubular instruments meant for seeing inside the throat

is of 10 angulas (finger breadth) in length and half angula in diameter (thickness).

Sangrahini Nadi (Tubular instruments for holding the handles)

पञ्चमुखच्छिद्रा चतुष्कर्णस्य सङ्ग्रहे ॥ १३ ॥
वारङ्गस्य द्विकर्णस्य त्रिच्छिद्रा तत्प्रमाणतः ।
वारङ्गकर्णसंस्थानानाहदैर्घ्यानुरोधतः ॥ १४ ॥

To hold the four eared handle or bolt / wedge / arrow, the tubular instruments with five openings and five orifices may be used.

To hold the two eared handle / bolt / arrow , the tubular instruments having three orifices and dimensions in accordance to the handle / bolt which it holds should be used.

Depending on the shape, thickness and length of the handle of the arrow etc. or bolt, the tubular instruments should be designed so as to grip them.

These instruments were used to hold the arrow etc. weapons which had pierced the body, to grip them and remove them.

Designing various instruments depending on the dimensions of parts to be observed:

नाडीरेवंविधाश्चान्या द्रष्टुं शल्यानि कारयेत् ।

Many similar types of tubular instruments may be prepared
to observe the foreign bodies located in other organs / channels of the body.

Nirghatini Yantra (Instrument to remove foreign body):

पद्मकर्णिकया मूर्ध्नि सदृशी द्वादशाङ्गुला ॥ १५ ॥
चतुर्थसुषिरा नाडी शल्यनिर्घातिनी मता ।

The tubular instrument resembling padma karnika (the round, flat, central portion of the lotus, studded with small holes) at its top, 12 angulas (finger breadth) in length, having a hollow portion in its one fourth length, is called shalya nirghatini yantra because it is useful for catching and removing the foreign bodies.

Arsho Yantra (Proctoscope):

अर्शसां गोस्तनाकारं यन्त्रकं चतुरङ्गुलम् ॥ १६ ॥ नाहे पञ्चाङ्गुलं पुंसां प्रमदानां षडङ्गुलम् ।
द्विच्छिद्रं दर्शने व्याधेरेकच्छिद्रं तु कर्मणि ॥ १७ ॥ मध्येऽस्य त्र्यङ्गुलं छिद्रं अङ्गुष्ठोदरविस्तृतम् ।

अर्धाङ्गुलोच्छ्रितोद्वृत्तकर्णिकं च तदूर्ध्वतः ॥ १८ ॥

The arshoyantra is of the shape of udder of a cow (cylindrical), is of four finger breadth in length and 5 finger breadth in circumference (thickness) for men, 6 finger breadth circumference for women (length being the same) with two orifices for the purpose of visualizing the pile masses, with one orifice for conducting (surgical, cauterization etc.) procedures, right at the center of it there is a slit / orifice of 3 finger breadth length. And with a width equivalent to the middle portion of a thumb, half angula above the slit / orifice there is a karnika i.e. rim of the instrument.

Shami Yantra (Instrument to squeeze / compress the pile mass) (variant of proctoscope):

शम्याख्यं तादृगच्छिद्रं यन्त्रं अर्शःप्रपीडनम् ।

The instrument known as Shami yantra is similar to the above instrument (arsho yantra), but is devoid of orifices. It is used for squeezing / compressing the pile masses.

Bhagandara yantra (Instrument to see and operate fistula in ano):

सर्वथापनयेदोष्ठं छिद्रादूर्ध्वं भगन्दरे ॥ १९ ॥

In Bhagandara yantra, the rim / edge above the slit should always be removed (in proctoscope, if the brim present half finger breadth above the slit is removed, it becomes a fistula instrument).

Tubular instruments used to see nasal polyps, piles etc.:

घ्राणार्बुदार्शसामेकच्छिद्रा नाड्यङ्गुलद्वया ।

प्रदेशिनीपरीणाहा स्यात् भगन्दरयन्त्रवत् ॥ २० ॥

The tubular instruments to see nasal polyps and pile-like masses developing in the nose, shall have only one orifice, two angulas (finger breadth) in length, of the thickness equivalent to that of index finger and resembles instrument designed for rectal fistula.

Anguli Tranaka Yantra (Finger protector):

अङ्गुलीत्राणकं दान्तं वार्क्षं वा चतुरङ्गुलम् ।

द्विच्छिद्रं गोस्तनाकारं तद्वक्त्रविवृतौ सुखम् ॥ २१ ॥

The Anguli Tranaka Yantra is made up of ivory or wood, is of 4 angulas (finger breadth) in length, has two orifices, and is of the shape of cow udder. It helps in dilating the mouth easily (while protecting the finger from contact with teeth and consequent injury).

Yoni Vrana Vikshana Yantra (Instrument to look into wounds in vagina):
योनिव्रणेक्षणं मध्ये सुषिरं षोडशाङ्गुलम् । मुद्राबद्धं चतुर्भित्तं अम्भोजमुकुलाननम् ॥ २२ ॥
चतुःशलाकं आक्रान्तं मूले तद्विकसेन्मुखे ।
The instrument used to look into the vagina and wounds (or wounds in vagina) shall be hollow in the middle (of the instrument), 16 angulas in length, with four flaps held tightly in position by a ring, resembling the bud of a lotus flower in shape, fixed with four rods at its root (where the instrument is held to handle) and its mouth opened like that of a flower bud.

Instrument to oil the sinuses and to wash them:
यन्त्रे नाडीव्रणाभ्यङ्गक्षालनाय षडङ्गुले ॥ २३ ॥ वस्तियन्त्राकृती मूले मुखेऽङ्गुष्ठकलायखे
।
अग्रतोऽकर्णिके मूले निबद्धमृदुचर्मणी ॥ २४ ॥
Two instruments, one for oiling the sinus ulcer and the other one for washing the sinus ulcer are both 6 finger breadth (angula) in length. Its shape resembles the nozzle of an enema apparatus with an orifice at its root allowing the entry of the thumb, and another orifice at its tip allowing the entry of a round pea, without any edge / rim at its tip and fixed with a soft leather bag at its root.

Dakodara Yantra (Instrument for ascites):
द्विद्वारा नलिका पिच्छनलिका वोदकोदरे ।
The Dakodara Yantra shall have two orifices, one at each end, alternatively the tube of a peacock feather can be used.

Dhumayantra (netra) / vastiyantra (Instruments for medicated smoking, enema etc.):
धूमवस्त्यादियन्त्राणि निर्दिष्टानि यथायथम् ॥ २५ ॥
The tubular instruments used in medicated smoking, enema etc. therapies are explained in the related contexts.

Animal Horn as an instrument:
त्र्यङ्गुलास्यं भवेच्छृङ्गं चूषणेऽष्टादशाङ्गुलम् ।
अग्रे सिद्धार्थकच्छिद्रं सुनद्धं चूचुकाकृति ॥ २६ ॥
The animal horn used for sucking (liquids) will be of 18 angulas in length,

having orifice of 3 finger breadth at its root and orifice of the size of mustard seed at the tip, is properly bound. The tip resembles the shape of a nipple.

Alabu yantra (The hollowed gourd as an instrument):

स्याद्द्वादशाङ्गुलोऽलाबुर्नाहे त्वष्टादशाङ्गुलः ।
चतुस्त्र्यङ्गुलवृत्तास्यो दीप्तोऽन्तः श्लेष्मरक्तहृत् ॥ २७ ॥

The hollowed gourd will be 12 angulas (1 angula = 1 finger breadth) in length, 18 angulas in diameter, with a round orifice of 4 angulas or 3 angulas. In which a burning wick placed in its interior (vacuum is created) is used for extraction of vitiated kapha and blood.

Ghati Yantra (Pot as an instrument):

तद्वत् घटी हिता गुल्मविलयोन्नमने च सा ।

Pot is also similar (to hollowed gourd) and is useful in making the abdominal tumors soft and elevate it to the surface from its low level.

Shalaka Yantra (Rod shaped instruments):

शलाकाख्यानि यन्त्राणि नानाकर्मांकृतीनि च ॥ २८ ॥ यथायोगप्रमाणानि

Rod like instruments serve many functions and have various shapes and sizes suitable to the purpose for which they are used.

Gandupadamukha Shalaka Yantra (Probing rod like instruments):

तेषां एषणकर्मणी । उभे गण्डूपदमुखे

Among them (rod like instruments), two are for probing. Both these instruments have their mouth resembling that of an earthworm.

Masuradala vaktra Shalaka Yantra (Rod like instruments having lentil like mouth):

स्रोतोभ्यः शल्यहारिणी ॥ २९ ॥ मसूरदलवक्त्रे द्वे स्यातां अष्टनवाङ्गुले ।

Two of those rod like instruments having lentil shaped mouths are used for removing the foreign bodies from the channels. One is 8 angulas and the other is 9 angulas in length.

Shanku Yantra (Number of hook like instruments):

शङ्कवः षड्

The hook-like instruments are six in number.

Ahiphana vaktra shanku (Hooks resembling the shape of serpent):

उभौ तेषां षोडशद्वादशाङ्गुलौ ॥ ३० ॥ व्यूहनेऽहिफणावक्त्रौ

Two (hook instruments) among them, one of 16 angulas and the other 12 angulas in length. Their mouths, resembling the hood of the serpent, are used for joining (the edges of the wound etc).

Sharapunkhasya shanku (Hooks resembling the shape of arrow bottom):

द्वौ दशद्वादशाङ्गुलौ । चालने शरपुङ्खास्यौ

Two more (hook like instruments), one of 10 and the other of 12 angula length, having their mouth resembling the bottom of the arrow, are used for loosening the hard objects (which are to be removed or extracted).

Badisha shanku yantr (Hooks used for extraction):

आहार्ये बडिशाकृती ॥ ३१ ॥

The hooks used for extraction resemble the shape / size of a fish hook.

Garbha Shanku (Hook instrument resembling conch):

नतोऽग्रे शङ्कुना तुल्यो गर्भशङ्कुरिति स्मृतः ।
अष्टाङ्गुलायतस्तेन मूढगर्भं हरेत् स्त्रियाः ॥ ३२ ॥

The hook instrument resembling a conch is called Garbha shanku and is bent at its tip, is 8 angulis in length. Using it, the impacted fetus is pulled out in women.

Sarpaphanakhya (Instrument for extracting urinary stones):

अश्मर्याहरणं सर्पफणावत् वक्रमग्रतः ।

The instrument meant for extracting the stones from the urinary bladder, will have the shape of the hood of a snake, bent inwards at the tip.

Instruments for extracting tooth and clearing sinuses:

शरपुङ्खमुखं दन्तपातनं चतुरङ्गुलम् ॥ ३३ ॥
कार्पासविहितोष्णीषाः शलाकाः षट् प्रमार्जने ।

Instrument used for extracting the tooth will have the shape of base of an arrow and is of 4 angulas in length. The 6 rod like instruments meant for clearing and cleansing sinuses etc. should have their tip covered with a cap of cotton wool.

Payu Pramarjini Shalaka (Instruments for manipulating rectum):

पायावासन्नदूरार्थं द्वे दशद्वादशाङ्गुले ॥ ३४ ॥

Two other rod like instruments, one of 10 angulas and the other one of 12 angula length are used for drawing the rectum closer and extending it farther respectively.

Instruments for nose and ears:

द्वे षट्सप्ताङ्गुले घ्राणे द्वे कर्णेऽष्टनवाङ्गुले ।

Two other instruments of 6 and 7 angulas length each are meant to be used in the nose

द्वे कर्णे अष्ट नव अङ्गुले

Two similar instruments are used in the ears, one of 8 and the other of 9 angula length.

Instruments for cleaning the ears:

कर्णशोधनं अश्वत्थपत्रप्रान्तं सुवाननम् ॥ ३५ ॥

The instrument meant for clearing the ears will have its edges resembling the leaf of Ashvattha tree (Sacred Fig) and its face resembling a ladle.

Jambavoushta (Cylindrical smooth stones):

शलाकाजाम्बवौष्ठानां क्षारेऽग्नौ च पृथक् त्रयम् । युञ्ज्यात् स्थूलाणुदीर्घाणां

The rod like instruments known as Jambavaushtha i.e. cylindrical smooth stones are each three in number, thick, thin and long in shape are used for application of caustic alkalis and fire cauterization therapies.

Rod like instruments used for inguinal hernia:

शलाकां अन्त्रवर्धमनि ॥ ३६ ॥ मध्योर्ध्ववृत्तदण्डां च मूले चार्धेन्दुसन्निभाम् ।

The rod-like instruments used in inguinal hernia, will have a rod which is rounded in the middle and upper portions and has its root shaped like a half moon.

Instrument used for cauterization of nasal polyps:

कोलास्थिदलतुल्यास्या नासार्शोऽबुददाहकृत् ॥ ३७ ॥

The instrument having its mouth resembling the cotyledon of the stone of jujube fruit is used for cauterizing the polyps and tumors of the nose.

Instrument for applying caustic alkali therapy:

अष्टाङ्गुला निम्नमुखास्तिस्रः क्षारौषधक्रमे । कनीनीमध्यमानामीनखमानसमैर्मुखैः ॥ ३८

||

The three instruments for applying caustic alkali shall be eight angulas in length and their mouths bent downwards. Their mouths resemble the nails of the index, middle and ring fingers in size respectively.

Instruments for clearing / cleansing urethra and applying eye salves:

स्वं स्वमुक्तानि यन्त्राणि मेढ्रशुद्ध्यञ्जनादिषु ।

The instruments meant for clearing / cleansing the penis (urethra) and for applying collyrium (eye salves) are explained in the related contexts (chapters) respectively.

Anu Yantrani (Accessory Instruments):

अनुयन्त्राण्ययस्कान्तरज्जूवस्त्राश्ममुद्गराः ॥ ३९ ॥ वध्रान्त्रजिह्वावालाश्च शाखानखमुखद्विजाः ।

कालः पाकः करः पादो भयं हर्षश्च तत्क्रियाः ॥ ४० ॥

उपायवित् प्रविभजेदालोच्य निपुणं धिया ॥ ४०a ॥

The accessory instruments are –

ayaskanta – magnet

rajju – rope

vastra – cloth

ashma – stone

mudgara - hammer

vadhra – leather strap

antra – intestines of the animals

jihva – tongue

bala – and hairs

shakha – branches of trees

nakha – nails

mukha – mouth

dvija - teeth

kala - time

paka - digestion

kara - hands

pada – feet

bhaya - fear

harsha – pleasure

A skillful and intelligent physician should use them judiciously based on the assessment of the disease and the patient.

Different functions of the instruments:

निर्घातनोन्मथनपूरणमार्गशुद्धिसंव्यूहनाहरणबन्धनपीडनानि ।
आचूषणोन्नमननामनचालभङ्गव्यावर्तनर्जुकरणानि च यन्त्रकर्म ॥ ४१a ॥

The functions of the blunt instruments are as below mentioned –

nirghatana – pulling out something after crushing it

unmathana – pulling out something after twisting it

poorana – filling

margashuddhi – cleansing the passages

samvyoohana – bringing together

aaharana – extraction

bandhana – binding

peedana – rubbing

aachooshana – sucking / suction

unnamana – lifting up

naamana – pushing down / bending down

chaala – moving / shaking something

bhanga – breaking something

vyaavartana – over-turning

rujukarana – and straightening etc.

Appraisal of Kankamukha instrument:

विवर्तते साध्ववगाहते च ग्राह्यं गृहीत्वोद्धरते च यस्मात् ।
यन्त्रेष्वतः कङ्कमुखं प्रधानं स्थानेषु सर्वेष्वधिकारि यच्च ॥ ४२b ॥

It can be twisted easily, dipped deep, can be held firmly, catches the objects firmly and removes them, and is the authority in all places. Therefore, among all the blunt instruments, the Kankamukha instrument is considered as the best.

इति श्री वैद्यपति सिंहगुप्त सूनु श्रीमत् वाग्भट विरचितायां अष्टाङ्गहृदयसंहितायां सूत्रस्थाने यन्त्रविधिर्नाम पञ्चविंशतितमो अध्यायः॥२५॥

Thus ends the 25th chapter of Ashtangahridaya Samhita Sutrasthana, named Yantra Vidhim Adhyayam, written by Shrimad Vagbhata, son of Shri Vaidyapati Simhagupta.

26

शस्त्रविधिमध्यायम् (shastravidhim adhyayam)

The 26th chapter of Sutrasthanam of Ashtanga Hridayam is named as Shastra Vidhi Adhyayam. This chapter deals with the detailed procedure of administration of usage of sharp instruments in different conditions.

अथातो शस्त्रविधिमध्यायं व्याख्यास्याम: इति ह स्माहुरात्रेयादयो महर्षय:॥

Atreya and other sages pledge that henceforth they will be explaining the chapter named Shastra vidhim adhyaya.

Features of Shastra (Sharp Instruments):

षड्विंशतिः सुकर्मारैर्घटितानि यथाविधि । शस्त्राणि रोमवाहीनि बाहुल्येनाङ्गुलानि षट् ॥ १ ॥

सुरूपाणि सुधाराणि सुग्रहाणि च कारयेत् । अकरालानि सुध्मातसुतीक्ष्णावर्तितेऽयसि ॥ २ ॥

समाहितमुखाग्राणि नीलाम्भोजच्छवीनि च । नामानुगतरूपाणि सदा सन्निहितानि च ॥ ३ ॥

स्वोन्मानार्धचतुर्थांशफलान्येकैकशोऽपि च । प्रायो द्विवत्राणि युञ्जीत तानि स्थानविशेषतः ॥ ४ ॥

मण्डलाग्रं वृद्धिपत्रमुत्पलाध्यर्धधारके । सर्पैषण्यौ वेतसाख्यं शरार्यास्यत्रिकूर्चके ॥ ४+(१) ॥

कुशास्यं साटवदनमन्तर्वक्त्रार्धचन्द्रके । व्रीहिमुखं कुठारी च शलाकाङ्गुलिशस्त्रके ॥ ४+(२) ॥

बडिशं करपत्राख्यं कर्तरी नखशस्त्रकम् । दन्तलेखनकं सूच्यः कूर्चा नाम खजाह्वयम् ॥ ४+(३) ॥

आरा चतुर्विधाकारा तथा स्यात्कर्णवेधनी ॥ ४+(४) ॥

Generally, the sharp instruments are 6 angulas (finger breadth) in length. They are 26 in number. The ideal sharp instruments should be prepared by skilled metal smiths following traditional methods of preparing sharp instruments.

They should be capable of cutting/shaving hairs (including body hair). They should be prepared in a way that they are good looking, have well defined sharp edges and can be held firmly. They should be prepared from metals like iron which have been well blown (to remove impurities from the metal), stirred well and shaped into sharpness.

They (finished products) should not be ugly in appearance and shape. The finished front portion i.e., blade of the instrument (edges of the instrument, hammered well and made sharp) should have the color blue variety of lotus, with shape in accordance to their names and always available at hand (accessible), ready to be used.

The cutting blades of these sharp instruments should be $1/4^{th}$ of half of their own size (total length) i.e. $1/8^{th}$ of the instrument.

Generally, each of these instruments, two or three in number should be made (as back up) and should be made use of in surgical methods as suitable to the site of operation.

Name of the instruments –
mandalagra, vriddhipatra, utpala, ardha dharaka, sarpa, eshani, vetasakhya
sharari, trikoorchajka, kusha, satavadana, antarvaktra, ardhachandraka
vreehimukha, kuthari, shalaka, angulishastraka, badisha
kharapatra, kartari, nakshashastraka, dantalekhanaka, soochi
koorcha, khajahvaya, four types of aara and the last one is karnavedhini.

Mandalagra Shastra (Round edged knife):
मण्डलाग्रं फले तेषां तर्जन्यन्तर्नखाकृति । लेखने छेदने योज्यं पोथकीशुण्डिकादिषु ॥ ५ ॥
Among these shastras, the knife with a round edge, at its tip, has its blade resembling the shape of the nail of the index finger.

It is used for scraping and excision in diseases like cyst in the eyelid/ trachoma, tonsils etc.

Vridhipatra Shastra (Scalpel):
वृद्दिधपत्रं क्षुराकारं छेदभेदनपाटने । ऋज्वग्रमुन्नते शोफे गम्भीरे च तदन्यथा ॥ ६ ॥
नताग्रं पृष्ठतो दीर्घह्रस्ववक्त्रं यथाश्रयम् ।
Vridhipatra Shastra is shaped like a razor,
and is useful for excision, incision and for tearing (separating).
The one with a straight pointed edge is meant for use in elevated (bulging) swellings.
The same instrument (another form of scalpel) with its tip bent backwards is meant for use in deep seated swellings. It bears long or short edge (long bladed or short bladed) depending on the dimension of the swelling (part of the body) it is put into use

Utpalapatra & Ardhadhara Shastra (Lancets):
उत्पलाध्यर्धधाराख्ये भेदने छेदने तथा ॥ ७ ॥
Utpalapatra & Ardhadhara Shastra are used for the purpose of splitting and cutting (excision).

Sarpasya/Sarpamukha Shastra (hooked knife):
सर्पास्यं घ्राणकर्णार्शश्छेदनेऽर्धाङ्गुलं फले ।
The instrument whose blade is of the shape of a snake hoodie, Serpent bladed scalpel or a hooked knife is used for excising polyps in the nose and ears and has an edge of half angula.

Eshani (probes):
गतेरन्वेषणे श्लक्ष्णा गण्डूपदमुखैषणी ॥ ८ ॥ भेदनार्थेऽपरा सूचीमुखा मूलनिविष्टखा ।
The probe shaped like the mouth of an earthworm is smooth and meant for exploring sinuses. Another kind of probe is meant for splitting, has blade like a needle, with a slit hole at its root

Vetasapatra (probes):
वेतसं व्यधने
The instrument with a pointed end like a bamboo leaf (scalpel) is used for puncturing.

Shararimukhi and Trikurchaka (scissors pointed like heron's beak and three toothed brush):
स्राव्ये शरार्यास्यत्रिकूर्चके ॥ ९ ॥

Shararimukhi shastra and trikurchika (instrument looking like a three toothed brush) are meant for draining out fluids.

Kushapatra and Atimukha Shastra – scissors pointed like heron's beak and three toothed brush:

कुशाटावदने स्राव्ये द्व्यङ्गुलं स्यात्तयोः फलम् ।

Kushapatra i.e., razor resembling the blade of kusha grass (Graef's cataract knife) & aateevadana/aatavadana razor resembling the beak of aati bird i.e., hawk – lancet, are meant for draining. Their edges measure 2 angulas in length

Antarmukha Shastra (half moon shaped draining instrument):

तद्वदन्तर्मुखं तस्य फलमध्यर्धमङ्गुलम् ॥ १० ॥ अर्धचन्द्राननं चैतत्

Similar to those (kushapatra and atimukha shastras) is antarmukha instrument, used for draining fluids. Its blades measure ½ angula and have a half moon shape.

Vrihimukha Shastra (trocar):

तथाध्यर्धाङ्गुलं फले । व्रीहिवक्त्रं प्रयोज्यं च तत् शिरोदरयोर्व्यधे ॥ ११ ॥

The instrument with the blade resembling a grain of rice (trocar), having its edge of 1.5 angulas is used for puncturing the veins and abdomen

Kuthari Shastra (axe):

पृथुः कुठारी गोदन्तसदृशार्धाङ्गुलानना । तयोर्ध्वदण्डया विध्येदुपर्यस्थनां स्थितां शिराम् ॥ १२ ॥

The Kuthari Shastra is broad and resembles the tooth of a cow in shape. It has an edge of half angula length and bears a wooden handle. Using this, the vein situated on the bones should be cut keeping the handle of this axe vertically over it.

Shalaka (rod for piercing the lens in cataract):

ताम्री शलाका द्विमुखी मुखे कुरुबकाकृतिः । लिङ्गनाशं तया विध्येत्

The rod, made up of copper, bears two edges on either side, having the shape of the bud of kurubaka. It is meant for piercing the lens in linganasha (cataract)

Anguli Shastra (finger knife/ring scalpel):

कुर्यादङ्गुलिशस्त्रकम् ॥ १३ ॥ मुद्रिकानिर्गतमुखं फले त्वर्धाङ्गुलायतम् ।
योगतो वृद्धिपत्रेण मण्डलाग्रेण वा समम् ॥ १४ ॥ तत् प्रदेशिन्यग्रपर्वप्रमाणार्पणमुद्रिकम् ।
सूत्रबद्धं गलस्रोतोरोगच्छेदनभेदने ॥ १५ ॥

The Anguli Shastra should be prepared in such a way that it should bear a ring which can be fit on the finger (the ring of the instrument shall be worn on the index finger by the surgeon, he need not hold the instrument). Its blade is half angula in width. The instrument resembles either vriddhipatra i.e., scalpel or mandalagra shastra i.e., round edged knife. The ring of the instrument should be capable of permitting the entry of the first phalanx of the index finger. It is tied with a thread (to the wrist, to keep it in position, such that the instrument doesn't get dislodged during the process of operation) and is used for excision and splitting of the diseases parts in the diseases afflicting the passages of the throat.

Badisha (sharp hook):

ग्रहणे शुण्डिकार्मादेर्बडिशं सुनताननम् ।

Badisha is a sharp hook with a bent blade that is meant for holding enlarged uvula, pterygium etc.

Karapatra (saw):

छेदेऽस्थ्नां करपत्रं तु खरधारं दशाङ्गुलम् ॥ १६ ॥ विस्तारे द्व्यङ्गुलं सूक्ष्मदन्तं
सुत्सरुबन्धनम् ।

Karapatra is used for cutting the bones, and has rough and strong edge. It is of 10 angulas in length and 2 angulas in width and has fine-sharp, small teeth (serrated edge), and a handle to be held tight in position with the fist.

Kartari (scissors):

स्नायुसूत्रकचच्छेदे कर्तरी कर्तरीनिभा ॥ १७ ॥

Kartari i.e., Scissor is an instrument used to cut tendons, threads, hairs etc. It resembles scissors used by a common man

Nakha shastra (nail cutter/nail chip):

वक्रर्जुधारं द्विमुखं नखशस्त्रं नवाङ्गुलम् । सूक्ष्मशल्योद्धृतिच्छेदभेदप्रच्छानलेखने ॥ १८
॥

The Nakha shastra has either curved or straight edges (one edge is curved and the other edge is straight), and is two bladed. It is of 9 angulas in length. And it is used for removing small foreign bodies, excision, incision, splitting and scraping procedures.

Danta lekhana (dental lancet):

एकधारं चतुष्कोणं प्रबद्धाकृति चैकतः । दन्तलेखनकं तेन शोधयेद्दन्तशर्कराम् ॥ १९ ॥

The Danta lekhana has a single edge, four angles, and has knotted shape at one end. Using this instrument one should cleanse/scrape the tartar on the teeth.

Soochi (needles):

वृत्ता गूढदृढाः पाशे तिस्रः सूच्योऽत्र सीवने । मांसलानां प्रदेशानां त्र्यस्रा त्र्यङ्गुलमायता ॥ २० ॥

अल्पमांसास्थिसन्धिस्थव्रणानां द्व्यङ्गुलायता । व्रीहिवक्त्रा धनुर्वक्रा पक्वामाशयमर्मसु ॥ २१ ॥

सा सार्धद्व्यङ्गुला

Soochis used for suturing are of three types. They are –
One which is round, strong and stable, has a pass-through hole in their body near the root of the instrument and it is meant for use in fleshy parts, having three edges and length of three angulas (finger breadth).
And the other one for use in less muscular parts, bony joints and wounds on joints, with a length of 2 angulas.
The vrihi vaktra/vrihi mukha suchi i.e., curved needle is bent like a bow. It is used for suturing the intestines, stomach and vital parts of the body and measures 2 and half angulas in length.

Koorcha (brush):

सर्ववृत्तास्ताश्चतुरङ्गुलाः । कूर्चो वृत्तैकपीठस्थाः सप्ताष्टौ वा सुबन्धनाः ॥ २२ ॥
स योज्यो नीलिकाव्यङ्गकेशशातेषु कुट्टने ।

The same soochis when have rounded spikes (ends) and are fixed on one end of a rounded base, 7-8 in number and fastened well on the base are called as koorcha i.e., brush like instrument, each rounded spike fixed to the base is of 4 angulas length. It is used for scraping in blue patches, dark patches and loss of hairs etc.

Khaja (churner):

अर्धाङ्गुलमुखैर्वृत्तैरष्टाभिः कण्टकैः खजः ॥ २३ ॥ पाणिभ्यां मथ्यमानेन घ्राणातेन हरेदसृक्
।

The Khaja has blade of half angula length. It is round in shape and has eight spikes fixed in it. They are used for removing vitiated blood from the nose by churning with the hands

Karnapali Vyadhana (instrument for puncturing the ear lobe):

व्यधनं कर्णपालीनां यूथिकामुकुलाननम् ॥ २४ ॥

The Karnapali Vyadhana or instrument meant for puncturing the ear lobe should have its blade in the shape of a jasmine bud.

Ara (awl/cobbler's knife/shoemaker's knife):

आराधाङ्गुलवृत्तास्या तत्प्रवेशा तथोर्ध्वतः ।

चतुरस्रा तया विध्येच्छोफं पक्वामसंशये ॥ २५ ॥

कर्णपालीं च बहलां बहलायाश्च शस्यते ।

सूची त्रिभागसुषिरा त्र्यङ्गुला कर्णवेधनी ॥ २६ ॥

The Ara has a rounded blade of half angula below and four blades/edges above. Using this, one should puncture swellings when there is doubt whether the swelling is ripe or unripe and also to puncture the earlobe which is thick. In the case of thick earlobes, a ear piercing needle, hollow in three parts of it and of three angulas in length is best.

Anushastra (accessory instruments):

जलौकःक्षारदहनकाचोपलनखादयः । अलौहान्यनुशस्त्राणि तान्येवं च विकल्पयेत् ॥ २७ ॥

अपराण्यपि यन्त्रादीन्युपयोगं च यौगिकम् ।

The Anushastra or accessory instruments are -

jalauka – leeches,

kshara - caustic alkalis,

dahana – fire,

kacha – glass,

upala - cow dung cake,

nakha - nail etc. instruments which are non metallic (but can be used as instruments). The same shall be used in many procedures. Many other (similar) instruments may also be designed as needed for use in special operations and sites

Shastra karya (functions of sharp instruments):

उत्पाट्यपाट्यसीव्यैष्यलेख्यप्रच्छानकुट्टनम् ॥ २८ ॥ छेद्यं भेद्यं व्यधो मन्थो ग्रहो दाहश्च तत्क्रियाः

The functions shastra (of the sharp instruments) are as below enlisted) –

utpatana – extracting

patana – tearing/splitting

seevana – suturing

eshana – probing

lekhana – scraping

prcchana – scratching/incising/minute puncturing

kuttana – beating, hitting, pounding

chedana - excising/cutting

bhedana - breaking

vyadhasna - puncturing

manthana – churning

grahana – holding/grasping

dahana – burning, cauterization.

Shastra dosha (defects of sharp instruments):

कुण्ठखण्डतनुस्थूलह्रस्वदीर्घत्ववक्रताः ॥ २९ ॥ शस्त्राणां खरधारत्वमष्टौ दोषाः प्रकीर्तिताः ।

kuntha – bluntness

khanda – brokenness

thanu – thinness

sthoola – stoutness

hrisva – smallness/excessively small

deerghatva – lengthiness/excessively long

vakrata - curvedness/crookedness/irregular shape

khara dharatva – rough edge

These are considered to be eight defects of the sharp instruments.

Shastra grahana vidhi (method of holding different sharp instruments)

छेदभेदनलेख्यार्थं शस्त्रं वृन्तफलान्तरे ॥ ३० ॥ तर्जनीमध्यमाङ्गुष्ठैर्गृह्णीयात् सुसमाहितः ।

विस्रावणानि वृन्ताग्रे तर्जन्यङ्गुष्ठकेन च ॥ ३१ ॥ तलप्रच्छन्नवृन्ताग्रं ग्राह्यं व्रीहिमुखं मुखे ।

मूलेष्वाहरणार्थानि क्रियासौकर्यतोऽपरम् ॥ ३२ ॥

For doing cutting (excision), breaking (incision) and scraping, the instrument should be held between the handle and the edge (blade), with the help of index, middle fingers and thumbs, carefully for draining, the instrument shall be held at the tip of the handle, with the help of index finger and the thumb for scratching purpose, the tip of the handle should be held with the palm. Vrihimukha instrument i.e., trocar should be held at its mouth tip for extracting, the instrument shall be held at its root. Other instruments may be held in a convenient manner, as required in the surgical process (operation to be conducted).

Shastra kosha (instrument wallet):

स्यान्नवाङ्गुलविस्तारः सुघनो द्वादशाङ्गुलः । क्षौमपत्रोर्णकौशेयदुकूलमृदुचर्मजः ॥ ३३ ॥
विन्यस्तपाशः सुस्यूतः सान्तरोर्णास्थशस्त्रकः । शलाकापिहितास्यश्च शस्त्रकोशः सुसञ्चयः ॥ ३४ ॥

The Shastra kosha should be 9 angulas in width, 12 angulas in length and very dense (thick). It is made up of linen/silken linen, leaves, wool, silk, inner bark of trees or soft leather. It should be endowed with a net of threads, well stitched, having a compartment for instruments, kept wrapped in wool. Its opening is closed and held tight with a rod acting like a bolt and should be pleasing to look at.

Jalauka (leeches):

जलौकसस्तु सुखिनां रक्तस्रावाय योजयेत् ।

The leeches should be used for letting out blood (bloodletting) in people who live a comfortable life.

Indrayudha and poisonous type of leeches:

दुष्टाम्बुमत्स्यभेकाहिशवकोथमलोद्भवाः ॥ ३५ ॥ रक्ताः श्वेता भृशं कृष्णाश्चपलाः स्थूलपिच्छिलाः ।
इन्द्रायुधविचित्रोर्ध्वराजयो रोमशाश्च ताः ॥ ३६ ॥ सविषा वर्जयेत्

Leeches are born in dirty water contaminated by putrefying dead bodies of fishes, frogs and snakes or by their excreta.
Indrayudha type of leeches are red, white or dark black in color, very active, thick and slimy.
Poisonous leeches are those which have varied lines on their backs and are very hairy. These poisonous varieties of leeches should be rejected.

Effects of using poisonous leeches:

ताभिः कण्डूपाकज्वरभ्रमाः । विषपित्तास्रनुत् कार्यं तत्र

These (poisonous leeches, when used) cause itching, ulceration (suppuration), fever and giddiness. In these conditions treatment should be done by administering medicines which mitigate poison, pitta vitiation and blood vitiation.

Nirvisha jalauka (non-poisonous/safe leeches):

शुद्धाम्बुजाः पुनः ॥ ३७ ॥ निर्विषाः शैवलश्यावा वृत्ता नीलोर्ध्वराजयः ।
कषायपृष्ठास्तन्वङ्ग्यः किञ्चित्पीतोदराश्च याः ॥ ३८ ॥

Again, nirvisha jalaukas (which can be used for bloodletting therapy) are those which are born in clean water, dark as wood of wild Himalayan cherry, round in shape, have blue lines on their back, have hard backs/back resembling the bark of trees, have thin bodies and with slightly yellowish belly.

Conditions for rejecting nirvisha Jalauka:

ता अप्यसम्यग्वमनात् प्रततं च निपातनात् । सीदन्तिः सलिलं प्राप्य रक्तमत्ता इति त्यजेत्
॥ ३९ ॥

Even the nirvisha jalaukas, when they do not completely vomit out the sucked blood, when they fall off frequently and when they are inactive even after getting into the water, should be considered as suffering from blood intoxication and should be rejected.

Jalauka avacharana, upayoga (method of applying leeches, benefits):

अथेतरा निशाकल्कयुक्तेऽम्भसि परिप्लुताः । अवन्तिसोमे तक्रे वा पुनश्चाश्वासिता जले ॥
४० ॥

लागयेद्घृतमृत्स्तन्यरक्तशस्त्रनिपातनैः । पिबन्तीरुन्नतस्कन्धाश्छादयेन्मृदुवाससा ॥
४१ ॥

सम्पृक्ताद्दुष्टशुद्धास्राज्जलौका दुष्टशोणितम् । आदत्ते प्रथमं हंसः क्षीरं क्षीरोदकादिव ॥
४२ ॥

गुल्मार्शोविद्रधीन् कुष्ठवातरक्तगलामयान् । नेत्ररुग्विषवीसर्पान् शमयन्ति जलौकसः ॥
४२+(१) ॥

After examining the jalaukas, the non-poisonous leeches are immersed in the water mixed with paste of turmeric, in fermented grain water or grain washed water or buttermilk.

It should again be made comfortable by putting them in pure water and should be applied to the desired part of the body which has been rubbed/ anointed with ghee, mud, breast milk, blood or by making a wound on that part with a sharp instrument. When the leech starts drinking the blood by raising its shoulders, it should be covered with a soft cloth, thus stuck to the body (after holding to the afflicted part of the body being attracted to ghee, blood etc.). The leech will suck only the vitiated blood first from the mixture of vitiated and pure blood, just like the swan sucks the milk from a mixture of milk and water.

Application of leeches (bloodletting) mitigate diseases such as

gulma - abdominal tumors

arsha - haemorrhoids

vidhradi - abscess

kushtha - skin diseases

vatarakta - gout

galamaya - diseases of the neck

netra ruk - eye pain/eye diseases

visha - affliction of poisons/poisoning

visarpa - herpes etc.

Removal of leech, post leech application care and care of leeches used in the therapy:

दंशस्य तोदे कण्डुवां वा मोक्षयेत् वामयेच्च ताम् । पटुतैलाक्तवदनां श्लक्ष्णकण्डनरूषिताम् ॥ ४३ ॥

रक्षन् रक्तमदाद्भूयः सप्ताहं ता न पातयेत् । पूर्ववत् पटुता दाढर्य सम्यग्वान्ते जलौकसाम् ॥ ४४ ॥

क्लमोऽतियोगान् मृत्युर्वा दुर्वान्ते स्तब्धता मदः । अन्यत्रान्यत्र ताः स्थाप्या घटे मृत्स्नाम्बुगर्भिणि ॥ ४५ ॥

लालादिकोथनाशार्थं सविषाः स्युस्तदन्वयात् । अशुद्धौ स्रावयेद्दंशान् हरिद्रागुडमाक्षिकैः ॥ ४६ ॥

शतधौताज्यपिचवस्ततो लेपाश्च शीतलाः । दुष्टरक्तापगमनात् सद्यो रागरुजां शमः ॥ ४७ ॥

अशुद्धं चलितं स्थानात् स्थितं रक्तं व्रणाशये । व्यम्लीभवेत् पर्युषितं तस्मात् तत् स्रावयेत् पुनः ॥ ४८ ॥

At the site of bite (of leech), when pricking pain or itching develops, the leech should be removed.

After this, the leeches are made to vomit (the blood which they have sucked) by touching their mouth with salt and oil or by gently rubbing the leech in the direction of their mouth (from below upwards) after smearing fine rice flour over their body

After having made the leeches to vomit, they should be protected from blood intoxication and the same leeches should not be used for bloodletting again for the next seven days.

After proper vomiting, the leech regains its previous activities and becomes strong. By too much vomiting, the leeches become very weak or even may die

If vomiting occurs inadequately (improper), the leeches become lazy, inactive and intoxicated.

The leeches should be transferred from one pot to the other, filled with good mud and water.

In order to destroy (avoid) putrefaction by saliva, excreta of leeches, because the leeches become poisonous when they come into contact with these things. When there is a doubt of impurity (improper cleansing), the site of bite should be made to bleed by applying paste of turmeric, jaggery and honey.

Later, a piece of cloth soaked in ghee washed hundred times or coolant pastes prepared from herbs having cold potency should be applied (over the site) with removal of vitiated blood, the redness and pain will immediately subside.

The vitiated blood, displaced from its site and accumulating in the interior of the wounds would become immensely sour due to overnight stagnation, hence it should be expelled out again

Use of gourd (alabu) or pot (ghatika) for bloodletting – contraindications and indications:

युञ्ज्यान्नालाबुघटिका रक्ते पित्तेन दूषिते । तासामनलसंयोगात् युञ्ज्यात् तु कफवायुना ॥ ४९ ॥

A gourd or pot should not be used for removing the blood vitiated by pitta, because they (pitta and blood) are associated with fire. They can be used in case of blood vitiation caused by imbalanced kapha and vata

Use of horn (shringa) for bloodletting – contraindications and indications:

कफेन दुष्टं रुधिरं न शृङ्गेण विनिर्हरेत् । स्कन्नत्वात् वातपित्ताभ्यां दुष्टं शृङ्गेण निर्हरेत् ॥ ५० ॥

The blood vitiated by kapha should not be extracted by using a sucking horn, because of the thickness of the blood (the blood contaminated by kapha will be thick and will be clumpy and hence cannot be sucked by horns). The blood contaminated/vitiated by vata and pitta shall be removed using the sucking horn

Prachchana – scarifying to produce bleeding:

गात्रं बद्ध्वोपरि दृढं रज्ज्वा पट्टेन वा समम् । स्नायुसन्ध्यस्थिमर्माणि त्यजन् प्रच्छानमाचरेत् ॥ ५१ ॥

अधोदेश प्रविसृतैः पदैरुपरिगामिभिः । न गाढघनतिर्यग्भिर्न पदे पदमाचरन् ॥ ५२ ॥

The part of the body above the site selected for scarifying (so as to produce bleeding) should be tightly tied with the help of a rope or a leather strap.

The tendons, joints, bones and vital spots should be avoided and the scarifying therapy (scratching, incising) should be done by using a sharp scalpel from below upwards. Scarification should not be done too deep, too thick, in horizontal direction or repeatedly

Administration of various types of bloodletting in various conditions:

प्रच्छानेनैकदेशस्थं ग्रथितं जलजन्मभिः । हरेच्छृङ्गादिभिः सुप्तमसृग्व्यापि सिराव्यधैः ॥ ५३ ॥

The blood accumulated in any localized area (small area of the body) can be removed by scratching/scarifying therapy. The blood which has clotted and solidified (as in tumors, abscess etc.) can be removed by using leeches.

When loss of sensation has been caused by vitiated blood (at the site of accumulation of vitiated blood) shall be removed by using the sucking horn etc. (Including gourds, pots etc.) and when the vitiated blood has soared all over the body, it shall be removed by venesection.

Various types of bloodletting in various conditions:

प्रच्छानं पिण्डिते वा स्यात् अवगाढे जलौकसः । त्वक्स्थेऽलाबुघटीशृङ्गं शिरैव व्यापकेऽसृजि ॥ ५४ ॥

वातादिधाम वा शृङ्गजलौकोऽलाबुभिः क्रमात् ।

Scarification/scratching/incision for removal of blood is done when the blood has been solidified.

When the vitiated blood is deep seated, it is removed by leech application.

When the vitiated blood is localized in the skin, it is removed with the help of gourds, pots or horns.

When the vitiated blood is spread all over the body, it is removed through venesection

Horns, leech and gourds are used for bloodletting in that order, for the seats of vata and other doshas.

Various types of bloodletting in various conditions:
सूतासृजः प्रदेहाद्यैः शीतैः स्याद्वायुकोपतः ॥ ५५ ॥ सतोदकण्डुः शोफस्तं सर्पिषोष्णेन सेचयेत् ॥ ५५a ॥

After bloodletting when vata gets aggravated following the application of cold anointments/pastes etc., leading to the manifestation of symptoms like pricking pain, itching and swelling. The area should be bathed with warm ghee.

इति श्रीवैद्यपति सिंहगुप्तसूनु श्रीमत् वाग्भट विरचितायां अष्टाङ्गहृदयसंहितायां सूत्रस्थाने शस्त्रविधिर्नाम षड् विंशोऽध्यायः॥२६॥

Thus ends the 26th chapter of Ashtangahridaya Samhita Sutrasthana, named Shastra Vidhim Adhyayam, written by Shrimad Vagbhata, son of Shri Vaidyapati Simhagupta.

27

सिराव्यधविधिमध्यायम्
(siravyadha vidhim adhyayam)

The 27th chapter of Sutrasthanam of Ashtanga Hridayam is named as Siravyadha Vidhi Adhyayam. This chapter deals with the detailed procedure of administration of venesection form of bloodletting. Pledge by the author(s):

अथातो सिराव्यधविधिमध्यायं व्याख्यास्यामः इति ह स्माहुरात्रेयादयो महर्षयः॥
Atreya and other sages pledge that henceforth they will be explaining the chapter named Siravyadha vidhim adhyaya.

Features of shuddha rakta (pure blood):
मधुरं लवणं किञ्चिदशीतोष्णमसंहतम् । पद्मेन्द्रगोपहेमाविशशलोहितलोहितम् ॥ १ ॥
लोहितं प्रभवः शुद्धं तनोस्तेनैव च स्थितः ।
Shuddha rakta is slightly sweet and salty in taste, neither too cold nor hot, liquid in nature, resembling the color of lotus, indragopa insect (firefly), gold and blood of sheep and rabbit.
It (pure blood) is the cause of origin of the body, by determining the healthy and unhealthy condition (nature of existence) of the body.

Vitiation of blood by doshas:
तत्पित्तश्लेष्मलैः प्रायो दूष्यते

Blood usually gets vitiated by pitta and kapha.

Effects of dushta rakta (vitiated blood):
कुरुते ततः ॥ २ ॥ विसर्पविद्रधिप्लीहगुल्माग्निसदनज्वरान् ।
मुखनेत्रशिरोरोगमदतृइलवणास्यताः ॥ ३ ॥ कुष्ठवातास्रपित्तास्रकट्वम्लोद्गिरणभ्रमान् ।
शीतोष्णस्निग्धरूक्षाद्यैरुपक्रान्ताश्च ये गदाः ॥ ४ ॥ सम्यक् साध्या न सिध्यन्ति ते च
रक्तप्रकोपजाः ।

The blood (thus vitiated by kapha and pitta) causes –
visarpa - herpes
vidradhi – abscesses
pleeha – diseases of spleen/splenomegaly
gulma – abdominal tumors
agnisadana – dyspepsia/weak digestive power
jvara - fever
mukha netra shiroroga – diseases of mouth, eyes and head
mada – intoxication
thrit - thirst
lavanasyata - salty taste in the mouth
kushtha – skin diseases
vatasra – gout
pittasra – bleeding disorders/discharge of blood contaminated by pitta from
various orifices of the body
katu amla udgeerana – belching with pungent and sour tastes in the mouth
bhrama – dizziness/giddiness
Those curable diseases, not getting cured even after appropriate cold or hot,
unctuous or dry treatments, they too should be understood as being caused
from aggravated blood
Purpose of siravyadha (venesection)
तेषु स्रावयितुं रक्तमुद्रिक्तं व्यधयेत्सिराम् ॥ ५ ॥
In these diseases (mentioned above), in order to drain out the vitiated
blood, the veins should be cut/punctured (venesection should be done).

Siravyadha anarha (Persons unsuitable for venesection):
न तूनषोडशातीतसप्तत्यब्दसुतासृजाम् ।
अस्निग्धास्वेदितात्यर्थस्वेदितानिलरोगिणाम् ॥ ६ ॥
गर्भिणीसूतिकाजीर्णपित्तास्रश्वासकासिनाम् ।
अतीसारोदरच्छर्दिपाण्डुसर्वाङ्गशोफिनाम् ॥ ७ ॥

स्नेहपीते प्रयुक्तेषु तथा पञ्चसु कर्मसु ।
नायन्त्रितां सिरां विध्येन्न तिर्यङ्नाप्यनुत्थिताम् ॥ ८ ॥
नातिशीतोष्णवाताभ्रेष्वन्यत्रात्ययिकाद्गदात् ।

Siravyadha should not be done in those -

who are less than 16 and more than 70 years of age,

who have not experienced bleeding previously (due to any cause),

who have undergone deficit oleation and sudation therapies and also excessive sudation therapy,

who are suffering from diseases caused by vitiated vata,

pregnant women, the woman in parturition,

who are suffering from indigestion, bleeding disorders, dyspnoea, cough,

who are suffering from diarrhoea, ascites/abdominal disorders (enlargement of abdomen, intestinal obstruction), vomiting, anemia and swelling all over the body (dropsy),

who have been given fat (ghee, oil) to drink as a part of oleation therapy,

who are undergoing Panchakarma treatments (five purifying treatments),

The vein should not be cut without enforcing control on the body, venesection should not be done on the vein which is horizontal, that has not been raised up (not full), venesection should not be done on days which are very cold, very hot, very windy or cloudy, venesection should not be done in emergency and life threatening diseases.

Sites for sirayvadha in Shiro netra vikara:

शिरोनेत्रविकारेषु ललाट्यां मोक्षयेत् सिराम् ॥ ९ ॥ अपाङ्ग्यामुपनास्यां वा

In diseases of the head and eyes, the veins situated on the forehead, outer angle of the eyes or the area around the nose should be cut

Sites for siravyadha in Karnarogas:

कर्णरोगेषु कर्णजाम् ।

In the diseases of the ear, the veins near the ear should be cut.

Sites for siravyadha in Nasarogas:

नासारोगेषु नासाग्रे स्थितां

In the diseases of the nose, veins located at the tip of the nose should be cut.

Sites for siravyadha in Peenasa:

नासाललाट्योः ॥ १० ॥ पीनसे

In rhinitis, the veins located in the nose and forehead (should be cut)

Sites for siravyadha in Mukharogas:

मुखरोगेषु जिह्वौष्ठहनुतालुगाः ।

In diseases of the mouth (oral cavity), veins located in the tongue, lips, jaws and palate (should be cut).

Sites for siravyadha in cysts/tumors located above the shoulders:

जत्रूर्ध्वग्रन्थिषु ग्रीवाकर्णशङ्खशिरःश्रिताः ॥ ११ ॥

In cysts and tumors located above the level of the shoulders, the veins located in the neck, temples or head (should be cut).

Sites for siravyadha in insanity/lunacy/madness:

उरोऽपाङ्गललाटस्था उन्मादे

In insanity, the veins in the region of chest, angle of the eye and forehead (should be cut).

Sites for siravyadha in epilepsy/memory disorders:

ऽपस्मृतौ पुनः । हनुसन्धौ समस्ते वा शिरां भ्रूमध्यगामिनीम् ॥ १२ ॥

Again in epilepsy (loss of memory, memory disorders) and diseases located all over the body, the veins located in the jaw should be cut. Also the veins located in between the eyebrows shall be cut in epilepsy.

Sites for siravyadha in abscess and pain in the flanks:

विद्रधौ पार्श्वशूले च पार्श्वकक्षास्तनान्तरे ।

In abscesses and pain in the flanks, the veins located in the flanks, axilla and in between the breasts should be cut.

Sites for siravyadha in fevers occurring on every third day:

तृतीयकेऽसयोर्मध्ये

In case of intermittent fevers, especially those occurring on every third day, the veins located in between the scapulae i.e. in the centre of the upper back, between the shoulders (should be cut).

Sites for siravyadha in fevers occurring on every fourth day:

स्कन्धस्याधश्चतुर्थके ॥ १३ ॥

In fevers occurring on every fourth day, the veins located below the shoulder joints should be cut.

Sites for siravyadha in dysentery associated with pain:
प्रवाहिकायां शूलिन्यां श्रोणितो द्व्यङ्गुले स्थिताम् ।

In dysentery associated with pain, the veins located 2 angulas away from the pelvis should be cut.

Sites for siravyadha in diseases of semen and penis:
शुक्रमेढ्रामये मेढ्रे

In diseases of semen and penis, the veins in the penis should be cut.

Sites for siravyadha in goiter/swelling of the neck:
ऊरुगां गलगण्डयोः ॥ १४ ॥

In goitre/swellings of the neck, the veins located in the thighs should be cut.

Sites for siravyadha in sciatica:
गृध्रस्यां जानुनोऽधस्तादूर्ध्वं वा चतुरङ्गुले ।

In sciatica, the veins located 4 angulas above or below the knee joints should be cut.

Sites for siravyadha in glandular enlargement of the neck:
इन्द्रवस्तेरधोऽपच्यां द्व्यङ्गुले

In glandular enlargement of the neck (apachi disease), the veins located 2 angulas below the indravasti marma (vital point located in the middle of the forearm) should be cut.

Sites for siravyadha in pain in thigh and swelling of the knee joints:
चतुरङ्गुले ॥ १५ ॥
ऊर्ध्वं गुल्फस्य सक्थ्यर्तौ तथा क्रोष्टुकशीर्षके ।

In thigh pain and swelling of the knee joints, the veins located 4 angulas above ankle joints should be cut.

Sites for siravyadha in burning sole, gout, tingling feet, fissures of feet, ankle sprain and diseases of toenails:
पाददाहे खुडे हर्षे विपाद्यां वातकण्टके ॥ १६ ॥ चिप्पे च द्व्यङ्गुले विध्येदुपरि क्षिप्रमर्मणः ।

In burning sensation of the foot (soles), gout, tingling sensation of the foot, cracks and fissures in the sole of the foot, ankle/foot sprain and diseases of toenails, the veins located 2 angulas above the kshipra marma (vital spot located in between the big toe and the first toe) should be cut

Sites for siravyadha in vishwachi i.e. pain in the arm/upper limb:
गृध्रस्यामिव विश्वाच्यां
In pain in the arms/upper limb, the veins should be cut in the same way as explained in sciatica.
Sites for siravyadha in invisible veins
यथोक्तानामदर्शने ॥ १७ ॥ मर्महीने यथासन्ने देशेऽन्यां व्यधयेत् सिराम् ।
If the mentioned veins are not visible at the mentioned sites meant to be cut, another (different) vein/veins situated at a nearby place (of the mentioned vein), which is devoid of vital spots, should be cut.

Siravyadha vidhi:
Preparation for procedure of conducting venesection
अथ स्निग्धतनुः सज्जसर्वोपकरणो बली ॥ १८ ॥
कृतस्वस्त्ययनः स्निग्धरसान्नप्रतिभोजितः ।
अग्नितापातपस्विन्नो जानूच्चासनसंस्थितः ॥ १९ ॥
मृदुपट्टात्तकेशान्तो जानुस्थापितकूर्परः ।
मुष्टिभ्यां वस्त्रगर्भाभ्यां मन्ये गाढं निपीडयेत् ॥ २० ॥
दन्तप्रपीडनोत्कासगण्डाध्मानानि चाचरेत् ।
पृष्ठतो यन्त्रयेच्चैनं वस्त्रमावेष्टयन् नरः ॥ २१ ॥
कन्धरायां परिक्षिप्य न्यस्यान्तर्वामतर्जनीम् ।
एषोऽन्तर्मुखवर्ज्यानां सिराणां यन्त्रणे विधिः ॥ २२ ॥
After having decided the site for conducting venesection, all the necessary equipment needed for venesection should be kept ready. The patient who is strong should be given oleation therapy. The person (patient who is to undergo venesection) should perform auspicious rituals and should consume meat juice and boiled rice mixed with ghee.
The person should then be exposed to the heat of the fire or sunlight for sweating (as a part of sudation). The patient should now be made to sit on a chair/stool of the height of his knee. A band of soft cloth should be tied around his head at the lower border of the hairs. He should be made to keep his elbows over his knees (while sitting on the stool) with the help of fists of the physician in which a pad of cloth is held, the neck of the patient should be pressed (massaged) briskly. Grinding the teeth, coughing, inflating the

mouth to enlarge the cheeks should also be allowed to be done. The back of the patient should be tied with a band of cloth, to keep him in control by covering the neck with a band of cloth kept in position with the help of left index finger. This is the method of raising the deep seated veins, excluding the veins located over and in the depth of the face

Siravyadha vidhi – method of bloodletting through venesection:
ततो मध्यमयाङ्गुल्या वैद्योऽङ्गुष्ठविमुक्तया । ताडयेत् उत्थितां ज्ञात्वा स्पर्शाद्वाङ्गुष्ठपीडनैः ॥ २३ ॥

कुठार्या लक्षयेन्मध्ये वामहस्तगृहीतया । फलोद्देशे सुनिष्कम्पं सिरां तद्वच्च मोक्षयेत् ॥ २४ ॥

ताडयन् पीडयंश्चैनां

Then the physician should tap the raised vein with his middle finger ripped off by the thumb. After noticing the elevation, by touching the vein or after raising it, once again by kneading the vein with the thumb, holding the axe with his left hand, without shaking his hand, the physician should place the edge of the axe on the middle portion of the vein (marking the vein supposed to be cut) and aiming good results (out of the procedure), should cut the vein likewise (as marked). Tapping and kneading the vein to discharge more (vitiated) blood should be done again

Method of siravyadha through venesection at various sites of the body:
Siravyadha of siras of nose and surrounding areas
विध्येद्व्रीहिमुखेन तु । अङ्गुष्ठेनोन्नमय्याग्रे नासिकामुपनासिकाम् ॥ २५ ॥
The vein of the nose and the surrounding area of the nose should be cut with a Vrihimukhi sharp instrument i.e. lancet having its face (blade) resembling grain of rice, after raising the tip of the nose with the thumb.

Venesection of veins underneath the tongue:
अभ्युन्नतविदष्टाग्रजिह्वस्याधस्तदाश्रयाम् ।
The vein situated underneath the tongue should be cut by instructing the patient to keep the tip of the tongue raised and biting it by holding the tongue firmly by the upper row of teeth.
Venesection of veins of the neck

यन्त्रयेत्स्तनयोरूर्ध्वं ग्रीवाश्रितसिराव्यधे ॥ २६ ॥
पाषाणगर्भहस्तस्य जानुस्थे प्रसृते भुजे ।
कुक्षेरारभ्य मृदिते विध्येद्बद्धोर्ध्वपट्टके ॥ २७ ॥

To perform venesection on the neck veins, the veins should be raised by manipulating the area above the breasts, the patient is made to hold a stone in each of his fists and made to keep his shoulders on his knees and outstretched. The patient's body is then massaged (pressed) starting from the belly upwards. Then the vein is cut after having tied a strap in the upper region.

Siravyadha of siras of the hand:

विध्येद्धस्तशिरां बाहावनाकुञ्चितकूर्परे ।
बद्ध्वा सुखोपविष्टस्य मुष्टिमङ्गुष्ठगर्भिणम् ॥ २८ ॥
ऊर्ध्वं वेध्यप्रदेशाच्च पट्टिकां चतुरङ्गुले ।

The veins of the hand are cut when the patient is sitting comfortably, keeping his arm straight without bending his elbows, clenching his fist with the fingers folded inwards, with a band of cloth tied four angulas above the site of cutting.

Siravyadha of siras of the flanks:

विध्येदालम्बमानस्य बाहुभ्यां पार्श्वयोः सिराम् ॥ २९ ॥

The veins of the flanks should be cut by keeping the arms hanging loose.

Siravyadha of siras of the penis:

प्रहृष्टे मेहने

The veins of the penis shall be cut when it is erected.

Siravyadha of siras of the calves:

जङ्घासिरां जानुन्यकुञ्चिते ।

The veins of the legs i.e. calf muscles shall be cut keeping the knee joints flexed.

Siravyadha of siras of the feet

पादे तु सुस्थितेऽधस्ताज्जानुसन्धेर्निपीडिते ॥ ३० ॥
गाढं कराभ्यामागुल्फं चरणे तस्य चोपरि ।
द्वितीये कुञ्चिते किञ्चिदारूढे हस्तवत्ततः ॥ ३१ ॥ बद्ध्वा विध्येत् सिराम्

The veins of the feet should be cut, when the patient's feet are kept steady, after having briskly massaged/pressed the leg from knee downwards up to the ankle joint and foot with the hands (of the physician), while keeping the other leg (foot) slightly bent (flexed) slightly overlapped and pressed over it, tying a band similar to the method described in the venesection for the hand.

Skills of the physician (surgeon) in conducting Venesection:

इत्थमनुक्तेष्वपि कल्पयेत् । तेषु तेषु प्रदेशेषु तत्तद्यन्त्रमुपायवित् ॥ ३२ ॥

In the similar way, a wise physician (surgeon having precise and comprehensive knowledge about various instruments and surgical wisdom) should adopt similar methods of raising the veins (to be cut) appropriate to the places, by the techniques not even mentioned here.

Siravyadha of siras fleshy and bony parts:

मांसले निक्षिपेद्देशे व्रीह्यास्यं व्रीहिमात्रकम् ।
यवार्धमस्थ्नामुपरि सिरां विध्यन् कुठारिकाम् ॥ ३३ ॥

On fleshy parts of the body the vrihimukha sharp instrument i.e., lancet should be used and the vein cut to the size of a rice grain only. The veins on the bones should be cut to a size of half a barley by using the kutharika sharp instrument i.e., an axe.

Signs of properly done Siravyadha:

सम्यग्विद्धा स्रवेद्धारां यन्त्रे मुक्ते तु न स्रवेत् ।

When the vein is cut properly, the blood flows out in a steady stream and does not flow (bleeding stops) when the tourniquet control is removed.

Signs of inadequately and excessively done Siravyadha:

अल्पकालं वहत्यल्पं दुर्विद्धा तैलचूर्णनैः ॥ ३४ ॥
सशब्दमतिविद्धा तु स्रवेद्दुःखेन धार्यते ।

When the vein is inadequately cut (improper vensection), the blood flows for a short time and is less in quantity, in this case, the site of vensection should be rubbed with a mixture of oil and lime powder to promote proper bleeding.

When the vein is cut excessively, blood flows out with a sound and stops with great difficulty.

Causes for absence of blood flow:

भीमूर्च्छायन्त्रशैथिल्यकुण्ठशस्त्रातितृप्तयः ॥ ३५ ॥
क्षामत्ववेगितास्वेदा रक्तस्यासृतिहेतवः ।

Causes of absence of blood flow are –

bhee - fear
moorcha – fainting/loss of consciousness
yantra shaithilya – loose tourniquet
kuntha shastra – blunt instruments
ati tripti - excessively satiated
kshaamatva - debility
vegita – presence of urges of urine, feces etc
asveda – absence of/not having done sweating therapy

Measures to be taken when there is inadequate blood flow:

असम्यगस्रे स्रवति वेल्लव्योषनिशानतैः ॥ ३६ ॥

सागारधूमलवणतैलैर्दिह्यात् सिरामुखम् ।

When the blood is not flowing properly (in sufficient quantity),
The cut end of the vein should be applied (smeared) with Embelia ribes,
three pungent herbs (Trikatu - black pepper, long pepper and ginger)
turmeric – Curcuma longa, Valeriana wallichi, house soot, salt and oil.

Promoting easy blood flow following siravyadha:

सम्यक्प्रवृत्ते कोष्णेन तैलेन लवणेन च ॥ ३७ ॥

When the blood is flowing properly (following venesection), the site should
be smeared with warm oil and salt.

Observations to be made in the blood flowing following siravyadha:

अग्रे स्रवति दुष्टास्रं कुसुम्भादिव पीतिका ।

सम्यक् सुत्वा स्वयं तिष्ठेच्छुद्धं तदिति नाहरेत् ॥ ३८ ॥

The vitiated blood flows out first, just like the yellow-juice flows from
the safflower seeds before its oil flows out. After properly bleeding (in
sufficient quantity), if the blood stops by itself, it should be considered as
pure, un-vitiated blood and further bleeding should not be encouraged.

Measures to be taken when the person faints following siravyadha:

यन्त्रं विमुच्य मूर्छायां वीजिते व्यजनैः पुनः ।

स्रावयेन् मूर्छति पुनस्त्वपरेद्युस्त्र्यहेऽपि वा ॥ ३९ ॥

If the patient faints during the time of bleeding, then the tourniquet should
be released. He should be fanned (given air) with fans to bring him back to
consciousness and the bloodletting should be continued. If he faints again,
bloodletting should be postponed to the next day or third day.

Characteristics of impure/contaminated blood:

वाताच्छ्यावारुणं रूक्षं वेगस्राव्यच्छफेनिलं ।
पित्तात् पीतासितं विस्रमस्कन्द्यौष्ण्यात् सचन्द्रिकम् ॥ ४० ॥
कफात् स्निग्धमसृक् पाण्डु तन्तुमत् पिच्छिलं घनम् ।
संसृष्टलिङ्गं संसर्गात् त्रिदोषं मलिनाविलम् ॥ ४१ ॥

The blood vitiated by vata will be bluish black or crimson in color, dry, flowing with force, clear and frothy.

The blood vitiated by pitta will be yellow or black, have a foul smell, not thick because of increase of heat, and mixed with shining particles.

The blood vitiated by kapha will be unctuous, pale-yellowish/yellowish-white in color, has small thread suspensions in it, and is slimy and thick.

When the blood gets vitiated by combination of two doshas, there will be mixed features of both doshas.

When the blood vitiated by all three doshas will be dirty and thick/cloudy.

Quantity of blood flow during siravyadha:

अशुद्धौ बलिनोऽप्यस्रं न प्रस्थात् स्रावयेत् परम् ।
अतिस्रुतौ हि मृत्युः स्याद्दारुणा वा चलामयाः ॥ ४२ ॥
तत्राभ्यङ्गरसक्षीररक्तपानानि भेषजम् ।

The vitiated blood should not be allowed to flow for more than 768 ml, even in a strong person. Excessive bleeding will lead to either death or dreadful diseases of vata origin. In such conditions, oil massage, drinking of meat soup, milk and blood are the ideal treatments.

Post-operative procedures to be done after siravyadha:

सुते रक्ते शनैर्यन्त्रमपनीय हिमाम्बुना ॥ ४३ ॥
प्रक्षाल्य तैलप्लोताक्तं बन्धनीयं सिरामुखम् ।
अशुद्धं स्रावयेद्भूयः सायमह्न्यपरेऽपि वा ॥ ४४ ॥
स्नेहोपस्कृतदेहस्य पक्षाद्वा भृशदूषितम् ।

After the flow of blood (has occurred properly following venesection), the controls (tourniquet) should be gradually removed. The site of venesection should be washed with cold water. The cut end of the vein should be covered with a cotton swab soaked in oil and bandaged. The vitiated blood should be removed once again either in the same evening or on the following day. If the blood is found to be excessively vitiated with more quantity of doshas, the vitiated blood should be removed again after a fortnight after administering oleation.

Residual vitiated blood in the body post siravyadha:

किञ्चिदिद्ध शेषे दुष्टास्त्रे नैव रोगोऽतिवर्तते ॥ ४५ ॥

सशेषमप्यतो धार्यं न चातिस्रुतिमाचरेत् ।

If a small residue of vitiated blood remains inside the body, diseases do not get worsened. Therefore it can be allowed to stay inside the body. But excessive flow of blood should not be attempted.

Management of residual vitiated blood in the body post siravyadha:

हरेच्छृङ्गादिभिः शेषं प्रसादमथवा नयेत् ॥ ४६ ॥

शीतोपचारपित्तास्रक्रियाशुद्धिविशोषणैः ।

दुष्टं रक्तमनुद्रिक्तमेवमेव प्रसादयेत् ॥ ४७ ॥

Such residual blood (left out in the body following venesection) may be removed by making use of horns etc. or it can be purified of its doshas by administration of cold comforts, therapies prescribed for bleeding disorders (bleeding due to simultaneous contamination of blood and the pitta residing in the blood), purification therapies (panchakarma therapies) etc. and by methods of making the body thin. Even the blood which is mildly vitiated by doshas but not increased in quantity, should be treated with the above mentioned methods.

Management of excessive bleeding:

रक्ते त्वतिष्ठति क्षिप्रं स्तम्भनीमाचरेत् क्रियाम् ।

लोध्रप्रियङ्गुपत्तङ्गमाषयष्ट्याह्वगैरिकैः ॥ ४८ ॥

मृत्कपालाञ्जनक्षौममषीक्षीरित्वगङ्कुरैः ।

विचूर्णयेद्व्रणमुखं पद्मकादिहिमं पिबेत् ॥ ४९ ॥

तामेव वा सिरां विध्येद्व्यधात् तस्मादनन्तरम् ।

सिरामुखं वा त्वरितं दहेत् तप्तशलाकया ॥ ५० ॥

If the bleeding does not stop, measures to check the bleeding should be adopted immediately. The orifice of the wound (at the site of venesection) should be smeared/sprinkled with the powder of either Symplocos racemosa, Callicarpa macrophylla, Sappan wood - Caesalpinia sappan, black gram (Vigna mungo), licorice (Glycyrrhiza glabra), red ochre, pot shred, collyrium, linen ash of flax or the bark and sprouts of latex yielding trees. Cold infusion prepared from the herbs of Padmakadi group of herbs should be taken as a drink.

The same vein should be cut again. After cutting the vein, the ends of the vein should be quickly touched with a red-hot rod (cauterization).

Displacement of doshas due to binding by tourniquet, its management:

उन्मार्गगा यन्त्रनिपीडनेन स्वस्थानमायान्ति पुनर्न यावत् ।
दोषाः प्रदुष्टा रुधिरं प्रपन्नास्तावद्धिताहारविहारभाक् स्यात् ॥ ५१ ॥

Due to the application of tourniquet (for venesection), the aggravated doshas which have entered the blood may move to other parts of the body. After the tourniquet is removed, the doshas will come back again to their normal seats until then (until the doshas return back to their places), one should adhere to only healthy foods and activities.

Annapana after siravyadha:

नात्युष्णशीतं लघु दीपनीयं रक्तेऽपनीते हितं अन्नपानम् ।
तदा शरीरं ह्यनवस्थितासृगग्निर्विशेषादिति रक्षितव्यः ॥ ५२ ॥

Foods and drinks which are neither very hot, very cold, light (easy to digest) and appetite stimulants are suitable after venesection. This is because, after the bloodletting procedure, the body will be unstable, especially the digestion activity will be unstable (low digestion activity) and the mentioned foods are intended to protect the digestive fire (and to balance the digestion).

Features of persons with vishuddha rakta (healthy blood)

प्रसन्नवर्णेन्द्रियमिन्द्रियार्थान् इच्छन्तमव्याहतपक्तृवेगम् ।
सुखान्वितं पुष्टिबलोपपन्नं विशुद्धरक्तं पुरुषं वदन्ति ॥ ५३ ॥

Desire for obtaining (and having) excellence of color and complexion, improved power of sense organs, good perception of sense objects by sense organs, good digestive activity, enjoyment of comforts (comfortable life), being endowed with good nutrition and immunity - are the characteristics of the person having pure blood (the person with above said virtues is said to be one with non-vitiated and healthy blood).

इति श्रीवैद्यपति सिंहगुप्तसूनु श्रीमद्वाग्भटविरचितायामष्टाङ्गहृदयसंहितायां सूत्रस्थाने शिराव्यधविधिर्नाम सप्तविंशोऽध्यायः ॥ २७ ॥

Thus ends the 27th chapter of Ashtangahridaya Samhita Sutrasthana, named Siravyadha Vidhim Adhyayam, written by Shrimad Vagbhata, son of Shri Vaidyapati Simhagupta.

28

शल्याहरणविधिमध्यायम् (shalyaharana vidhim adhyam)

The 28th chapter of Sutrasthanam of Ashtanga Hridayam is named as Shalyaharana Vidhi Adhyayam. This chapter deals with the detailed procedure of removal of foreign bodies from the body.

अथातो शल्याहरणविधिमध्यायं व्याख्यास्यामः इति ह स्माहुरात्रेयादयो महर्षयः॥

Atreya and other sages pledge that henceforth they will be explaining the chapter named Shalyaharana vidhim adhyaya.

Shalya Gati (Directions of entry of foreign bodies):
वक्रर्जुतिर्यगूर्ध्वाधः शल्यानां पञ्चधा गतिः ।

vakra – irregular/curved

ruju – straight

tiryak – oblique/horizontal

urdhwa - upward and

adha - downward

These are the five directions of movement of the shalya (foreign bodies)

Recognition of vrana with shalya inside them:
ध्यामं शोफरुजावन्तं स्रवन्तं शोणितं मुहुः ॥ १ ॥

अभ्युद्गतं बुद्बुदवत् पिटिकोपचितं व्रणम् ।

मृदुमांसं च जानीयादन्तःशल्यं समासतः ॥ २ ॥

The wound having a foreign body inside it should be recognized with the help of the below mentioned features in the wound –
dhyama - bluish black discoloration/dark colored
shopha – swelling
rujavanta - pain
muhur shonita srava - frequent bleeding
abhudgatam budbudavat – elevated like a bubble
pitikopachita - studded with eruptions/boils/lumps
mrudu mamsa – and softness of muscles.

Twak gata shalya lakshana (Signs of Shalya in the skin):
विशेषात् त्वग्गते शल्ये विवर्णः कठिनायतः ।
शोफो भवति
Specifically, when the foreign body is located in the skin,
There is discoloration with the presence of hard and large swelling is seen.

Mamsa gata shalya lakshana (Signs of foreign body in mamsa):
मांसस्थे चोष शोफो विवर्द्धते ॥ ३ ॥
पीडनाक्षमता पाकः शल्यमार्गो न रोहति ।
When the foreign body is in the flesh, there will be sucking pain, increase in swelling (gradual progression in swelling), tenderness/hypersensitivity, suppuration, non healing of the wounds formed at the entry of foreign body. Peshyantara gata shalya lakshana (Signs of foreign body in between the peshis)
When the foreign body is present in between two muscles, the signs will be similar to the signs of foreign body residing inside the flesh (muscle mass), except swelling.

Snayu gata shalya lakshana (Signs of foreign body in the tendons):
आक्षेपः स्नायुजालस्य संरम्भस्तम्भवेदनाः । स्नायुगे दुर्हरं चैतत्
When the foreign body is located in the tendons, convulsions (tremors), angriness/irritation in the network of tendons, stiffness and pain occur. And it is difficult to remove (the foreign body cannot be easily removed when stuck in the network of tendons).

Signs of foreign body in the veins – sira gata shalya lakshana:
सिराध्मानं सिराश्रिते ॥ ५ ॥

When the foreign body is localized in the veins, there is distension of the veins.

Sroto gata shalya lakshana (Signs of foreign body in the srotas):
स्वकर्मगुणहानिः स्यात्स्रोतसां स्रोतसि स्थिते ।
When the foreign body is localized in the channels of the body, there is loss of their respective functions and qualities in the respective channels.

Dhamani gata shalya lakshana (Signs of foreign body in the dhamani):
धमनीस्थेऽनिलो रक्तं फेनयुक्तमुदीरयेत् ॥ ६ ॥ निर्याति शब्दवान् स्याच्च हृल्लासः साङ्गवेदनः ।
When the foreign body is located in the arteries, the vitiated vata/air (in the arteries) will cause bleeding with froth (air mixed with blood causing frothing of blood) and the blood to flow with sounds, presence of nausea and body pains.

Asthi-sandhi gata shalya lakshana (Signs of foreign body in the bony joints):
सङ्घर्षो बलवानस्थिसन्धिप्राप्तेऽस्थिपूर्णता ॥ ७ ॥
When the foreign body is localized in the bony joints of the body, there is severe collision/severe rubbing of the edges of the bones/severe irritation in the joints and filling of the bones with fluids.

Asthi gata shalya lakshana (Signs of foreign body in the bones):
नैकरूपा रुजोऽस्थिस्थे शोफः
When the foreign body is located in the bones, there occurs not just a single type of pain (many types of pain occur) and swelling.

Sandhi gata shalya lakshana (Signs of foreign body in the body joints):
तद्वच्च सन्धिगे । चेष्टानिवृत्तिश्च भवेत्
When the foreign body is located in the joints of the body (junction of structures), the symptoms similar to the foreign body located in the bones occur and the activities of related joints cease (destroyed).

Koshta gata shalya lakshana (Signs of foreign body in the abdomen):
आटोपः कोष्ठसंश्रिते ॥ ८ ॥ आनाहोऽन्नशकृन्मूत्रदर्शनं च व्रणानने ।
When the foreign body is stuck in the abdomen (abdomen cavity), there occurs flatulence of abdomen, distension of abdomen (bloating, swelling)

and discharge/appearance of food, fecal material and urine from the orifice of the wound.

Marma gata shalya lakshana (Signs of foreign body in the abdomen):
विद्यान्मर्मगतं शल्यं मर्मविद्धोपलक्षणैः ॥ ९ ॥
When the foreign body is located in the vital spots of the body, the signs of injury to such spots appear.

Parisrava (discharge of related fluids) from the body parts:
यथास्वं च परिस्रावैस्त्वगादिषु विभावयेत् ।
In addition to the general signs enumerated above, the foreign body in the body structures will cause discharge of fluids related to (from) skin etc. related structure/tissue (example lymph from skin, blood from veins and arteries, bone marrow from the bones etc.)

Healing of the wounds caused by shalya in a person who had undergone purification therapies:
रूह्यते शुद्ध देहानामनुलोम स्थितं तु तत्॥१०॥ दोषकोपाभिघातादिक्षोभाद्भूयोऽपि बाधते
।
If the wound caused by the foreign body is located in the body (even after removal of the foreign body) of the person who has undergone purification therapies and if it is located in the line of the passage of purification, the wounds get healed spontaneously. The wounds (or foreign body) left out in the body of those who have not undergone purification therapy will trouble the person once again due to the irritation caused by dosha aggravation or trauma (yet again).

Recognizing the site of foreign body disappeared/vanished beneath the skin:
त्वङ्नष्टे यत्र तत्र स्युरभ्यङ्गस्वेदमर्दनैः ॥ ११ ॥ रागरुग्दाहसंरम्भा यत्र चाज्यं विलीयते ।
आशु शुष्यति लेपो वा तत्स्थानं शल्यवद्वदेत् ॥ १२ ॥
When there is the appearance of redness, pain, burning sensation and tenderness, after anointing with oil/massaging the region, fomentation or rubbing in the region (skin) wherein the foreign body is concealed beneath the skin. When there is melting of solid ghee placed at the site and when there is quick drying of the pastes (of sandalwood etc.) applied over that region, one can tell that the foreign body is located exactly in that region

(beneath the skin).

Identifying the location of a shalya hidden in the mamsa:
मांसप्रणष्टं संशुद्ध्या कर्शनाच्छलथतां गतम् । क्षोभाद्रागादिभिः शल्यं लक्षयेत्

The foreign body concealed in the flesh can be recognized by seeing the looseness/flaccidity of the muscles following the administration of cleansing treatments (panchakarma treatments) or by other treatments/ methods for thinning the body. And by seeing the redness etc. symptoms due to irritation (at the place where the foreign body is concealed).

Identifying the location of a shalya hidden in the muscles, bony joints and abdomen:
तद्वदेव च ॥ १३ ॥
पेश्यस्थिसन्धिकोष्ठेषु नष्टम्

The foreign bodies concealed in the muscles, bony joints and abdomen will present with similar signs (as explained in the foreign body concealed in flesh).

Identifying the location of a shalya hidden in the bones:
अस्थिषु लक्षयेत् ।
अस्थ्नामभ्यञ्जनस्वेदबन्धपीडनमर्दनैः ॥ १४ ॥

The site of the foreign body concealed in the bones is recognized by anointing/massaging with oil, sudation, tying a rope or bandage, squeezing and pressing on the afflicted bones (these methods will worsen pain and other symptoms and help in identifying the underlying foreign body).

Identifying the location of a shalya hidden in the joints:
प्रसारणाकुञ्चनतः सन्धिनष्टं तथास्थिवत् ।

The site of foreign bodies concealed in the joints are recognized by extending or flexion of joints and also by signs similar to those explained in case of foreign bodies concealed in the bones.

Identifying the location of a shalya hidden in the tendons/ligaments, veins, channels of the body and arteries:
नष्टे स्नायुसिरास्रोतोधमनीष्वसमे पथि ॥ १५ ॥
अश्वयुक्तं रथं खण्डचक्रमारोप्य रोगिणम् ।
शीघ्रं नयेत् ततस्तस्य संरम्भाच्छल्यमादिशेत् ॥ १६ ॥

The sites of the foreign body concealed in the ligaments/tendons, veins, channels of the body and arteries are recognized when irritation, pain occurs (at the site of impaction of foreign body) due to the speed of the horse wagon, when a chariot pulled by a horse (horse wagon) having broken wheels on which the patient (having the foreign body concealed in one or more of the above said structures) is seated is driven with great speed on uneven roads.

Identifying the location of a shalya hidden in the vital spots:

मर्मनष्टं पृथङ् नोक्तं तेषां मांसादिसंश्रयात् ।

The features of foreign body concealed in the vital/vulnerable spots of the body are not described separately, because these spots are composed of muscles and other tissues (and the features of foreign body located in muscles and other tissues have already been enumerated above).

General principle of identifying the location of a shalya hidden in any part of the body:

Generally, the site of the foreign body (wherein the foreign body is concealed) is recognized by the appearance of distressing symptoms (irritation caused by the foreign body) after doing some activity (including some abnormal movements of the body parts wherein the foreign body is concealed) and the presence of pain (in the place where foreign body is located).

Recognizing the shape of the foreign body concealed in the body:

वृत्तं पृथु चतुष्कोणं त्रिपुटं च समासतः ।
अदृश्यशल्यसंस्थानं व्रणाकृत्या विभावयेत् ॥ १८ ॥

The shape of the invisible foreign body (concealed in some body part) is determined by the shape of the wound such as round, wide, with four angles, with 3 edges etc.

Method of removing the shalya entering the body from above and below:

तेषामाहरणोपायौ प्रतिलोमानुलोमकौ ।
अर्वाचीनपराचीने निर्हरेत् तद्विपर्ययात् ॥ १९ ॥

The method of removal of the foreign bodies entering the body from above, reaching downwards and from below, reaching upwards are through opposite routes (removed through opposite routes). i.e., the foreign body should be removed from upward direction (when the foreign body is located below, having entered from above and moved downward) and from downward direction (when the foreign body is located above, having entered from below and moved upwards).

Method of removing the tiryaggata shalyas (foreign bodies which have entered the body from sideward):

सुखाहार्यं यतश्छित्त्वा ततस्तिर्यग्गतं हरेत् ।

The foreign bodies which have entered obliquely should be removed by cutting them in a convenient way (without troubling the patient)

Restrictions to remove foreign bodies:

शल्यं न निर्घात्यमुरःकक्षावङ्क्षणपार्श्वगम् ॥ २० ॥

प्रतिलोममननुतुण्डं छेद्यं पृथुमुखं च यत् ।

नैवाहरेद्विशल्यघ्नं नष्टं वा निरुपद्रवम् ॥ २१ ॥

The foreign bodies lodged in chest, axillae, groins and flanks, those which have entered upwards, which are not elevated like a bubble of water, which are fit to be cut and having broad blades should not be removed (not be pulled out).

Similarly those foreign bodies which lead to death soon after their removal, which are lost/invisible (absorbed by the body) and those which do not produce any complications - should not be removed.

Means and methods of removal of shalya:

अथाहरेत् करप्राप्यं करेणैवेतरत् पुनः ।

दृश्यं सिंहाहिमकरवर्मिकर्कटकाननैः ॥ २२ ॥

अदृश्यं व्रणसंस्थानाद्ग्रहीतुं शक्यते यतः ।

कङ्कभृङ्गाह्वकुररशरारिवायसाननैः ॥ २३ ॥

Those (foreign bodies) which can be held with the hand should be removed by the hand itself. While others (foreign bodies) which are visible should be held by lion faced, snake faced, crocodile faced, fish faced, crab faced instruments. Those (foreign bodies) which are invisible but can be grasped by instruments, through the wound,

should be pulled out by instruments having faces like heron, shrike, osprey, a kind of heron and crow.

Removal of Shalyas lodged in the skin and other tissues:

सन्दंशाभ्यां त्वगादिस्थम् ।

Foreign bodies lodged in the skin and other tissues should be removed using forceps.

Removal of hollow foreign bodies:

तालाभ्यां सुषिरं हरेत् ।

Those foreign bodies which are hollow should be removed using instruments with flat discs.

Removal of foreign bodies lodged in hollow spaces:

सुषिरस्थं तु नलकैः शेषं शेषैर्यथायथम् ॥ २४ ॥

Those (foreign bodies) which are lodged in hollow spaces should be removed using tubular instruments

and the other (foreign bodies) should be removed using other convenient instruments, as and when needed.

Removal of shalya which cannot be held by instruments:

शस्त्रेण वा विशस्यादौ ततो निर्लोहितं व्रणम् ।

कृत्वा घृतेन संस्वेद्य बद्धाचारिकमादिशेत् ॥ २५ ॥

Those foreign bodies which cannot be held by instruments, should be removed by cutting open the site with sharp instruments. Then after the blood has been discharged (wound cleared of the blood), the wound is fomented with ghee (warm ghee), bandaged and the patient is advised to follow the prescribed regimen (related to diet).

Removal of shalya which cannot be held by instruments:

सिरास्नायुविलग्नं तु चालयित्वा शलाकया ।

Foreign bodies lodged in the veins and ligaments (tendons, nerves) should be pulled out after loosening them with the help of rod like instruments.

Removal of shalyas embedded in the chest/heart:

हृदये संस्थितं शल्यं त्रासितस्य हिमाम्बुना ॥ २६ ॥

ततः स्थानान्तरं प्राप्तं आहरेत् तद्यथायथम् ।

यथामार्गं दुराकर्षम् ।

If the foreign body is embedded in the heart/chest, in a person, chilled water should be sprinkled. Later, after knowing that it has reached a distant place (different site in chest), it should be removed by situational usage of instrumentation as apt to that site and shape, size and shape of the foreign body and the pathway in which it has been impacted. The foreign body located in the heart is difficult to extract/remove.

Removal of un-removable Shalyas embedded in other sites of the body:

अन्यतोऽप्येवमाहरेत् ॥ २७ ॥

The un-removable (difficult to remove) foreign bodies located elsewhere in the body too should be removed just as mentioned in case of heart (they should be removed when they move away to a distant place).

Removal of shalyas embedded in the bones:

अस्थिदष्टे नरं पद्भ्यां पीडयित्वा विनिर्हरेत् ।
इत्यशक्ये सुबलिभिः सुगृहीतस्य किङ्करैः ॥ २८ ॥

Foreign bodies lodged in the bones should be removed by holding the patient tightly (in position) with the help of the legs of the physician. If it is not possible to remove the foreign body even by this method, it should be pulled out by attendants who are strong.

Measures taken to remove the shalyas when they cannot be pulled out:

तथाप्यशक्ये वारङ्गं वक्रीकृत्य धनुर्ज्यया ।
सुबद्धं वक्त्रकटके बध्नीयात्सुसमाहितः ॥ २९ ॥
सुसंयतस्य पञ्चाङ्ग्या वाजिनः कशयाऽथ तम् ।
ताडयेदिति मूर्धानं वेगेनोन्नमयन् यथा ॥ ३० ॥
उद्धरेच्छल्यमेवं वा शाखायां कल्पयेत् तरोः ।
बद्ध्वा दुर्बलवारङ्गं कुशाभिः शल्यमाहरेत् ॥ ३१ ॥

When it is not possible to extract the foreign body even by the above said method, the tail end of the foreign body (example, arrow) should be bent and fastened tight to the string of a bent bow. And the bow should be tied perfectly to the bridle bit of a horse whose all four limbs and face are tied aptly. The horse should then be whipped, so that it raises its head suddenly and with force exerted on the foreign helps in removal of the foreign body. Similarly, the branches of the trees may be made use of, in case of arrows with thin/fragile tail ends, thin bamboo poles are tied to the arrow and removed.

Other measures to remove the stubborn shalya/arrows:

श्वयथुग्रस्तवारङ्गं शोफमुत्पीड्य युक्तितः ।

मुद्गराहतया नाड्या निर्घात्योतुण्डितं हरेत् ॥ ३२ ॥
तैरेव चानयेन्मार्गममार्गोत्तुण्डितं तु यत् ।
मृदित्वा कर्णिनां कर्ण नाड्यास्येन निगृह्य वा ॥ ३३

If the tail end of the foreign body (arrow) is surrounded by an elevation, it should be pulled out after squeezing/pressing out the bulged part suitably. If the arrow head has caused a bulging on the body, it should be removed with the help of a tubular instrument after hitting (shaking) the bulge with a hammer by the hammer, the arrow which does not have a clear exit passage, should be brought into a passage, such that it is suitable to pull it out. Those (foreign bodies) which have ear-like projection, should be pulled out after loosening off their ears or by fixing them inside with the help of tubular instruments.

Use of magnets to remove shalya:
अयस्कान्तेन निष्कर्णं विवृतास्यमृजुस्थितम् ।

The arrow heads without ear-like projections, which have caused a wide opening in the body and have lodged straight, can be removed by making use of a magnet.

Removal of shalya which have entered the colon:
पक्वाशयगतं शल्यं विरेकेण विनिर्हरेत् ॥ ३४ ॥

The foreign bodies which have entered the large intestine can be removed by giving purgation.

Removal of shalya by sucking apparatus:
दुष्टवातविषस्तन्यरक्ततोयादि चूषणैः ।

Bad air (flatus), poison, breast milk, blood, fluids etc. (which have become foreign bodies due to stagnation) are removed by sucking (with the help of animal horns etc. equipment).

Removal of shalya impacted in the throat:
कण्ठस्रोतोगते शल्ये सूत्रं कण्ठे प्रवेशयेत् ॥ ३५ ॥
बिसेनात्ते ततः शल्ये बिसं सूत्रं समं हरेत् ।

When the foreign body has gone into the passage of the throat (and has impacted therein), a lotus stalk tied with a thread should be passed into the throat and when the foreign body gets stuck to the stalk, the thread should be pulled out slowly.

Removal of shalyas made up of lac impacted in the throat:

नाड्याग्नितापितां क्षिप्त्वा शलाकामप्स्थिरीकृताम् ॥ ३६ ॥

आनयेज्जातुषं कण्ठात् जतुदिग्धामजातुषम् ।

If the foreign body in the throat is made up of lac, a heated iron rod should be passed through a tubular instrument (into the throat) and made to touch the foreign body and then the foreign body is removed from the throat. Those (foreign body) not made out of lac should be removed by making use of rods smeared with lac at its tip.

Removal of thorny shalyas impacted in the throat:

केशोन्दुकेन पीतेन द्रवैः कण्टकमाक्षिपेत् ॥ ३७ ॥

सहसा सूत्रबद्धेन वमतस्तेन चेतरत् ।

Thorny (hook like) foreign bodies impacted in the throat should be removed by inserting a ball of hair fastened with a thread (into the throat), consumed along with water (or before insertion of the ball). The foreign body stuck to the ball of hair is removed by pulling the thread quickly when the person vomits the consumed fluid. Similarly the hair and other foreign bodies should be removed by making use of a hook.

Removal of shalya stuck in the mouth and nose and food stuck in the throat:

अशक्यं मुखनासाभ्यां आहर्तुं परतो नुदेत् ॥ ३८ ॥

अप्पानस्कन्धघाताभ्यां ग्रासशल्यं प्रवेशयेत् ।

If the foreign bodies lodged/impacted in the mouth and nose, if not possible to be removed out through their respective orifices, should be pushed back, making them enter into the wider tract (so that they can be removed from a wider tract). If the consumed bolus of food is stuck in the form of foreign body in the throat, it should be pushed back into the stomach, by making the person drink water or by tapping over the shoulder with fists (gently).

Removal of small shalya stuck in the eyes and wounds:

सूक्ष्माक्षिव्रणशल्यानि क्षौमवालजलैर्हरेत् ॥ ३९ ॥

Small sized foreign bodies located in eyes or wounds should be removed with the help of linen, hairs or water

Removal of water swallowed during drowning:

अपां पूर्णं विधुनुयादवाक्क्शिरसमायतम् ।
वामयेच्चामुखं भस्मराशौ वा निखनेन्नरम् ॥ ४० ॥

The person who has swallowed water to his full stomach (due to drowning), should be held upside down, with his legs up, and shaken well, or made to vomit all water or the person should be immersed in a heap of ash till the level of head.

Removal of water which has entered the ears:

कर्णेऽम्बुपूर्णे हस्तेन मथित्वा तैलवारिणी ।
क्षिपेदधोमुखं कर्णं हन्याद्वाऽऽचूषयेत वा ॥ ४१ ॥

If the ears are full of water, it should be removed by putting the oil removers churned with hands of the physician, into the ears (of the patient) or the ears should be kept facing downwards and the head should be given a blow from the side or the water can be sucked out with the help of tubular instruments.

Removal of insects which have entered the ears:

कीटे स्रोतोगते कर्णं पूरयेद्लवणाम्बुना ।
शुक्तेन वा सुखोष्णेन मृते क्लेदहरो विधिः ॥ ४२ ॥

If any insect has entered into the passage of the ear, the ears should be filled with warm salt water or sour gruel, when the insect is dead, dehydration measures (measures to remove the fluid) should be adopted.

Melting of certain shalyas by the body heat:

जातुषं हेमरूप्यादिधातुजं च चिरस्थितम् ।
ऊष्मणा प्रायशः शल्यं देहजेन विलीयते ॥ ४३ ॥

Foreign bodies like lac, and metals like gold, silver etc.
remaining for long time inside the body probably get dissolved due to the heat of the body.

Shalyas which do not melt in the body and its effect:

मृद्वेणुदारुशृङ्गास्थिदन्तवालोपलानि न ।
विषाणवेण्वयस्तालदारुशल्यं चिरादपि ॥ ४४ ॥
प्रायो निर्भुज्यते तद्धि पचत्याशु पलासृजी ।

The foreign bodies of the likes of mud, bamboo, wood, horn, bone, tooth and hairs of animals or man, stone etc. do not get dissolved by the heat of the body. Those composed of horn, bamboo, iron, wood of palm tree remaining inside the body for longer time duration, usually get distorted, remain undissolved and quickly produce putrefaction in the muscles and blood.

Measures taken to remove deep concealed shalyas:

शल्ये मांसावगाढे चेत्स देशो न विदह्यते ॥ ४५ ॥
ततस्तं मर्दनस्वेदशुद्धिकर्षणबृंहणैः ।
तीक्ष्णोपनाहपानान्नघनशस्त्रपदाङ्कनैः ॥ ४६ ॥
पाचयित्वा हरेच्छल्यं पाटनैषणभेदनैः ।

If the foreign body is concealed deep inside the fleshy parts, and if the site having the foreign body has not undergone suppuration (the foreign body being in place, not causing suppuration). Purification/suppuration (ripening of the part of the body consisting of the foreign body) of such parts should be done by the measures like squeezing, fomentation, cleansing/purifying therapies, thinning measures, nourishing therapies, application of strong poultices, strong drinks and foods, by application of incising etc methods of sharp instrumentation, trampling by feet etc. And then the foreign bodies be removed by excision, probing or splitting/cutting methods.

Wisdom of physician in removing different types of shalya:

शल्यप्रदेशयन्त्राणामवेक्ष्य बहुरूपताम् ॥ ४७ ॥
तैस्तैरुपायैर्मतिमान् शल्यं विद्यात्तथाहरेत् ॥ ४७ऊअब् ॥

Keeping in mind the different and peculiar features of the foreign bodies, their place of lodgment and instruments which should be preferred to remove them, the brilliant physician should recognize them and remove the foreign bodies by adopting appropriate methods (of removal).

इति श्रीवैद्यपति सिंहगुप्तसूनु श्रीमद्वाग्भट विरचितायां अष्टाङ्गहृदयसंहितायां सूत्रस्थाने शल्याहरणविधिर्नाम अष्टाविंशोऽध्यायः ॥२८॥

Thus ends the 28th chapter of Ashtanga Hridaya Samhita Sutrasthana, named Shalyaharana Vidhim Adhyayam, written by Shrimad Vagbhata, son of Shri Vaidyapati Simhagupta.

29

शस्त्रकर्मविधिमध्यायम् (shastra karma vidhim adhyayam)

The 29th chapter of Sutrasthanam of Ashtanga Hridayam is named as Shastrakarma Vidhi Adhyayam. This chapter deals in detail with the surgical procedures and the way of conducting them.Pledge by the author(s):

अथातो शस्त्रकर्मविधिमध्यायं व्याख्यास्यामः इति ह स्माहुरात्रेयादयो महर्षयः॥

Atreya and other sages pledge that henceforth they will be explaining the chapter named Shastrakarma vidhim adhyaya.

Need and urgency to treat Shvayathu (swelling):

व्रणः सञ्जायते प्रायः पाकाच्छ्वयथुपूर्वकात् ।

तमेवोपचरेत्तस्मादरक्षन् पाकं प्रयत्नतः ॥ १ ॥

सुशीतलेपसेकास्रमोक्षसंशोधनादिभिः ।

The ulcers may develop due to the suppuration on the backdrop of swelling (swelling suppurates and then ulcers occur). Therefore (to prevent suppuration of swelling and subsequent formation of ulcers), the swelling should be treated first and the suppuration (formation of pus) should be prevented by all means and efforts by application of cold poultices, sprinkling / showering the part with cold decoction of the herbs, bloodletting and purifying therapies (Panchakarma treatments).

Ama Shopha (Unripe swelling):

शोफोऽल्पोऽल्पोष्मरुक् सामः सवर्णः कठिनः स्थिरः ॥ २ ॥

The unripe swelling is mild (less swollen) with mild heat and pain, has the same color of the skin, hard in consistency and immovable.

Pachyamana Shopha (A swelling in the process of ripening):

पच्यमानो विवर्णस्तु रागी बस्तिरिवाततः ।
स्फुटतीव सनिस्तोदः साङ्गमर्दविजृम्भिकः ॥ ३ ॥
संरम्भारुचिदाहोषातृइज्वरानिद्रतान्वितः ।
स्त्यानं विष्यन्दयत्याज्यं व्रणवत् स्पर्शनासहः ॥ ४ ॥

The swelling which is in the process of ripening is discolored, usually red colored, distended like a urinary bladder, feels as if the swelling is going to burst open, has pricking pain aches all over the body, excessive yawning, agitation or irritation in the swelling, tastelessness / anorexia, burning sensation, increased temperature, thirst, fever, loss of sleep, quick melting of solid ghee placed on the swelling (due to high temperature), tenderness (intolerance on touching) just as in an ulcer.

Pakwa Shopha (Swelling which has ripened):

पक्वेऽल्पवेगता म्लानिः पाण्डुता वलिसम्भवः ।
नामोऽन्तेषून्नतिर्मध्ये कण्डूशोफादिमार्दवम् ॥ ५ ॥
स्पृष्टे पूयस्य सञ्चारो भवेद्बस्ताविवाम्भसः ।

In pakwa shopha, the swelling / symptoms are less severe, swelling is reduced in size with pale color, appearance of wrinkles on it (swelling). The swelling is depressed all around the periphery and is elevated at the center. Itching, swelling etc. symptoms are mild in nature. On touch of the swelling, the movement of pus can be known, resembling the movement of water within the bladder.

Symptoms of involvement of doshas in swelling and suppuration:

शूलं नर्तेऽनिलाद्दाहः पित्ताच्छोफः कफोदयात् ॥ ६ ॥
रागो रक्ताच्च पाकः स्यादतो दोषैः सशोणितैः ।

In swelling, pain doesn't occur without the involvement of vata, burning sensation doesn't occur without the involvement of pitta, swelling doesn't occur without the involvement of kapha, redness doesn't occur without the involvement of rakta. The suppuration of swelling occurs due to the involvement of all the three doshas along with the blood.

Symptoms of ati paka (excessive suppuration in the swelling):

पाकेऽतिवृत्तेऽतिसुषिरस्तनुत्वग्दोषभक्षितः ॥ ७ ॥

वलीभिराचितः श्यावः शीर्यमाणतनूरुहः ।

When there is excessive suppuration (formation of pus) in the swelling, cavity forms inside the swelling (hollowed inwards). The skin over the swelling becomes thin and gets destroyed by the vitiated doshas. It gets covered with wrinkles, becomes dark / black in color and there is fall of body hairs (in the region of the suppurated swelling).

Raktapaka (Suppuration of blood in swelling caused by kapha):

कफजेषु तु शोफेषु गम्भीरं पाकमेत्यसृक् ॥ ८ ॥

पक्वलिङ्गं ततोऽस्पष्टं यत्र स्याच्छीतशोफता ।

त्वक्सावर्ण्यं रुजोऽल्पत्वं घनस्पर्शत्वमश्मवत् ॥ ९ ॥

रक्तपाकमिति ब्रूयात्तं प्राज्ञो मुक्तसंशयः ।

In the swelling caused by predominance of kapha dosha, the blood gets suppurated / ripened deep inside the swelling, in a concealed way. Therefore, the signs of ripening / suppuration are not clearly seen. Such conditions can be made out by the presence of cold swelling (swelling which is cold on touch), is of the same color as that of surrounding skin, has mild pain, is hard to touch, just like a stone (stony hardness). The wise without any doubt, call this condition as rakta paka i.e. suppuration of blood.

Darana - Tearing (bursting, splitting) and
Patana - Cutting (incise) of swelling:

अल्पसत्त्वेऽबले बाले पाकाद्वात्यर्थमुद्धते ॥ १० ॥

दारणं मर्मसन्ध्यादिस्थिते चान्यत्र पाटनम् ।

Bursting / tearing the swelling (abscess – pus filled swelling) should be done (by application of alkalis etc.) in persons having weak mind, who are debilitated, in children or when the swelling is elevated due to excessive accumulation of pus and when the swelling is located in the vital spots of the body and on the joints of the body. In other cases (apart from the above said conditions), the swelling should be cut open by using sharp instruments.

Contraindication of darana and patana of the swelling in ama condition of the shopha:

आमच्छेदे सिरास्नायुव्यापदोऽसृग्गतिस्रुतिः ॥ ११ ॥

रुजोऽतिवृद्धिर्धर्देरणं विसर्पो वा क्षतोद्भवः ।

Cutting (bursting) an unripe swelling leads to diseases and complications of veins and ligaments (tendons), profuse bleeding, severe increase in pain or herpes / spreading skin ulcers due to tearing of skin or injury.

Effect of not opening and discharging the pus in mature swelling / suppurated swelling:

तिष्ठन्नन्तः पुनः पूयः सिरास्नाय्वसृगामिषम् ॥ १२ ॥
विवृद्धो दहति क्षिप्रं तृणोल्पमिवानलः ।

The pus remaining inside (the swelling) and getting increased in quantity, once again quickly burns the veins, ligaments, tendons, blood and muscles, just as a spark of fire burns away a hay stack.

Effect of early / delayed opening and discharging the pus:

यश्छिनत्त्यामज्ञानाद्यश्च पक्वमुपेक्षते ॥ १३ ॥
श्वपचाविव विज्ञेयौ तावनिश्चितकारिणौ ।

Due to ignorance, the one (physician) who breaks open an unripe swelling and the one who neglects a ripe swelling (and doesn't open it) is considered to be equivalent to a dog keeper / feeder (mean / unwise surgeon). Both being considered doing indiscriminate acts (doing things without reasoning).

Purvakarma (Pre-operative procedures):

प्राक् शस्त्रकर्मणश्चेष्टं भोजयेदन्नमातुरम् ॥ १४ ॥
पानपं पाययेन्मद्यं तीक्ष्णं यो वेदनाक्षमः ।
न मूर्छत्यन्नसंयोगान्मत्तः शस्त्रं न बुध्यते ॥ १५ ॥
अन्यत्र मूढगर्भाश्ममुखरोगोदरातुरात् ।

Before conducting the main procedure i.e., opening of an abscess, the patient should be given the food he likes. The person who is accustomed to drinking alcohol may be given a drink of strong wine which should enable him to withstand the pain of the surgical process.

Due to intake of food, the person doesn't lose consciousness / faint (during the surgical procedure). Being sedated by consumption of strong wine, he doesn't have sense of the sharp instrument being operated over him (on the swelling) with exception of those patients suffering from obstructed delivery (impacted fetus), renal stones, those suffering from diseases of mouth and abdominal disorders (these patients should not be given food or wine before surgery).

Pradhana karma (Operative procedure):

अथाहृतोपकरणं वैद्यः प्राङ्मुखमातुरम् ॥ १६ ॥
संमुखो यन्त्रयित्वाशु न्यस्येन्मर्मादि वर्जयन् ।
अनुलोमं सुनिशितं शस्त्रमापूयदर्शनात् ॥ १७ ॥
सकृदेवाहरेत्तच्च

Next, keeping ready all the surgical equipment required, the physician should make the patient sit facing east. Sitting in front of the patient facing him, the physician should incise the swelling quickly with a well sharpened instrument. Incision should be made in the direction of the hairs (from above downward), avoiding vulnerable parts, deep enough till the pus is seen and then removing the instrument quickly.

Method of incising, probing and evacuating the pus in a suppurated (mature) swelling:

पाके तु सुमहत्यपि ।
पाटयेद्द्व्यङ्गुलं सम्यग्द्व्यङ्गुलत्र्यङ्गुलान्तरम् ॥ १८ ॥
एषित्वा सम्यगेषिण्या परितः सुनिरूपितम् ।
अङ्गुलीनालवालैर्वा यथादेशं यथाशयम् ॥ १९ ॥
यतो गतं गतिं विद्यादुत्सङ्गो यत्र यत्र च ।
तत्र तत्र व्रणं कुर्यात् सुविभक्तं निराशयम् ॥ २० ॥
आयतं च विशालं च यथा दोषो न तिष्ठति ।

If the area of suppuration is large, the incisions of 2 angula dimension shall be made properly either two or three angulas (1 angula = 1 finger breadth) apart (the incisions should not be made too close to each other).

After properly considering the entire interior of the swelling, suppurated area should then be thoroughly excavated / probed with either a probe, finger, tube or hairs of animals, as suitable to the site and area of the swelling The pus path is determined, wherever the bulge (of the suppurated swelling) is found, therein the cut is done (cutting through the bulge of the wounds), creating a well cut, well cleaned, long and deep, wide wound so that no vitiating material can remain inside the wound.

Characteristics of an ideal surgeon:

शौर्यमाशुक्रिया तीक्ष्णं शस्त्रमस्वेदवेपथू ॥ २१ ॥

असम्मोहश्च वैद्यस्य शस्त्रकर्मणि शस्यते ।

Courage, quickness of action, keeping the instruments very sharp, not sweating, not trembling, not getting confused are the qualities best desired of a surgeon who is about to conduct a surgical procedure.

Oblique or horizontally curved incision:

तिर्यक्छिन्द्याल्ललाटभ्रूदन्तवेष्टकजत्रुणि ॥ २२ ॥

कुक्षिकक्षाक्षिकूटौष्ठकपोलगलवङ्क्षणे ।

अन्यत्र छेदनात् तिर्यक् सिरास्नायुविपाटनम् ॥ २३ ॥

The incision (cut through the swelling) should be made horizontally curved (obliquely) in places such as forehead, eyebrows, gums of teeth, shoulders, abdomen, axillae, eye sockets, lips, cheeks, throat and groins. In other places, if a horizontal cut is made, it might lead to cutting of the veins, ligaments (tendons) etc.

Paschat Karma (Post operative procedures):

शस्त्रेऽवचारिते वाग्भिः शीताम्भोभिश्च रोगिणम् ।

आश्वास्य परितोऽङ्गुल्या परिपीड्य व्रणं ततः ॥ २४ ॥

क्षालयित्वा कषायेण प्लोतेनाम्भोऽपनीय च ।

गुग्गुल्वगुरुसिद्धार्थहिङ्गुसर्जरसान्वितैः ॥ २५ ॥

धूपयेत् पटुषड्ग्रन्थानिम्बपत्रैर्घृतप्लुतैः ।

तिलकल्काज्यमधुभिर्यथास्वं भेषजेन च ॥ २६ ॥

दिग्धां वर्तिं ततो दद्यात् तैरेवाच्छादयेच्च ताम् ।

घृताक्तैः सक्तुभिश्चोर्ध्वं घनां कवलिकां ततः ॥ २७ ॥

निधाय युक्त्या बध्नीयात् पट्टेन सुसमाहितम् ।

पार्श्वे सव्येऽपसव्ये वा नाधस्तान्नैव चोपरि ॥ २८ ॥

After removing the sharp instruments, the patient should be comforted with encouraging words and cold water. The area all around the wound should be squeezed with the help of fingers. The wound is washed with the decoction of medicinal herbs. The moisture is removed by wiping the area with cotton wool. The wound should be fumigated with the smoke of the below mentioned herbs mixed with plenty of ghee –

- guggulu – Commiphora mukul
- aguru – Aquilaria agallocha
- siddhartha – Brassica campestris
- hingu – Ferula asafoetida

- sarjarasa - Vateria indica
- patu – salt
- shad grantha – Acorus calamus
- nimbapatra - leaves of Azadirachta indica

Then a wick smeared with paste of sesame, ghee, honey and appropriate medicinal herbs should be placed inside the wound and should be covered. Over that, a thick plaster prepared from corn flour and ghee is put on and skillfully bandaged with a thick sheet of cloth in a well laden way winding the bandage either from right to left or from left to right, but not from either bottom or from top.

Nature of bandage cloth used in dressing:

शुचिसूक्ष्मदृढाः पट्टाः कवल्यः सविकेशिकाः ।
धूपिता मृदवः श्लक्ष्णा निर्वलीका व्रणे हिताः ॥ २९ ॥

The bandage cloth should be clean, thin and strong. The medicinal wicks should consist of cotton threads, which are fumigated, soft, smooth and devoid of folds. These are beneficial for dressing the ulcers

Oblations to protect the ulcers:

कुर्वीतानन्तरं तस्य रक्षां रक्षोनिषिद्धये ।
बलिं चोपहरेत् तेभ्यः

After the surgery, the ulcers should be protected from the invasion of bad evils (microbes), insects, flies which feed on blood. They should be offered oblations.

Wearing protective herbs on the head:

सदा मूर्ध्ना च धारयेत् ॥ ३० ॥
लक्ष्मीं गुहामतिगुहां जटिलां ब्रह्मचारिणीम् ।
वचां छत्रामतिच्छत्रां दूर्वां सिद्धार्थकानपि ॥ ३१ ॥

The patient should always wear on his head, potent herbs such as

lakshmee - Prosopis cineraria

guha – Desmodium gangeticum

atiguha - Uraria picta

jatila - Nardostachys jatamansi

brahmacharini – Bacopa monnieri

vacha - Acorus calamus

chatra – Anethum sowa

atichatra - Pistacia integerrima

doorva - Cynodon dactylon

siddharthaka - siddhārthakān api – and Brassica campestris.

Following measures mentioned in snehana and contraindication of divaswapna in post operative management of inflammatory swelling / ulcers:

ततः स्नेहदिनेहोक्तं तस्याचारं समादिशेत् ।

दिवास्वप्नो व्रणे कण्डूरागरुक्शोफपूयकृत् ॥ ३२ ॥

Later, the patient should be made to follow the regimen prescribed for the day of Snehana karma. Day sleep leads to production of symptoms like itching, redness, pain, swelling and pus in the ulcer (therefore, day sleep should be contraindicated in the post operative care of ulcer).

Contraindication of sexual intercourse and sexual thoughts:

स्त्रीणां तु स्मृतिसंस्पर्शदर्शनैश्चलितसुते ।

शुक्रे व्यवायजान् दोषानसंसर्गेऽप्यवाप्नुयात् ॥ ३३ ॥

Thoughts, touch, sight of women which leads to mobilization (from its seats) and ejaculation of semen, leads to other bad effects of intercourse, in spite of not getting indulged actually in the sexual act (therefore these should be avoided in the post operative care of ulcers).

Effects of doing the contraindicated things in the post operative care of ulcers:

व्रणे श्वयथुरायासात् स च रागश्च जागरात् ।

तौ च रुक् च दिवास्वापात्ताश्च मृत्युश्च मैथुनात् ॥ ३३+(१) ॥

In an ulcer, the swelling gets increased by strenuous activities. Redness increases by keeping awake at night, pain increases by day sleep and death occurs by indulging in copulation.

Aharakrama after shastrakarma;

भोजनं च यथासात्म्यं यवगोधूमषष्टिकाः ।

मसूरमुद्गतुवरीजीवन्तीसुनिषण्णकाः ॥ ३४ ॥

बालमूलकवार्ताकतण्डुलीयकवास्तुकम् ।

कारवेल्लककर्कोटपटोलकटुकाफलम् ॥ ३५ ॥

सैन्धवं दाडिमं धात्री घृतं तप्तहिमं जलम् ।

जीर्णशाल्योदनं स्निग्धमल्पमुष्णोदकोत्तरम् ॥ ३६ ॥
भुञ्जानो जाङ्गलैर्मांसैः शीघ्रं व्रणमपोहति ।

The food of the patient should be that which is congenial such as (those given below)

yava – barley – Hordeum vulgare

godhuma – wheat – Triticum aestivum

shashtika - rice ripened and harvested in 60 days

masura – lentils – Lens culinaris

mudga – green gram – Vigna radiata

tuvari – tur dal – Cajanus cajan

jivanti – Leptadenia reticulata

sunishannaka - Blepharis edulis

bala mulaka – tender radish

vartaka – eggplant / brinjal

tanduleeyaka – Amaranthus viridis

vastuka – Chenopodium album

karavellaka – bitter gourd - Momordica charantia

karkota – Momordica dioica

patola – Trichosanthes dioica

katukaphala – fruits of Picrorhiza kurroa

saindhava - rock salt

dadima - pomegranate / Punica granatum

dhatri – Emblica officinalis

ghruta - ghee

tapta hima jala – boiled and cooled water,

rice prepared from old rice, added with fats, consumed in little quantity along with meat of animals of desert regions followed by drinking of hot water. This helps in quick healing of ulcers

Reasons to consume less quantity of food after surgery, during recovery:
अशितं मात्रया काले पथ्यं याति जरां सुखम् ॥ ३७ ॥
अजीर्णात् त्वनिलादीनां विभ्रमो बलवान् भवेत्
ततः शोफरुजापाकदाहानाहानवाप्नुयात् ॥ ३८ ॥

The food which is to be consumed in limited quantity, at appropriate time meant for eating and that which is healthy and conducive undergoes digestion easily. Indigestion (caused due to excessive eating) leads to severe aggravation of vata and other doshas. Consequently swelling, pain, suppuration / putrefaction, burning sensation and distension of abdomen occurs.

Foods to be avoided post surgery:
नवं धान्यं तिलान् माषान् मद्यं मांसमजाङ्गलम् ।
क्षीरेक्षुविकृतीरम्लं लवणं कटुकं त्यजेत् ॥ ३९ ॥
यच्चान्यदपि विष्टम्भि विदाहि गुरु शीतलम् ।
वर्गोऽयं नवधान्यादिर्व्रणिनः सर्वदोषकृत् ॥ ४० ॥
nava dhanya - fresh grains
tila – sesame- Sesamum indicum
masha – black gram – Vigna mungo
madya - wines
ajangala mamsa – meat of animals other than those living in desert like regions
ksheera vikruti - products of milk
ikshu vikruti - products of sugarcane
amla lavana katuka – food substances which are predominantly sour, salty and pungent – all these foods should be avoided.
Any other food substances which cause constipation, burning sensation, which are heavy to digest and cold in nature (should be avoided). This group of substances consisting of new grains etc. (mentioned above) gives rise to aggravation of all the doshas in those suffering from ulcers.
Impact of strong wines / alcohol on ulcers
मद्यं तीक्ष्णोष्णरूक्षाम्लमाशु व्यापादयेद्व्रणम् ।
Strong penetrating wines / alcohol which is hot, dry (non unctuous) and sour in nature will quickly cause complications / death of the patient suffering from ulcers.

Dos and don'ts in ulcers:
वालोशीरैश्च वीज्येत न चैनं परिघट्टयेत् ॥ ४१ ॥
न तुदेन्न च कण्डूयेच्चेष्टमानश्च पालयेत् ।
स्निग्धवृद्धद्विजातीनां कथाः शृण्वन्मनःप्रियाः ॥ ४२ ॥
आशावान् व्याधिमोक्षाय क्षिप्रं व्रणमपोहति ।
The site of ulcer should be fanned with either tuft of hairs of animals or with that of Vetivaria zizanioides (vetiver grass). It should not be beaten, poked or scratched with nails. It should be protected from injury while doing other activities

The person who engages himself in hearing pleasant stories, about (from) virtuous elders and Brahmins, he who is hopeful of getting cured from the disease, gets cured of the ulcer quickly.

Care of ulcer on the third day, following surgery:
तृतीयेऽह्नि पुनः कुर्याद्व्रणकर्म च पूर्ववत् ॥ ४३ ॥
प्रक्षालनादि दिवसे द्वितीये नाचरेत्तथा ।
तीव्रव्यथो विग्रथितश्चिरात्संरोहति व्रणः ॥ ४४ ॥
On the third day (after surgery), the same treatment of the ulcers such as washing the ulcers etc. should be done again as explained earlier. These should not be done on the second day as that will give rise to severe pain, formation of tumors and delayed healing of the ulcers.

Nature and quality of wick and medicinal paste applied over the ulcer:
स्निग्धां रूक्षां श्लथां गाढां दुर्न्यस्तां च विकेशिकाम् ।
व्रणे न दद्यात् कल्कं वा स्नेहात् क्लेदो विवर्धते॥ ४५ ॥
मांसच्छेदोऽतिरुग्रौक्ष्याद्दरणं शोणितागमः ।
श्लथातिगाढदुर्न्यासैर् व्रणवर्त्मावघर्षणम् ॥ ४६ ॥
In the ulcers, the wick of cotton threads smeared with paste of herbs and also the paste of herbs should neither be too unctuous nor very dry, neither flabby (loose and thin) nor very thick (hard) and should not be improperly placed (over the ulcer). Because unctuousness (excessively oily or fatty) increases moistness, dryness causes tears in the muscles, severe pain, lacerations and bleeding, flabby, hard and improperly placed wicks produces friction of the edges of the ulcers.

Management of ulcer inside which the wick remains for long duration:
सपूतिमांसं सोत्सङ्गं सगति पूयगर्भिणम् ।
व्रणं विशोधयेच्छीघ्रं स्थिता ह्यन्तर्विकेशिका ॥ ४७ ॥
When the medicinal wick remains for a long duration inside the ulcer, it produces putrefaction of the muscles, elevated surface, loss of tissues and accumulation of pus inside (the ulcer). Then the ulcer should be cleared (cleaned) of its contents quickly.

Management of ignorantly cut unripe swelling:
व्यम्लं तु पाटितं शोफं पाचनैः समुपाचरेत् ।
भोजनैरुपनाहैश्च नातिव्रणविरोधिभिः ॥ ४८ ॥

When an unripe swelling has been cut open by ignorance, it should be treated with foods and poultices which bring about ripening of swelling. But which are, at the same time, not very much harmful to the ulcer.

Sadyovrana Chikitsa (Management of traumatic wounds):

सद्यः सद्योव्रणान् सीव्येदि्ववृतान् अभिघातजान् ।
मेदोजाल्लिखितान् ग्रन्थीन् ह्स्वाः पालीश्च कर्णयोः ॥ ४९ ॥
शिरोऽक्षिकूटनासौष्ठगण्डकर्णोरुबाहुषु ।
ग्रीवाललाटमुष्कस्फिइ्मेढ्रपायूदरादिषु ॥ ५० ॥
गम्भीरेषु प्रदेशेषु मांसलेष्वचलेषु च ।

Traumatic wounds which are caused due to recent injury (recently occurred) and those which are wide, should be sutured immediately.

So also the ulcers which are made by scraping fatty tumors, pinna of the ears which are very thin, ulcers located on the head, eye-sockets, nose, lips, cheeks, ears, thighs, arms, neck, forehead, scrotum, buttocks, penis, rectum, abdomen etc. which are situated on important and deep, fleshy and immovable parts should be sutured.

Wounds that should not be sutured immediately:

न तु वङ्क्षणकक्षादावल्पमांसे चले व्रणान् ॥ ५१ ॥
वायुनिर्वाहिणः शल्यगर्भान् क्षारविषाग्निजान् ।

The ulcers / wounds which are located on groins, axilla etc. which are less muscular and movable, ulcers which emit air (gas), which have foreign bodies inside them, which are produced by alkalis, poisons and fire should not be sutured.

Method of proper suturing of wounds and materials used therein:

सीव्येच्चलास्थिशुष्कास्रतृणरोमापनीय तु ॥ ५२ ॥
प्रलम्बि मांसं विच्छिन्नं निवेश्य स्वनिवेशने ।
सन्ध्यस्थि च स्थिते रक्ते स्नाय्वा सूत्रेण वल्कलैः ॥ ५३ ॥
सीव्येन् न दूरे नासन्ने गृह्णन्नाल्पं न वा बहु ।

Suturing should be done only after removing loose pieces of bones, dried blood clots, grass, hairs, etc. by placing the torn and hanging pieces of muscles in their proper places and also by keeping the joints of the bones and bones fractured in their normal positions and after the stoppage of bleeding,

by making use of tendons of animals, threads (of cotton, silk, flax etc) or inner fibers of bark of trees, suturing being done neither very far apart nor very close, holding neither very much of the tissues nor very little.

Measures to be taken after suturing the wounds:

सान्त्वयित्वा ततश्चार्त व्रणे मधुघृतद्रुतैः ॥ ५४ ॥

अञ्जनक्षौमजमषीफलिनीशल्लकीफलैः ।

सलोध्रमधुकैर्दिग्धे युञ्ज्याद्बन्धादि पूर्ववत् ॥ ५५ ॥

After suturing, having comforted the patient (with encouraging words, cold water, fanning etc.), the ulcer should be covered with cotton swab soaked in a mixture of honey, melted ghee, collyrium, ash of flax, Callicarpa macrophylla, fruits of Boswellia serrata, Symplocos racemosa, Madhuka longifolia. Then bandaging and other measures should be done as described previously.

Suturing the non bleeding ulcers:

व्रणो निःशोणितौष्ठो यः किञ्चिदेवावलिख्य तम् ।

सञ्जातरुधिरं सीव्येत् सन्धानं ह्यस्य शोणितम् ॥ ५६ ॥

The edges of the ulcer which are not bleeding should be scraped a little to induce bleeding and it should be sutured when the blood is flowing. Because the blood is the cause (agent) for healing of ulcers.

Bandhana (Bandages):

बन्धनानि तु देशादीन् वीक्ष्य युञ्जीत तेषु च ।

आविकाजिनकौशेयमुष्णं क्षौमं तु शीतलम् ॥ ५७ ॥

शीतोष्णं तुलासन्तानकार्पासस्नायुवल्कजम् ।

ताम्रायस्त्रपुसीसानि व्रणे मेदःकफाधिके ॥ ५८ ॥

भङ्गे च युञ्ज्यात् फलकं चर्मवल्ककुशादि च ।

After having analyzed the site of the ulcer, bandages suitable to the site of the ulcer / organs of the body should be made use of therein. Among them, the bandages prepared from skin of sheep and silk are hot, bandages made out of flax is cold, the bandages made from silk-cotton, cotton, tendons of the animals, sheaths, thin layers of tendons etc. and bark of trees is both hot and cold.

Wounds which have more of fat and kapha (caused by predominance of fat and kapha) should be covered with sheets of copper, iron, zinc or lead (also in fractures)

In case of fractures, bandaging should be done by using leather, barks of trees and splints, hard and flat pieces of bamboo, wood, metal etc.

Bandhana Prakara (Types of Bandages):
स्वनामानुगताकारा बन्धास्तु दश पञ्च च ॥ ५९ ॥
कोशस्वस्तिकमुत्तोलीचीनदामानुवेल्लितम् ।
खट्वाविबन्धस्थगिकावितानोत्सङ्गगोष्फणाः ॥ ६० ॥
यमकं मण्डलाख्यं च पञ्चाङ्गी चेति योजयेत् ।
यो यत्र सुनिविष्टः स्यात् तं तेषां तत्र बुद्धिमान् ॥ ६१ ॥
विदध्यात् तेषु तेष्वेव कोशमङ्गुलिपर्वसु ।
स्वस्तिकं कर्णकक्षादिस्तनेषूक्तं च सन्धिषु ॥ ६११+(१) ॥
खट्वां गण्डे हनौ शङ्खे विबन्धं पृष्ठकोदरे ।
अङ्गुष्ठाङ्गुलिमेढ्राग्रे स्थगिकामन्त्रवृद्धिषु ॥ ६११+(३) ॥
वितानं पृथुलाङ्गादौ तथा शिरसि चेरयेत् ।
विलम्बिनि तथोत्सङ्गं नासौष्ठचिबुकादिषु ॥ ६११+(४) ॥
गोष्फणं सन्धिषु तथा यमकं यमिके व्रणे ।
वृत्तेऽङ्गे मण्डलाख्यं च पञ्चाङ्गीं चोर्ध्वजत्रुषु ॥ ६११+(५) ॥
यो यत्र सुनिविष्टः स्यात्तं तेषां तत्र बुद्धिमान्॥६१॥

Bandages are of the same shapes implied in their very names and are fifteen in number.

They are sheath, cross shaped, winding, ribbon like, long roll shaped, spiral shaped, four tailed, noose like, betel box type, canopy shaped, loosely knotted, cow horn shaped, two tailed, ring shaped, and five tailed bandages - should be considered and administered in the relative sites of their usage (as mentioned below).

Sheath bandage should be used for the joints of the fingers,
cross shaped bandage should be used for ears, axilla etc., for breasts and bony joints, winding type of bandages should be used for the penis, neck etc. sites and ribbon like bandage should be used for the outer canthus of the eyes,

a long roll shaped bandage shall be used at the junction of body parts such as groins etc., and spiral shaped bandage for the extremities.

Four tailed bandage should be used over the cheeks, lower jaws and temples, noose like bandage is used for the back and abdomen, betel box shaped bandage should be used for the thumb, fingers, tip of penis, and in hernia, canopy type of bandage should be used for organs which are thick and also for the head, loosely knotted bandage is used for hanging parts of the body, cow horn shaped bandage should be used for the nose, lips, chin, joints etc. Two tailed bandages are used for places having two adjacent ulcers, ring shaped bandage should be used for parts of the body which are round,

Five tailed bandages are used for parts of the body above the shoulders, the brilliant physician should administer those types of bandages which are most suitable for particular parts of the body.

Tight, moderate and loose bandages:

बध्नीयाद्गाढमूरुस्फिक्ककक्षावङ्क्षणमूर्धसु ।
शाखावदनकर्णोरःपृष्ठपार्श्वगलोदरे ॥ ६२ ॥
समं मेहनमुष्के च नेत्रे सन्धिषु च श्लथम् ।
बध्नीयाच्छिथिलस्थाने वातश्लेष्मोद्भवे समम् ॥ ६३ ॥
गाढमेव समस्थाने भृशं गाढं तदाशये ।
शीते वसन्तेऽपि च तौ मोक्षणीयौ त्र्यहात् त्र्यहात् ॥ ६४ ॥
पित्तरक्तोत्थयोर्बन्धो गाढस्थाने समो मतः ।
समस्थाने श्लथो नैव शिथिलस्याशये तथा ॥ ६५ ॥
सायं प्रातस्तयोर्मोक्षो ग्रीष्मे शरदि चेष्यते ।

Bandages should be tied tight over the thighs, buttocks, axillae, groins, and head,

it should be moderately tight, over the extremities, face, ears, chest, back, flanks, neck, abdomen, penis and scrotum, over the eyes and joints, the bandage should be tied loose, so also on places which are flabby, on (flabby) places wherein the ulcers have been produced by vata and kapha, the bandage should be moderate, on places which are even neither hard nor flabby, it should be tight.

It should be very tight if the wound / ulcer is situated on the seats / organs belonging to vata and kapha.

Bandage should be removed once in three days during cold and spring seasons.

Bandage should be tied moderately tight on hard parts, if the ulcers / wounds on them are produced by pitta and kapha and on even parts, it should be loose.

In places where loose bandaging is prescribed, it should not be tied at all. During summer and autumn seasons, the bandage should be removed in the evening and morning.

Consequences of not bandaging the ulcers:

अबद्धो दंशमशकशीतवातादिपीडितः ॥ ६६ ॥
दुष्टीभवेच्चिरं चात्र न तिष्ठेत् स्नेहभेषजम् ।
कृच्छ्रेण शुद्धिं रूढिं वा याति रूढो विवर्णताम् ॥ ६७ ॥

If the ulcer is not bandaged, it gets contaminated by the bite of mosquitoes, cold breeze etc. The fats and medicines applied to the ulcer do not stay on for long. The ulcer gets clean with difficulty (requires longer time to become clean, without pus etc. contaminants) and also gets healed with difficulty. And even after healing, it will be discolored (the skin over the area around the wound / ulcer does not get back the normal color.

Benefits of bandaging the ulcers / wounds:
बद्धस्तु चूर्णितो भग्नो विश्लिष्टः पाटितोऽपि वा ।
छिन्नस्नायुसिरोऽप्याशु सुखं संरोहति व्रणः ॥ ६८ ॥
उत्थानशयनाद्यासु सर्वचासु न पीड्यते ।
उद्धृतौष्ठः समुत्सन्नो विषमः कठिनो ऽतिरुक् ॥ ६९ ॥
समो मृदुररुक् शीघ्रं व्रणः शुध्यति रोहति ।

Bandaging helps easy and quick healing of wounds, in which the bones are found crushed or fractured, joints are dislocated, which are cut up by the physician, in which tendons / ligaments and veins are severed.
By bandaging there will be no pain during getting up, lying down and such other acts. The ulcers which are uneven, elevated, having elevated edges, hard and very painful, even, soft, and painless, all become clean and also heal quickly.

Managing long standing and stubborn ulcers / wounds:
स्थिराणां अल्पमांसानां रौक्ष्यादनुपरोहताम् ॥ ७० ॥
प्रच्छाद्यमौषधं पत्रैर्यथादोषं यथर्तु च ।
अजीर्णतरुणाच्छिद्रैः समन्तात् सुनिवेशितैः ॥ ७१ ॥
धौतैरकर्कशैः क्षीरिभूर्जार्जुनकदम्बजैः ।

Ulcers which are persisting for long duration, which have very little muscular tissue, which do not heal to dryness (due to absence of moisture) should be applied with medicines which are wrapped in leaves of trees, appropriate to the doshas involved and the seasons. The leaves should not be ripened, should be young (tender), should not have holes, should be good in all respects, those washed well and not rough, should belong to the trees which have milky sap (latex yielding), Bhurja (Betula utilis), Arjuna or Kadamba.

Contraindication of bandaging:
कुष्ठिनां अग्निदग्धानां पिटिका मधुमेहिनाम् ॥ ७२ ॥
कर्णिकाश्चोन्दुरुविषे क्षारदग्धा विषान्विताः ।
बन्धनीया न मांस्पाके गुदपाके च दारुणे ॥ ७३ ॥
शीर्यमाणाः सरुग्दाहाः शोफावस्थाविसर्पिणः ।

Bandaging should not be done for ulcers occurring in those suffering from leprosy / skin diseases, caused due to fire burns, in ulcers having eruptions, those occurring in patients of diabetes mellitus, swelling which has occurred due to the rat bite, ulcers caused by burns caused by alkalis, caused by poison, having putrefaction of muscles, severe ulcerations of rectum, which are degenerating with loss of tissues, which are associated with pain and burning sensation, which retains the swelling over long period and ulcers which spread to other parts of the body.

Measures to manage infected ulcers:
अरक्षया व्रणे यस्मिन् मक्षिका निक्षिपेत् कृमीन् ॥ ७४ ॥
ते भक्षयन्तः कुर्वन्ति रुजाशोफास्रसंस्रवान् ।
सुरसादिं प्रयुञ्जीत तत्र धावनपूरणे ॥ ७५ ॥
सप्तपर्णकरञ्जार्कनिम्बराजादनत्वचः ।
गोमूत्रकल्कितो लेपः सेकः क्षाराम्बुना हितः ॥ ७६ ॥
प्रच्छाद्य मांसपेश्या वा व्रणं तानाशु निर्हरेत् ।

The flies deposit bacteria (worms) inside the ulcers which are not protected by bandaging, the bacteria by eating (destroying) the tissues cause pain, swelling and bleeding

For washing and filling of such infected ulcers, the herbs of Surasadi Gana group of herbs should be used, the paste of barks of Alstonia scholaris, Pongamia pinnata, Calotropis gigantean, Azadirachta indica and Vigna unguiculata made in (ground and made paste in) urine of cow should be pasted.

Bathing the ulcer with the solution of alkalis (alkaline water) is beneficial or scarification of the muscle tissue, by these measures, the worms should be removed from the ulcers, quickly.

Effects of Hasty healing of ulcers:
न चैनं त्वरमाणोऽन्तः सदोषमुपरोहयेत् ॥ ७७ ॥
सोऽल्पेनाप्यपचारेण भूयो विकुरुते यतः ।

Hasty healing of the ulcers having residue doshas inside, should not be attempted, because it will flare up greatly even with slight improper regimen.

Restrictions to be followed even after healing of ulcers:
रूढेऽप्यजीर्णव्यायामव्यवायादीन् विवर्जयेत् ॥ ७८ ॥
हर्षं क्रोधं भयं चापि यावदास्थैर्यसम्भवात् ।
आदरेणानुवर्त्योऽयं मासान् षट् सप्त वा विधिः ॥ ७९ ॥
Even after the ulcer has healed, the patient should avoid indigestion (foods and activities which cause indigestion), physical activities, copulation etc., rejoicing, anger, fear etc., till he attains his full strength.
He should follow these principles and regulations (lead a disciplined life) with sincere efforts, for at least six or seven months.

Management of similar conditions:
उत्पद्यमानासु च तासु तासु वार्तासु दोषादिबलानुसारी ।
तैस्तैरुपायैः प्रयतश्चिकित्सेदालोचयन् विस्तरमुत्तरोक्तम् ॥ ८० ॥
Similar other conditions which manifest should be treated with great efforts, using methods appropriate to the strength of the doshas etc., in the light of details furnished in the uttara tantra, the last section of this treatise (chapters 25-27).

इति श्री वैद्यपति सिंहगुप्तसूनु श्रीमद्वाग्भटविरचितायां अष्टाङ्गहृदयसंहितायां सूत्रस्थाने शस्त्रकर्मविधिर्नाम एकोनत्रिंशोऽध्यायः ॥२९॥
Thus ends the 29th chapter of Ashtangahridaya Samhita Sutrasthana, named Shastra Karma Vidhim Adhyayam, written by Shrimad Vagbhata, son of Shri Vaidyapati Simhagupta.

30

क्षाराग्निकर्मविधिमध्यायम् (kshara agnikarma vidhima dhyayam)

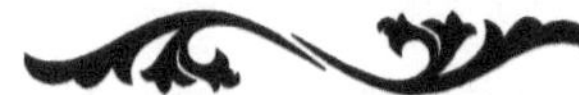

The 30th chapter of Sutrasthanam of Ashtanga Hridayam is named as Ksharagnikarma Vidhi Adhyayam. This chapter deals with the procedure and administration of alkali and fire cauterization.

अथातो क्षाराग्निकर्मविधिमध्यायं व्याख्यास्याम: इति ह स्माहुरात्रेयादयो महर्षय:॥

Atreya and other sages pledge that henceforth they will be explaining the chapter named Ksharagnikarma.

Advantages of kshara karma:

सर्वशस्त्रानुशस्त्राणां क्षार: श्रेष्ठो बहूनि यत् । छेद्यभेद्यादिकर्माणि कुरुते विषमेष्वपि ॥ १ ॥

दु:खावचार्यशास्त्रेषु तेन सिद्धिमयात्सु च । अतिकृच्छ्रेषु रोगेषु यच्च पानेऽपि युज्यते ॥ २ ॥

Among all the sharp instruments and accessory instruments, caustic alkali is the best. It performs many functions including incising, excising etc. It can be used even in inaccessible places

Success can be obtained by its (caustic alkali) use even in diseases which are very difficult to cure and also those conditions which cannot be easily treated by surgical interventions and also because alkali can be used even in the form of a drink.

Indications of drinkable alkali – Paniya Kshara:

स पेयोऽर्शोऽग्निसादाश्मगुल्मोदरगरादिषु ।

In a drinkable form, alkali is used in treating

arsha - hemorrhoids

agnisada – dyspepsia/sluggish digestion

ashma - renal calculus

gulma - abdominal tumors

udara - ascites/enlargement of abdomen

gara - chronic poisoning etc.

Indications for Pratisaraniya Kahara:

योज्यः साक्षान्मषशिवत्रबाह्यार्शःकुष्ठसुप्तिषु ॥ ३ ॥ भगन्दरार्बुदग्रन्थिदुष्टनाडीव्रणादिषु ।

In the form of direct application, alkali can be used in treating -

masha – moles, warts,

shvitra – leucoderma,

bahya arsha - external piles,

kushtha - skin diseases,

supti - anesthetic patches,

bhagandara - rectal fistula,

arbuda - cancerous growth,

granthi - tumor, fibroid,

dushta nadi vrana - foul and sinus ulcers etc.

Contraindications for administration of ksharas:

न तूभयोऽपि योक्तव्यः पित्ते रक्ते चलेऽबले ॥ ४ ॥ ज्वरेऽतीसारे हृन्मूर्धरोगे पाण्ड्वामयेऽरुचौ ।

तिमिरे कृतसंशुद्धौ श्वयथौ सर्वगात्रगे ॥ ५ ॥ भीरुगर्भिण्यृतुमतीप्रोद्धृतफलयोनिषु ।

अजीर्णेऽन्ने शिशौ वृद्धे धमनीसन्धिमर्मसु ॥ ६ ॥ तरुणास्थिसिरास्नायुसेवनीगलनाभिषु ।

देशेऽल्पमांसे वृषणमेढ्रस्रोतोनखान्तरे ॥ ७ ॥ वर्त्मरोगादृऋतेऽक्ष्णोश्च शीतवर्षोष्णदुर्दिने ।

Alkali should not be used in both ways i.e. externally or internally in (the below mentioned conditions) - aggravation of pitta and blood and diminished vata, fever, diarrhoea, diseases of heart and head, anaemia, anorexia, blindness, in those who have been recently administered with purifying therapies (Panchakarma therapies), swelling of the entire body, to people who are fearful/coward, pregnant woman, menstruating woman and woman who has displacement of vagina or uterus, when the food remains undigested, for infants and old people, on arteries, joints and vital spots, on the cartilages, veins, tendons (ligaments), sutures, throat and umbilicus (navel).

Places of the body with poor musculature, scrotum/testes, penis, orifices and passages of the body, interior of the nails, in the diseases of the eyes except those afflicting the eyelids, during cold, rainy and hot seasons and on days when the sun is not seen (cloudy days).

Madhyama kshara nirmana (Preparation of caustic alkalis of medium potency):

कालमुष्ककशम्याककदलीपारिभद्रकान् ॥ ८ ॥ अश्वकर्णमहावृक्षपलाशास्फोतवृक्षकान् ।

इन्द्रवृक्षार्कपूतीकनक्तमालाश्वमारकान्　　॥　　९　　॥ काकजङ्घामपामार्गमग्निमन्थाग्नितिल्वकान् ।

सार्द्रान् समूलशाखादीन् खण्डशः परिकल्पितान् ॥ १० ॥ कोशातकीश्चतस्रश्च शूकं नालं यवस्य च ।

निवाते निचयीकृत्य पृथक् तानि शिलातले ॥ ११ ॥ प्रक्षिप्य मुष्ककचये सुधाश्मानि च दीपयेत् ।

ततस्तिलानां कुतलैर्दग्ध्वाग्नौ विगते पृथक् ॥ १२ ॥ कृत्वा सुधाश्मनां भस्म द्रोणं त्वितरभस्मनः ।

मुष्ककोत्तरमादाय प्रत्येकं जलमूत्रयोः ॥ १३ ॥ गालयेदर्धभारेण महता वाससा च तत् ।

यावत् पिच्छिलरक्ताच्छस्तीक्ष्णो जातस्तदा च तम् ॥ १४ ॥ गृहीत्वा क्षारनिष्यन्दं पचेल्लौह्यां विघट्टयन् ।

पच्यमाने ततस्तस्मिंस्ताः सुधाभस्मशर्कराः　　॥　१५　॥　शुक्तीः　क्षीरपकं शङ्खनाभीश्चायसभाजने ।

कृत्वाग्निवर्णान् बहुशः क्षारोत्थे कुडवोन्मिते ॥ १६ ॥ निर्वाप्य पिष्ट्वा तेनैव प्रतीवापं विनिक्षिपेत् ।

श्लक्ष्णं शकृद्दक्षशिखिगृध्रकङ्ककपोतजम् ॥ १७ ॥ चतुष्पात्पक्षिपित्तालमनोह्वालवणानि च ।

परितः सुतरां चातो दर्व्या तमवघट्टयेत् ॥ १८ ॥ सबाष्पैश्च यदोत्तिष्ठेद्बुद्बुदैर्लेहवद्घनः ।

अवतार्य तदा शीतो यवराशावयोमये ॥ १९ ॥ स्थाप्योऽयं मध्यमः क्षारो

Moist roots, branches and other parts of the trees enlisted below,

kalamushkaka - Elaeodendron glaucum

shamyaka – Cassia fistula,

kadasli – Musa paradisiaca (banana, plantain)

paribhadraka – Erythrina variegata

Ashwakarna- Dipterocarpus turbinatus,

mahavriksha – Euphorbia neriifolia

palasha – Butea monosperma
asphota – Hemidesmus indicus
वृक्षकान् - vṛkṣakān – Ficus arnottiana
indravriksha – Holarrhena antidysenterica
arka – Calotropis porcera
pooteeka – Holoptelia integrifolia
naktamala – Pongamia pinnata
ashwamaraka – Nerium indicum
kaka jangha – Peristrophe bicalyculata
apamarga – Achyranthes aspera,
agnimanthā – Premna integrifolia
agni – Plumbago zeylanica
tilvaka – Symplocos racemosa - are cut into small pieces and placed separately segregated in heaps. Pieces of four kinds of Luffa acutangula plants, the spikes and reeds of Hordeum vulgare plants, are also (cut into pieces) and heaped separately, and placed on clean stone slabs, in a place devoid of breeze. Into the heap of Elaeodendron glaucum (and other herbs), pieces of limestone are put in. All the heaps are set on fire by making use of dried chaff of the Sesamum indicum plant.

After all the heaps have been well burnt and the fire has disappeared, after separating the ash of limestone, one drona (12,288 grams) of all the other herbs (except Elaeodendron glaucum) put together is taken and one forth of one drona of ash of Elaeodendron glaucum is taken.

They are mixed together (ashes), dissolved well in 48,000 ml of water and cow's urine taken separately and filtered through a thick cloth, till a slimy, reddish, clear and penetrating alkaline material is obtained.

Then that strained alkali is taken (transferred into) in an iron cauldron and cooked, stirring it constantly with a ladle. This filtered alkali is added with 192 grams of ash of limestone, shells of pearls, clay, spiral of conch shell, each made red hot over a pan, should be cooled by putting them into the alkaline liquid many times. Excreta of cock, peacock, falcon, heron and pigeon, bile of quadrupeds and birds, orpiment, realgar, and salts should be ground into fine powder (paste) dropped and admixed in the same boiling solution of alkali which is being cooked in the iron cauldron and the contents should be stirred with a stirrer, excessively, all the while, from all sides of the vessel. When it begins to emit fumes, bubbles come up and attains a solid consistency, like a confection, the cauldron should be taken out from the fire. When it gets cooled, it should be transferred into an iron vessel which is kept concealed in a heap of barley for some days. This is the mode of preparing the alkali of medium potency.

Preparation of mridu and teekshna ksharas (caustic alkalis of mild and strong potency):

न तु पिष्ट्वा क्षिपेन्मृदौ । निर्वाप्यापनयेत्तीक्ष्णे पूर्ववत् प्रतिवापनम् ॥ २० ॥

तथा लाङ्गलिकादन्तीचित्रकातिविषावचाः । स्वर्जिकाकनकक्षीरीहिङ्गुपूतिकपल्लवाः ॥ २१ ॥

तालपत्री बिडं चेति सप्तरात्रात् परं तु सः । योज्यः

For preparing the alkalis of mild potency, the admixture of ash of shells etc. should not be made into a paste and added. But they should be added in powder form, to the solution of alkali (being prepared in iron cauldron), filtered and discarded.

In preparing alkali of strong potency, the admixture should be same as that of previous preparation (alkali of medium potency) and also should include the paste of –

langalika – Gloriosa superba

danti – Baliospermum montanum

chitraka – Plumbago zeylanica

ativisha – Aconitum heterophyllum

vacha - Acorus calamus

svarjika – Fagonia cretica

kanaka ksheeri – Argemone mexicana

hingu – Ferula narthex

pooteeka pallava - pūtīka pallavāḥ - leaves of Holoptelea integrifolia,

talapatri – Chlorophytum borivilianum

bida – and bida salt (type of black salt).

Prepared as usual and used after a lapse of seven days.

Indications of three kinds of kshara:

तीक्ष्णोऽनिलश्लेष्ममेदोजेष्वर्बुदादिषु ॥ २२ ॥ मध्येष्वेष्वेव मध्योऽन्यः पितास्रगुदजन्मसु ।

बलार्थं क्षीणपानीये क्षाराम्बु पुनरावपेत् ॥ २३ ॥

Teekshna kshara (alkali of strong potency) should be used in diseases arising from vata, kapha, fat, cancerous growth (tumors and such others which are very difficult to treat.)

Madhyama kshara is useful in the same diseases of moderate strength (diseases not very difficult to cure).

The other one, i.e., mridu kshara is used in the diseases arising from pitta, blood and hemorrhoids. When the kshara loses its water content, some quantity of alkali solution should be added to strengthen it.

Properties and actions of kshara:

नातितीक्ष्णमृदुः श्लक्ष्णः पिच्छिलः शीघ्रगः सितः । शिखरी सुखनिर्वाप्यो न विष्यन्दी न चातिरुक् ॥ २४ ॥

क्षारो दशगुणः शस्त्रतेजसोरपि कर्मकृत् । आचूषन्निव संरम्भाद्गात्रमापीडयन्निव ॥ २५ ॥

सर्वतोऽनुसरन् दोषान् उन्मूलयति मूलतः । कर्म कृत्वा गतरुजः स्वयं एवोपशाम्यति ॥ २६ ॥

The ten ideal qualities of caustic alkali are -

na ati teekshna - it is neither too strong

na ati mridu – na ati mṛduḥ - not too mild

shlakshna - is smooth

picchila - is slimy

sheeghra - is quick in spreading

sita - is white in color

shikhari - remains like a mountain peak at the site of application

sukha nirvapya - is easily removable

na vishyandi - does not produce too much exudation/moistness

na cha atiruk - does not cause too much pain

It does all the functions of the sharp surgical instrument and also the fire (cauterization). By its sucking like actions, constricting like action all over the body owing to its quickness (quick action), healing effect over the body, spreading everywhere, it pulls out the doshas (morbid/vitiating materials, contaminants) by their roots. After such actions, when the diseases/painful conditions disappear, the alkali also subsides on its own accord (its action no longer happens).

Procedure of kshara karma (alkaline cauterization):

क्षारसाध्ये गदे छिन्ने लिखिते स्रावितेऽथवा ।

क्षारं शलाकया दत्वा प्लोतप्रावृतदेहया ॥ २७ ॥

मात्राशतमुपेक्षेत

The disease treatable by alkali should either be cut, scraped or made to exudate fluids first, then the alkali is taken in an iron rod and placed on the spot. The other spots (healthy areas) in the surrounding area are kept covered and protected by cotton swabs and a time period of 100 matra is awaited.

Application of kshara in various conditions:

तत्रार्शःस्वावृताननम् । हस्तेन यन्त्रं कुर्वीत वर्त्मरोगेषु वर्त्मनी ॥ २८ ॥

निर्भुज्य पिचुनाच्छाद्य कृष्णभागं विनिक्षिपेत् । पद्मपत्रतनुः क्षारलेपो घ्राणार्बुदेषु च ॥ २९ ॥

प्रत्यादित्यं निषण्णस्य समुन्नम्याग्रनासिकाम् । मात्रा विधार्यः पञ्चाशत् तद्वदर्शसि कर्णजे ॥ ३० ॥

In hemorrhoids, if the tip of the pile mass is concealed, it should be manipulated by hand (in such a way so as to place the alkali on them, inside the anal canal) and alkali applied.

In diseases of the eyelids, the lids are to be everted, the black area should be covered with cotton swab (and protected and then), the alkali should be applied as thin as the thickness of a lotus petal (to the interior of the eyelids).

In the tumors of the nose, the patient is made to sit facing the sun, the tip of the nose is raised up and the alkali is applied into the nostril and a time of fifty matra kala (counts) is awaited.

In case of polyps of the ears also it (method of application of alkali) shall be similar.

Measures to be taken after application of kshara:

क्षारं प्रमार्जनेनानु परिमृज्यावगम्य च । सुदग्धं घृतमध्वक्तं तत् पयोमस्तुकाञ्जिकैः ॥ ३१ ॥

निर्वापयेत् ततः साज्यैः स्वादुशीतैः प्रदेहयेत् । अभिष्यन्दीनि भोज्यानि भोज्यानि क्लेदनाय च ॥ ३२ ॥

यदि च स्थिरमूलत्वात् क्षारदग्धं न शीर्यते । धान्याम्लबीजयष्ट्याह्वतिलैरालेपयेत् ततः ॥ ३३ ॥

तिलकल्कः समधुको घृताक्तो व्रणरोपणः ।

After the prescribed time, the alkali is wiped off with a cotton swab etc. and considering that the site has been properly burnt by the alkali, a mixture of ghee and honey should be applied, made cool by pouring milk, whey or sour gruel, and then applying a paste of herbs of predominantly sweet taste and cold potency admixed in ghee.

The patient should consume foods which produce more secretions in the cells in order to moisten the site of burn (burnt by alkali). If the site of the burn does not get torn from an ulcer due to it being deep seated, then a paste of active essence of dhanyamla i.e., fermented sour gruel, Glycyrrhiza glabra and Sesamum indicum should be applied.

Paste of tila and Madhuka mixed with ghee heals the ulcer.

Symptoms of proper burning by kshara:

पक्वजम्ब्वसितं सन्नं सम्यग्दग्धं विपर्यये ॥ ३४ ॥ ताम्रतातोदकण्ड्वाद्यैर्दुर्दग्धं तं पुनर्दहेत् ।

Symptoms of good burning due to alkali are attaining black color similar to ripe fruit of Jamun (Syzygium cumini) and depression of the site. The opposite of it, that is the appearance of coppery red color, pricking pain, itching etc. are the features of improper/inadequate burning. Such an area should be burnt again.

Symptoms of excessive burning by kshara:

अतिदग्धे स्रवेद्रक्तं मूर्छादाहज्वरादयः ॥ ३५ ॥ गुदे विशेषादिवण्मूत्रसंरोधोऽतिप्रवर्तनम् । पुंस्त्वोपघातो मृत्युर्वा गुदस्य शातनाद्ध्रुवम् ॥ ३६ ॥ नासायां नासिकावंशदरणाकुञ्चनोद्भवः ।
भवेच्च विषयाज्ञानं तद्वच्छ्रोत्रादिकेष्वपि ॥ ३७ ॥

Over burning (by alkalis) produces bleeding, fainting, burning sensation, fever etc.

Excessive burning of the anus/rectum produces obstruction for passing of feces and urine or their excessive elimination, loss of/destruction of sexual power (impotence) and sure death due to prolapsed of rectum.

In case of nose, the nasal bridge will fall off, contraction of the nasal bridge and loss of sense of smell. Similar complaints occur in the case of ears and other sense organs.

Management of excessive burning by kshara:

विशेषादत्र सेकोऽम्लैर्लेपो मधु घृतं तिलाः । वातपित्तहरा चेष्टा सर्वैव शिशिरा क्रिया ॥ ३८ ॥ अम्लो हि शीतः स्पर्शन क्षारस्तेनोपसंहितः । यात्याशु स्वादुतां तस्मादम्लैर्निर्वापयेत्तराम् ॥ ३९ ॥

In such conditions, pouring the part with sour fluids, applications of paste of honey, ghee and sesame, activities, foods and other comforts which mitigate vata and pitta and all others which produce cold should be adopted (cold foods and comforts).

Sour taste is cold to touch, when combined with alkali, the sour taste will quickly attain the properties of sweet taste. Hence the burns caused by alkali should be quickly washed with sour substances.

Effects of wrongly administered kshara:

विषाग्निशस्त्राशनिमृत्युतुल्यः क्षारो भवेदल्पमतिप्रयुक्तः ।
रोगान् निहन्यादचिरेण घोरान् स धीमता सम्यगनुप्रयुक्तो ॥ ३९+(१) ॥

Alkali administered in less or excessive proportions (by the physician of poor intellect) is like death caused by poison, fire, sharp weapons or thunderbolt, whereas when done properly by an intelligent physician, it cures even the dreaded diseases quickly.

Thermal/fire cauterization, Branding – Agnikarma:

अग्निः क्षारादपि श्रेष्ठस्तद्दग्धानामसम्भवात् । भेषजक्षारशस्त्रैश्च न सिद्धानां प्रसाधनात् ॥ ४० ॥

Fire cauterization is better than even alkali cauterization. The diseases that are treated by fire cauterization do not recur and it can be used even in diseases which have not been successfully treated by herbs, alkali or surgical methods.

Indications and contraindications for agnikarma:

त्वचि मांसे सिरास्नायुसन्ध्यस्थिषु स युज्यते । मषाङ्गग्लानिमूर्धार्तिमन्थकीलतिलादिषु ॥ ४१ ॥
त्वग्दाहो वर्तिगोदन्तसूर्यकान्तशरादिभिः ।

It is used on the skin, muscle, vein, tendon, joints and bones, in diseases like black moles, weakness of body parts, headache, glaucoma, warts, cysts etc.
Burning of the skin should be done either with a lighted wick, tooth of a cow, rock crystal, arrow head (or others such as Piper longum, excreta of goat, iron rod, piece of bangles).

Different materials used for agnikarma in different conditions:

अर्शोभगन्दरग्रन्थिनाडीदुष्टव्रणादिषु ॥ ४२ ॥ मांसदाहो मधुस्नेहजाम्बवौष्ठगुडादिभिः ।
शिलष्टवर्त्मन्यसृक्स्रावनील्यसम्यग्व्यधादिषु ॥ ४३ ॥ सिरादिदाहस्तैरेव

Hemorrhoids, rectal fistula, tumors/cysts, sinus ulcers and bad septic, long standing and foul ulcers etc., should be treated by burning of the muscles with hot honey, fats, an iron instrument with a spoon shaped tip (jambavoshta), jaggery etc.
In exudative disease of the eyelids, bleeding, blue mole, improper cutting – surgical wound etc., burning of the veins should be done by using the same

materials enumerated in the previous verse.

Contraindications for agnikarma:

न दहेत् क्षारवारितान् । अन्तःशल्यासृजो भिन्नकोष्ठान् भूरिव्रणातुरान् ॥ ४४ ॥

Burning should not be done for those who are not suitable for alkali cauterization, wounds which have foreign body (in them) or accumulation of blood inside, persons who have perforation of abdominal viscera and those who are suffering from severe wounds.

Care of site of properly done agnikarma:

सुदग्धं घृतमध्वक्तं स्निग्धशीतैः प्रदेहयेत् ।

The site which has been properly burnt by fire should be given a coating of ghee and honey and an application of paste of herbs which are unctuous and cold in potency.

Features of proper and improper agnikarma (fire cauterization):

तस्य लिङ्गं स्थिते रक्ते शब्दवल्लसिकान्वितम् ॥ ४५ ॥

पक्वतालकपोताभं सुरोहं नातिवेदनम् ।

The signs of proper burning are stoppage of bleeding, emergence of crackling sound accompanied with plasma, the area having color resembling a ripe toddy palm fruit or pigeon dark grey the wound healing easily and not much of pain.

Signs of inadequate and excessive agnikarma:

प्रमाददग्धवत्सर्वं दुर्दग्धात्यर्थदग्धयोः ॥ ४६ ॥ चतुर्धा तनु तुच्छेन

All the signs of inadequate burning and excessive burning are similar to those of careless/negligent burning . The burning is of four types together with poor/insignificant (tuchcha) burning.

Signs of insignificant/inadequate improper and excessively done agnikarma:

सह तुच्छस्य लक्षणम् । त्वग्विवर्णोष्यतेऽत्यर्थं न च स्फोटसमुद्भवः ॥ ४७ ॥

सस्फोटदाहतीव्रोषं दुर्दग्धमतिदाहतः । मांसलम्बनसङ्कोचदाहधूपनवेदनाः ॥ ४८ ॥

सिरादिनाशस्तृणमूर्छाव्रणगाम्भीर्यमृत्यवः ।

The signs of inadequate burns are discoloration of the skin, severe burning sensation and absence of manifestation of boils/blisters.

In case of improper burning, there is the appearance of blisters, burning sensation, and severe burning pain.

In case of excessive burning there occurs (below mentioned signs)

- mamsa lambana - dropping down of the muscles

- samkocha - constriction

- daha - burning sensation

- dhoopana - feeling of hot fumes coming out,

- vedana – pain

- siradi nasha - destruction of veins etc,

- trut - excessive thirst

- moorcha - fainting, loss of consciousness

- vrana gambhirya - worsening of the wound

- mrutyu - and death.

Management of insignificant/inadequately done agnikarma:

तुच्छस्याग्निप्रतपनं कार्यमुष्णं च भेषजम् ॥ ४९ ॥ स्त्यानेऽस्रे वेदनात्यर्थं विलीने मन्दता रुजः ।

In case of less/inadequate burning, the site should be burnt once again and paste of herbs which have hot potency should be used. When the blood is coagulated there is severe pain and when it is dissolved, pain is mild.

Management of durdagdhga (bad burning):

दुर्दग्धे शीतमुष्णं च युञ्ज्यादादौ ततो हिमम् ॥ ५० ॥

In case of bad burning, cold and hot treatments should be administered, the cold therapy should be done first, the hot therapy next.

Care following samyak dagdha (proper burning):

सम्यग्दग्धे तवक्षीरिप्लक्षचन्दनगैरिकैः । लिम्पेत् साज्यामृतैरूर्ध्वं पित्तविद्रधिवत् क्रिया ॥ ५१ ॥

In case of proper burning, a paste of Curcuma angustifolia, Ficus lacor, Santalum album, Red Ochre and Tinospora cordifolia,mixed with ghee should be applied on the area of burn and then therapies indicated for an abscess of pitta origin should be adopted.

Management of ati dagdha (excessive burning):

अतिदग्धे द्रुतं कुर्यात्सर्वं पित्तविसर्पवत् । स्नेहदग्धे भृशतरं रूक्षं तत्र तु योजयेत् ॥ ५२ ॥

In case of excessive burning, all the therapeutic measures prescribed for herpes caused by pitta origin should be done quickly, in case of burning by fats i.e. hot oil, ghee etc, measures which are very dry (causes severe dryness) should be adopted.

Advice of caution in shastrakarma and agnikarma (surgical and cauterization procedures):

शस्त्रक्षाराग्नयो यस्मान्मृत्योः परममायुधम् ।
अप्रमत्तो भिषक् तस्मात्तान् सम्यगवचारयेत् ॥ ५२+(१) ॥

The sharp instrument (like knife), alkali and fire are the chief weapons of the lord of death, hence the vigilant physician should administer them with great care.

Advice of caution in shastrakarma and agnikarma (surgical and cauterization procedures):

समाप्यते स्थानमिदं हृदयस्य रहस्यवत् । अत्रार्थाः सूत्रिताः सूक्ष्माः प्रतन्यन्ते हि सर्वतः ॥ ५३ ॥

Thus, this section of Ashtanga Hridaya which is full of secrets, codifies all the chief doctrines which are described in detail everywhere (in the entire treatment).

इति श्रीवैद्यपति सिंहगुप्तसूनु श्रीमद्वाग्भट विरचितायां अष्टाङ्गहृदयसंहितायां सूत्रस्थाने क्षाराग्निकर्मविधिर्नाम त्रिंशत्तमोऽध्यायः ॥३०॥

Thus ends the 30th chapter of Ashtangahridaya Samhita Sutrasthana, named Ksharagnikarma Vidhim Adhyayam, written by Shrimad Vagbhata, son of Shri Vaidyapati Simhagupta.

Easy Ayurveda Publications

English Books:
Easy Ayurveda Home Remedies
Living Easy With Ayurveda
Tridosha Made Easy
Ayurveda Tarka
    Kannada Books
Sugama Jivanakkagi Ayurveda
Ayurveda Santvana

Hindi Book
Ayurved Samadhan

Malayalam Books on Ayurveda
Ayurveda asvasam
Jeevitha Soukhyathinu Ayurvedam

Buy them at
EasyAyurveda.com/Books